*Dedicated to*

*James Charles Jenkins*

*1952-1979*

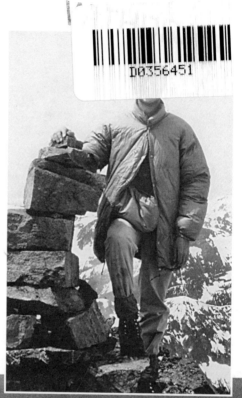

*Coauthor of the first*

*three editions of this book*

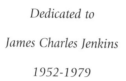

Ruby Johnson Jenkins

Mount Jenkins, named for former coauthor

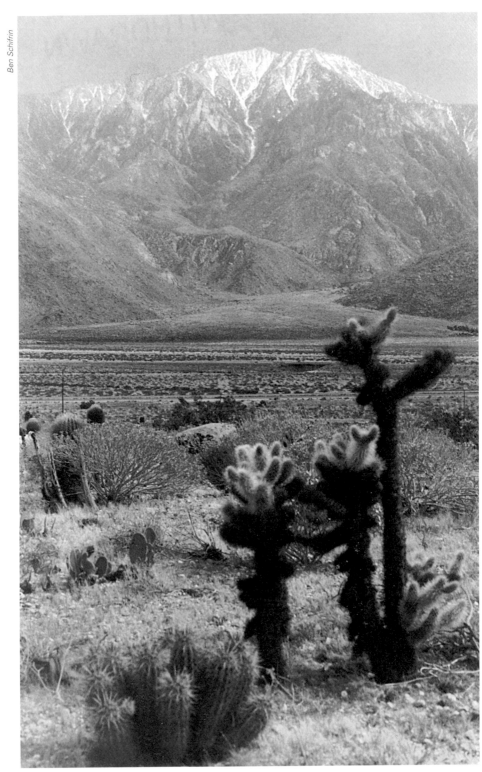

# CALIFORNIA

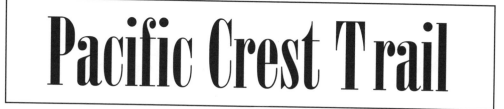

## Pacific Crest Trail

### From the Mexican Border to Yosemite's Tuolumne Meadows

Ben Schifrin

Ruby Johnson Jenkins

Thomas Winnett

Jeffrey P. Schaffer

**WILDERNESS PRESS** . . . *on the trail since 1967*

FIRST EDITION June 1973
SECOND EDITION September 1977
THIRD EDITION June 1982
FOURTH EDITION January 1989
FIFTH EDITION July 1995
**SIXTH EDITION** January 2003
Copyright © 1973, 1977, 1982, 1989, 1995, 2003 by Wilderness Press

Formerly published as *The Pacific Crest Trail, Volume 1: California.* Now the California section of the trail is covered in two books: *Pacific Crest Trail Southern California* (From the Mexican border to Yosemite's Tuolumne Meadows) and *Pacific Crest Trail Northern California* (From Tuolumne Meadows to the Oregon Border). A third book, *The Pacific Crest Trail, Volume 2: Oregon & Washington* (6th edition, August 2000) is also published by Wilderness Press; it covers the Northwestern part of the PCT and is co-authored by Jeffrey P. Schaffer and Andy Selters.

Cover and book design: Jaan Hitt
Compositor: Jaan Hitt
Original topographic maps: Jeffrey P. Schaffer and Bruce Appleyard
Original section maps: Barbara Jackson
(We also thank Glenn M. Bock, Tom Ekman, formerly of TOPO! National Geographic, Ben Pease, and Tom Reynolds; they all assisted us in our our efforts to digitize the maps for future editions.)
Editors: Paul Backhurst and Kris Kaiyala
Proofreaders: Jessica Lage and Jannie M. Dresser
Managing editor: Jannie M. Dresser
Publisher: Mike Jones

Cover photo: © 2003 Jane Dove Juneau, "Minaret Falls" (Section H)
Frontispiece photo: © 2003 Ben Schifrin, "Mt. San Jacinto from San Gorgonio Pass"
Back cover photo: © 2003 Jim Lundgren, "Sand Verbana, Anza-Borrego Desert Park"
Other photographs used in this book are through the courtesy of:
    U. S. Bureau of Land Management; Lyn Haber; J.C. Jenkins; Ruby Johnson Jenkins; John W. Robinson; Jeffrey P. Schaffer; Ben Schifrin; and Thomas Winnett.

International Standard Book Number 978-0-89997-316-6
Manufactured in the United States of America
Published by **Wilderness Press**
        **Keen Communications**
        **PO Box 43673**
        **Birmingham, AL 35243**
        **Phone (800) 443-7227; FAX (205) 326-1012**
        **www.wildernesspress.com**
Visit our website for a complete listing of our books and for ordering information.
Distributed by Publishers Group West

**Library of Congress Cataloging-in-Publication Data**
NEW CIP IN APPLICATION
Pacific Crest Trail—6th ed.
    p.  cm.
    Includes bibliographical references and index.
    Contents: Southern California / Ben Schifrin ...[et al.]
    1. Hiking—Pacific Crest Trail—Guidebooks. 2. Hiking—California—Guidebooks. 3. Pacific Crest Trail—Description and travel—Guidebooks. 4. California—Description and travel.
I. Schifrinr, Ben.
GV 199.42.P3P3  2003
796.5'1'0979—dc20            95-9325
                    CIP            ISBN 978-0-89997-316-6

# Disclaimer

Hiking in the backcountry entails unavoidable risk that every hiker assumes and must be aware of and respect. The fact that a trail is described in this book is not a representation that it will be safe for you. Trails vary greatly in difficulty and in the degree of conditioning and agility one needs in order to enjoy them safely. On some hikes, routes may have changed—or conditions may have deteriorated—since the descriptions were written. Also, trail conditions can change from day to day, or even hour to hour, owing to weather and other factors. A trail that is safe on a dry day or for a highly conditioned, agile, properly equipped hiker may be completely unsafe for someone else or unsafe under adverse weather conditions.

Minimize your risks on the trail by being knowledgeable, prepared, and alert. There is not space in this book for a general treatise on safety in the mountains. Fortunately, there are many good books and courses on the subject: use them to increase your knowledge. Just as important, take note of your own limitations and familiarize yourself in advance about what conditions you may face when and where you want to hike. If conditions are dangerous, or if you're not prepared to deal with them safely, choose a different hike! It's better to have wasted a drive than to be the subject of a mountain rescue.

Millions of people have safe and enjoyable hikes every year. However, one element of the beauty, freedom, and excitement of the wilderness is the presence of risks that do not confront us at home. When you hike, you assume those risks. They can be met safely, but only if you take time to inform yourself, then exercise your independent judgment and common sense while hiking or backpacking along any trail.

The following sections of the trail were researched and described by the authors named below:

Ben Schifrin         Section A –   Mexican Border
                     Section E     Tehachapi Pass

Ruby Johnson Jenkins  Sections F –  Highway 58 near Tehachapi Pass
                     Section G     Mt. Whitney

Tom Winnett          Section H     Mt. Whitney to Devils Postpile

Jeffrey P. Schaffer  Section H     Devils Postpile to Tuolumne Meadows

## Other books by these authors:

**Ruby Johnson Jenkins, with J.C. Jenkins**
*Exploring the Southern Sierra: East Side*
*Exploring the Southern Sierra: West Side*

**Jeffrey P. Schaffer**
*Carson-Iceberg Wilderness*
*Desolation Wilderness and the South Lake Tahoe Basin*
*Hiker's Guide to the High Sierra: Tuolumne Meadows (with Thomas Winnett)*
*Hiker's Guide to the High Sierra: Yosemite*
*Hiking the Big Sur Country*
*Lassen Volcanic National Park*
*The Geomorphic Evolution of the Yosemite Valley and Sierra Nevada Landscapes*
*The Pacific Crest Trail: Oregon-Washington (with Andy Selters)*
*The Tahoe Sierra*
*Yosemite National Park*

**Ben Schifrin**
*Emigrant Wilderness and Northwestern Yosemite*

**Thomas Winnett**
*Backpacking Basics (with Melanie Findling)*
*Guide to the John Muir Trail (with Kathy Morey)*
*Hiker's Guide to the High Sierra: Mt. Whitney*
*Hiker's Guide to the High Sierra: Tuolumne Meadows (with Jeffrey P. Schaffer)*
*Sierra North (co-author)*
*Sierra South (co-author)*

# Contents

Acknowledgments . . . . . . . . . . . . . . . . . . . . . . . . . . . . . . . . . . . . . . . . . . . .ix

# INTRODUCTORY CHAPTERS

**Locator Map**. . . . . . . . . . . . . . . . . . . . . . . . . . . . . . . . . . . . . . . . . . . . . . . .xii

**Chapter 1: The PCT, Its History and Use**. . . . . . . . . . . . . . . . . . . . . . . .1

**Chapter 2: Planning Your PCT Hike**. . . . . . . . . . . . . . . . . . . . . . . . . . . .7
Trekking Days or Weeks versus Trekking Months . . . . . . . . . . . . . . . . . . . 7
Organizations Relevant to the Pacific Crest Trail. . . . . . . . . . . . . . . . . . . . 9
Mailing Tips (including post offices along or near the route) . . . . . . . . . 14
Federal Government Agencies (with south-to-north listing) . . . . . . . . . . 15
Hiking the Pacific Crest Trail—Dayhiking/Backpacking . . . . . . . . . . . . . 18
Trail Advice . . . . . . . . . . . . . . . . . . . . . . . . . . . . . . . . . . . . . . . . . . . . . . . . 18
Items to consider for your backpack . . . . . . . . . . . . . . . . . . . . . . . . . . . . . 19
Animal and Plant Problems on the PCT . . . . . . . . . . . . . . . . . . . . . . . . . .23
Weather. . . . . . . . . . . . . . . . . . . . . . . . . . . . . . . . . . . . . . . . . . . . . . . . . . . .29
Hypothermia. . . . . . . . . . . . . . . . . . . . . . . . . . . . . . . . . . . . . . . . . . . . . . . 31
High Altitude Problems. . . . . . . . . . . . . . . . . . . . . . . . . . . . . . . . . . . . . . .32

**Chapter 3: PCT Natural History** . . . . . . . . . . . . . . . . . . . . . . . . . . . . . .33
Geology. . . . . . . . . . . . . . . . . . . . . . . . . . . . . . . . . . . . . . . . . . . . . . . . . . . .33
Biology . . . . . . . . . . . . . . . . . . . . . . . . . . . . . . . . . . . . . . . . . . . . . . . . . . . 42
Plant Communities of California's Pacific Crest Trail . . . . . . . . . . . . . . . .50

**Chapter 4: Using This Guide** . . . . . . . . . . . . . . . . . . . . . . . . . . . . . . . . .57
Our Route Description. . . . . . . . . . . . . . . . . . . . . . . . . . . . . . . . . . . . . . . .57
Icons Used in this Book. . . . . . . . . . . . . . . . . . . . . . . . . . . . . . . . . . . . . . .59
Following the Trail . . . . . . . . . . . . . . . . . . . . . . . . . . . . . . . . . . . . . . . . . . 60
Map Legend . . . . . . . . . . . . . . . . . . . . . . . . . . . . . . . . . . . . . . . . . . . . . . . 61
California PCT Mileage Table . . . . . . . . . . . . . . . . . . . . . . . . . . . . . . . 62-63

# TRAIL SECTIONS

Section A: **Mexican Border to Warner Springs** . . . . . . . . . . . . . . . . . . .64

Section B: **Warner Springs to San Gorgonio Pass** . . . . . . . . . . . . . . . . .96

Section C: **San Gorgonio Pass to Interstate 15 near Cajon Pass** . . . . .124

Section D: **Interstate 15 near Cajon Pass to Agua Dulce** . . . . . . . . . .160

Section E: **Agua Dulce to Highway 58 near Mojave** . . . . . . . . . . . . . .190

Section F: **Highway 58 near Tehachapi Pass to
Highway 178 at Walker Pass** . . . . . . . . . . . . . . . . . . . . . . . .226

Section G: **Highway 178 to Mt. Whitney** . . . . . . . . . . . . . . . . . . . . . .254

Section H: **Mt. Whitney to Tuolumne Meadows** . . . . . . . . . . . . . . . . .296

**Recommended Reading and Source Books** . . . . . . . . . . . . . . . . . . . . .342

**Index** . . . . . . . . . . . . . . . . . . . . . . . . . . . . . . . . . . . . . . . . . . . . . . . .345

# Acknowledgments

Each of the four authors of *The Pacific Crest Trail: Southern California* was responsible for describing a particular length of trail. Their individual acknowledgments are listed below:

**Ben Schifrin** (Sections A–E): Even though most of the PCT's route in California has been constructed, a dedicated legion of hikers remains passionately involved with maintaining the trail and offering continually updated reports on its condition. None is more committed than Pete Fish, a one-man trail-maintenance army for the PCTA in southern California. Along with Valerie Sing, Jack Yates, Carrol Barrett, Tim Connors and Laraine Kate Downer, also of the PCTA, he has also given frequent helpful notifications of changing trail conditions.

Brick Robbins has changed the face of PCT trip planning more than anyone, even Ray Jardine. By presiding over the Internet's PCT-List, he has maintained a democratic forum that offers all hikers, from neophyte to grizzled Triple-Crown veterans, the opportunity to discuss safe long-distance hiking techniques and to get vital, up-to-the-minute information on trail weather and all-important water supplies.

Numerous others have offered valuable comments, including Charlie Jones, Lynn Foss, John Hlavac, Karen Elder, Karl Duff, Bruce Gilbert, David Craft, Kevin Corcoran, and the tireless Supreme Hostess of the PCT, Donna Saufley. Chris Landa, in particular, provided extensive and accurate corrections. Ginny Owen provided a valuable perspective on the philosophy of trail guides.

Greg "Strider" Hummel, grand pooh-bah of ADZPCTKOP, throws the best hikers' parties and, along with the irrepressible Monte Dodge, reminds me every week why we Old Guys continue to love the Trail, even in our heavy leather boots. Nancy Kerr and Todd Fitzgibbon are my best hiking partners; they have shared most of this book's miles, more than once.

Finally I must remember two who are no longer with us: Alice Krueper was an inspiration of selfless devotion to development of the Trail. Jack Fair epitomized the quirkiness and color of the American desert and possessed a tireless generosity that was inspired by the Grand Idea of the PCT. They will be missed.

**Ruby Johnson Jenkins** (Sections F and G): An elderly man in failing health was responsible for a freeway accident in 1979 that took the life of J. C. Jenkins, the former author of these sections. Jenkins' mother, Ruby, assumed the field work and update for the succeeding editions to honor his memory. Ruby has hiked these sections many times and would like to thank her husband, Bill, and her friends from the Kern River Valley Hiking Club who often accompanied her.

**Thomas Winnett** (Section H, Mt. Whitney to Devils Postpile): Jason Winnett rehiked parts of the John Muir Trail section of the Pacific Crest Trail. Kathy Morey did the same.

**Jeffrey P. Schaffer** (Devils Postpile, in Section H): In addition to the people I've acknowledged in previous editions, I would like to mention those who sent helpful comments to us more recently, in particular, William M. Lane, William McCanna, Jr.,

Bruce Ohlson, David Shimek, and Thomas Zurr. Some others who have offered useful information are Scott Anderson, Bob Ellinwood, Bruce and Sharon Gilbert, John Olley, Steve Queen, Linda Spaulding, Jeff Stone, Gary Suttle, Taylor Wind Set, and Ben York. I have not had the time to check every detail all these fine folks have mentioned, but where I have, their notes have been quite accurate. I apologize to anyone who has sent me constructive comments but was not acknowledged here.

All the authors gratefully acknowledge the hard work and dedication of those at Wilderness Press who have been instrumental in creating this new edition. Paul Backhurst got the ball rolling by dividing the original PCT California volume, then coordinating with the authors about updates and changes. Jannie Dresser managed the project from beginning to printing. Jaan Hitt designed and did the lay-out on the book. Kris Kaiyala and Jessica Lage shared the proofreading and final editorial tasks. Mike Jones, as publisher of Wilderness Press, has remained devoted to keeping this book in print even when it meant tackling the costly and difficult task of modernizing old styles, formats, and production methods.

Jane Dove Juneau, Mammoth Lakes, California, and Jim Lundgren, Hillsboro, Oregon, contributed the beautiful front and back cover photographs (respectively) for this edition. Lyn Haber and Ralph Haber contributed additional photographs and thanks to them as well. And, finally, much appreciation goes to several gentlemen who moved us closer to the goal of digitizing all the maps. Thank you to Glenn M. Bock, Tom Ekman of TOPO! National Geographic, Ben Pease, and Tom Reynolds.

# About this Book

Wilderness Press first published its book on the Pacific Crest Trail in June 1973, over 30 years ago. Since then, the book has sold nearly 100,000 copies, or roughly 3,000 a year, and has earned the reputation as "the PCT Bible" from backpackers and thru-hikers on the trail. It is the most essential resource available to anyone who is planning a PCT trek, and its importance to those who are dreaming of hiking the PCT became all too clear the summer of 2002 when we let the old edition go out of print as we updated, corrected, and digitized the new edition. We received numerous phone calls and emails from folks who needed the book, and, to them, we do apologize. At last report, the old edition of *The Pacific Crest Trail* was being auctioned on eBay for over $75 a copy. Of such things, are legends made.

We made the decision in 2001 to split *The Pacific Crest Trail, Volume 1: California* into two separate volumes, and to take the time to bring the book into the 1990s. Times had changed and the way books and maps are produced for print media has undergone a tremendous revolution with the digital age. Many of Wilderness Press' books have needed to be transformed through the alchemical process of turning old mechanicals (the original topographic maps, art work and pasted-up boards) into digital files. For years we could get by doing things the old way, but now few printers can accommodate mechanically-prepared books: it's all disk-to-plate now and that required a complete republishing of the book.

We now present the California PCT book in two volumes. By splitting the original book, we were able to redesign it in order to enhance readability and make it a *bit* more portable. We also added some new photos and improved the quality of the old ones. The maps are as they were originally, with the changes that have been made to them in prior editions; we expect to have them completely digitized within the next five years. As many readers know or have heard, our maps are critically important since they supply much information that is not available anywhere else.

Formerly published as *The Pacific Crest Trail, Volume 1: California*, now the California section of the PCT is covered by two books: *Pacific Crest Trail: Southern California* (From the Mexican border to Yosemite's Tuolumne Meadows) and *Pacific Crest Trail: Northern California* (From Tuolumne Meadows to the Oregon Border). A third book, *The Pacific Crest Trail: Oregon & Washington* (6th edition, August 2000) is also published by Wilderness Press; it covers the Northwestern part of the PCT and is authored by Jeffrey P. Schaffer and Andy Selters. Since only a few users of the Pacific Crest Trail are complete thru-hikers, the division of these texts should make it easier for planning the kind of shorter two-to-three week treks that most folks do.

As Wilderness Press enters its 36th year of publishing, it intends to keep alive some of its classic older books, which means we are investing in the new technology and redesigning many of them. We would love to hear your comments or suggestions on how our books can be improved. Contact us at *mail@wildernesspress.com*, or write to Managing Editor, Wilderness Press, 1200 5th Street, Berkeley, CA 94710.

Thank you for buying and using this book. We hope it serves you well as you prepare for and set off on an incredible journey along the Pacific Crest Trail.

- Jannie M. Dresser, Managing Editor, Wilderness Press
January 2003

# The Pacific Crest Trail in California

Letters A-H on this map refer to trail chapters in this book. Letters I-R are covered in *Pacific Crest Trail: Northern California.*

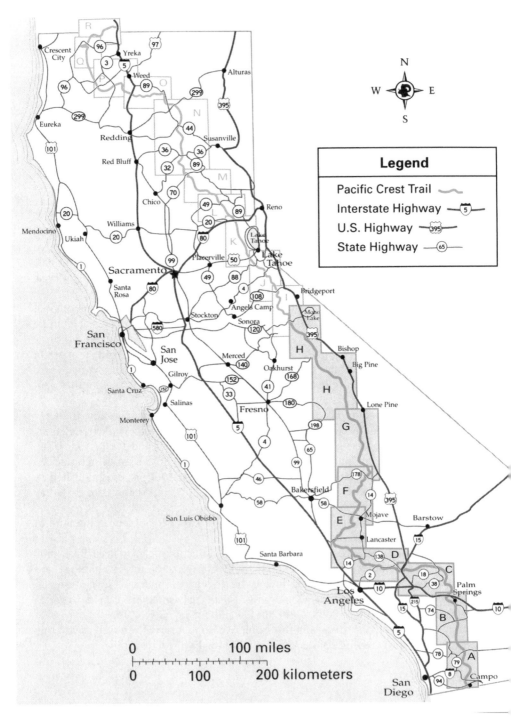

# Chapter 1

# The PCT, Its History and Use

During the 1800s, Americans traveling west toward the Pacific States were confronted with mountain barriers such as the Cascades and the Sierra Nevada. The idea of making a recreational trek along the crest of these ranges probably never entered anyone's mind, and probably did not occur until the 1890s, if that. However, relatively early in the 1900s, a party did make a recreational multi-day crest traverse of a part of the Sierra Nevada. From July 8-25, 1913, Charles Booth, accompanied by his wife, Nora, and two friends, Howard Bliss and Elmer Roberts, made a pack trip from Tuolumne Meadows north to Lake Tahoe. Today's Pacific Crest Trail closely follows much of their trek.

## Conception of the PCT

The first proposal for the creation of a Pacific Crest Trail that we have been able to discover is contained in the book *Pacific Crest Trails*, by Joseph T. Hazard (Superior Publishing Co.). He says that in 1926 a Catherine Montgomery at the Western Washington College of Education in Bel-

lingham suggested to him that there should be:

> "A high trail winding down the heights of our western mountains with mile markers and shelter huts—like those pictures I'll show you of the 'Long Trail of the Appalachians'—from the Canadian Border to the Mexican Boundary Line!"

To go back six years in time, the Forest Service had by 1920 routed and posted a trail from Mt. Hood to Crater Lake in Oregon, named the Oregon Skyline Trail, and with hindsight we can say that it was the first link in the PCT. (For brevity in this book, we refer to the Pacific Crest Trail as the "PCT." Technically the official name is the Pacific Crest National Scenic Trail, abbreviated as the PCNST. However, this abbreviation is more cumbersome, and essentially no one uses it.)

Hazard says that on that very night, he conveyed Miss Montgomery's suggestion to the Mt. Baker Club of Bellingham, which was enthusiastic about it. He says that soon a number of other mountain clubs and outdoor organizations in the Pacific Northwest adopted the idea and set about promoting it. Then, in 1928, Fred W. Cleator became Supervisor of Recreation for Region 6 (Oregon and Washington) of the US Forest Service. Cleator proclaimed and began to develop the Cascade Crest Trail, a route down the spine of Washington from Canada to the Columbia River. Later, he extended the Oregon Skyline Trail at both ends so that it too traversed a whole state. In 1937 Region 6 of the Forest Service developed a design for PCT trail markers and posted them from the Canadian border to the California border.

But the Forest Service's Region 5 (California) did not follow this lead, and it remained for a private person to provide the real spark not only for a California segment of the PCT but indeed for the PCT itself. In the early 1930s the idea of a Pacific Crest Trail entered the mind of Clinton C. Clarke of Pasadena, California, who was then chairman of the Executive Committee of the Mountain League of Los Angeles County. "In March 1932," wrote Clarke in *The Pacific Crest Trailway*, he "proposed to the United States Forest and National Park services the project of a continuous wilderness trail across the United States from Canada to Mexico. . . . The plan was to build a trail along the summit divides of the mountain ranges of these states, traversing the best scenic areas and maintaining an absolute wilderness character."

The proposal included formation of additional Mountain Leagues in Seattle, Portland, and San Francisco by representatives of youth organizations and hiking and mountaineering clubs similar to the one in Los Angeles. These Mountain Leagues would then take the lead in promoting the extension of the John Muir Trail northward and southward to complete a pathway from border to border. When it became evident that more than Mountain Leagues were needed for such a major undertaking, Clarke took the lead in forming the Pacific Crest Trail System Conference, with representatives from the three Pacific Coast states. He served as its President for 25 years.

As early as January 1935 Clarke published a handbook-guide to the PCT giving the route in rather sketchy terms ("the Trail goes east of Heart Lake, then south across granite fields to the junction of Piute and Evolution Creeks"—this covers about nine miles).

In the summer of 1935—and again the next three summers—groups of boys under the sponsorship of the YMCA explored the PCT route in relays, proceeding from Mexico on June 15, 1935, to Canada on August 12, 1938. This exploration was under the guidance of a YMCA secretary, Warren L. Rogers, who served as Executive Secretary of the Pacific Crest Trail System Conference from 1932 until 1957, when Clarke died (at age 84), and the conference disappeared. (Rogers was an enthusiastic hiker—and mountaineer—which is remarkable considering that he limped because as a child he had been stricken with polio.) On his own, Rogers more or less kept the idea of the PCT alive until hiking and trails were receiving national attention in the Sixties. He stayed active in promoting the trail and its joys almost to the time of his death in 1992 at age 83.

### National Trail System

In 1965 the Bureau of Outdoor Recreation, a federal agency, appointed a commission to make a nationwide trails study. The commission, noting that walking for pleasure was second only to driving for pleasure as the most popular recreation in America, recommended establishing a national system of trails of two kinds—long National Scenic Trails in the hinterlands and shorter National Recreation Trails in and near metropolitan areas. The commission recommended that Congress establish four Scenic Trails—the already existing Appalachian Trail, the partly existing Pacific

Crest Trail, a Potomac Heritage Trail and a Continental Divide Trail. Congress responded by passing, in 1968, the National Trails System Act, which set the framework for a system of trails and specifically made the Appalachian and the Pacific Crest trails the first two National Scenic trails.

### The Proposed Route

Meanwhile, in California, the Forest Service in 1965 had held a series of meetings about a route for the PCT in the state. These meetings involved people from the Forest Service, the Park Service, the State Division of Parks and Beaches, and other government bodies charged with responsibility over areas where the trail might go. These people decided that so much time had elapsed since Clarke had drawn his route that they should essentially start all over. Of course, it was pretty obvious that segments like the John Muir Trail would not be overlooked in choosing a new route through California. By the end of 1965 a proposed route had been drawn onto maps. (We don't say "mapped," for that would imply that someone actually had covered the route in the field.)

When Congress, in the 1968 law, created a citizens Advisory Council for the PCT, it was the route devised in 1965 which the Forest Service presented to the council as a "first draft" of a final PCT route. This body of citizens was to decide all the details of the final route; the Forest Service said it would adopt whatever the citizens wanted. The Advisory Council was also to concern itself with standards for the physical nature of the trail, markers to be erected along the trail, and the administration of the trail and its use.

In 1972 the Advisory Council agreed upon a route, and the Forest Service put it onto maps for internal use. Since much of the agreed-upon route was cross-country, these maps were sent to the various national forests along the route, for them to mark a temporary route in the places where no

trail existed along the final PCT route. This they did—but not always after field work. The result was that the maps made available to the public in June 1972 showing the final proposed route and the temporary detours did not correspond to what was on the ground in many places. A common flaw was that the Forest Service showed a temporary or permanent PCT segment following a trail taken from a pre-existing Forest Service map, when in fact there *was no trail* where it was shown on that map in the first place.

Perfect or not, the final proposed route was sent to Washington for publication in the Federal Register, the next step toward its becoming official. A verbal description of the route was also published in the Federal Register on January 30, 1973. But the material in the register did not give a precise route which could be unambiguously followed; it was only a *general* route, and the details in many places remained to be settled.

### Private Property Glitches

As construction on PCT trail segments began, many hikers were optimistic that the entire trail could be completed within a decade. Perhaps it could have, if it weren't for private property located along the proposed route. While some owners readily allowed rights-of-way, many others did not, at least initially, and years of negotiations passed before some rights were finally secured. While negotiations were in progress, the Forest Service sometimes built new trail segments on both sides of a parcel of private land, expecting to extend a trail segment through it soon after. At times this approach backfired, such as in the northern Sierra Nevada in the Gibraltar environs (Map M3 in *Pacific Crest Trail: Northern California*). The owners of some property never gave up a right-of-way, and so a new stretch of trail on Gibraltar's south slopes was abandoned for a snowier, costlier stretch on its north slopes, completed in

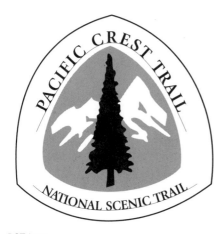

*PCT logo*

fall 1985. But at least the stretch was built, which was not true for a short stretch northwest of Sierra Buttes (Map M1, Section 7 also in the Northern California volume), where the PCT route is a road.

The major obstacle to the trail's completion had been the mammoth Tejon Ranch, which began in Civil War days as a sheep ranch, then later became a cattle ranch, and in 1936 became a public corporation that diversified its land use and increased its acreage. This "ranch," about the size of Sequoia National Park, straddles most of the Tehachapi Mountains. An agreement between the ranch's owners and government representatives finally was reached, and in 1993 this section of the PCT was completed. However, rather than traversing the length of the Tehachapi Mountains as intended by Congress, the PCT for the most part follows miles of roads along the west side of the high desert area of Antelope Valley before ascending to the edge of ranch property in the north part of the range.

Finally, there is another stretch in Northern California, covered in *The Pacific Crest Trail: Northern California* (Section Q and the start of Section R), where a trail will not replace existing roads. Private property was part of the problem, but also building a horse bridge across the Klamath River

proved economically unfeasible. One still treads 7.3 miles along roads, which is a blessing in disguise, for if the trail and bridge had been built, you would have bypassed Seiad Valley, a very important resupply point.

### "Golden Spike" Dedication

The Pacific Crest National Scenic Trail officially was dedicated on National Trails Day, June 5, 1993, a lengthy 25 years after Congress passed the National Trails System Act that had mandated it. The dedication was touted as the "Golden Spike" Completion Ceremony, in which a "golden" spike was driven into the trail, a reenactment of the 1869 ceremony at Promontory Point, near Ogden, Utah, where the converging Central Pacific and Union Pacific railroad companies joined to complete the transcontinental railroad. For the PCT, there were no competing trail crews, and the completion site should have been in the Tehachapi Mountains. However, the public was (and is) not welcome on the Tejon Ranch, and since that area is out of the way, a PCT site closer to metropolitan Southern California was chosen: a flat at the mouth of a small valley on the north side of Soledad Canyon (Map D13). Protected under a canopy to shelter them from the unseasonably cold, windy, drizzly weather, Secretary of the Interior Bruce Babbitt and others spoke to an unsheltered audience of about 300 hearty souls (and a dozen or so others protesting various unrelated environmental issues). The trail was proclaimed to be 2638 miles long officially, though the *accuracy* of this mileage may be questionable, since this number existed as early as 1990, *before* the completion of several stretches in Southern California and in the southern Sierra Nevada, and *before* the major relocation of the Hat Creek Rim stretch north of Lassen Volcanic National Park. Future relocations are likely, and so the authors of the Pacific Crest Trail books, for better or for worse, have used mileages that they have measured either directly along the trail or indirectly along the route they accurately drew on topographic maps.

## Some Who Walked and Rode

No doubt hikers did parts of the Pacific Crest Trail in the 19th Century— though that name for it didn't exist. It may be that someone walked along the crest from Mexico to Canada or vice versa many years ago. But the first person to claim he did the whole route in one continuous journey—in 1970—was Eric Ryback, in *The High Adventure of Eric Ryback*. Actually, he accepted rides for some of the approximately 2500-mile route, and so his claim was not quite true. Nevertheless, he hiked *most* of the route, which was quite an accomplishment for a 130-pound 18-year-old, hiking solo in the more difficult north-to-south direction *sans* guidebook or detailed maps. His 1971 book focused attention on the PCT, and other people began to plan end-to-end treks. Actually, the first documented hiker to complete the entire three-state trek was Martin Papendick (1922-2000), who did so way back in 1952 when a tri-state trail was still a dream.

As mentioned earlier, in June 1972 the Forest Service maps of the PCT route became available to the public, and the race was on. The first person to hike this entire route, as it then existed, was Richard Watson, who finished it on September 1, 1972. No one knew of Papendick, so for years Watson was considered the first *thru-hiker*, as backpackers who did the trail in one continuous, multi-month effort would come to be called. Barely behind him, finishing four days later, were Wayne Martin, Dave Odell, Toby Heaton, Bill Goddard and Butch Ferrand. Very soon after them, Henry Wilds went from Mexico to Canada solo. In 1972 Jeff Smukler did the PCT with Mary Carstens, who became the first woman to make it. The next year, Gregg Eames and Ben Schifrin set out to follow the official route as closely

as possible, no matter whether trail or cross country. Schifrin had to drop out with a broken foot at Odell Lake, Oregon (he finished the route the next year), but Eames got to Canada, and is probably the first person to have walked the official route almost without deviation.

In 1975, at least 27 people completed the PCT, according to Chuck Long, who was one of them and who put together a book of various trekkers' experiences. Perhaps as many as 200–300 hikers started the trail that year, intending to do it all. In 1976, one who made it all the way was Teddy Boston, the first woman to solo the trail, so far as we know. Teddy, then a 49-year-old mother of four, like Eric, made the trek the hard way, north to south.

Fascination with the trail steadily dropped, so that by the late 1980s perhaps only a dozen or so thru-hikers completed the entire trail in a given year. However, as completion of the trail approached, interest in it waxed, and some notable hikes were done. Perhaps some day a trekker's PCT anthology will be written, and in it many can be given due credit for their accomplishments. However, in a trail guide, space is limited, so we will mention only a (subjectively) select few who set "higher" goals. In the past we recommended that the thru-hiker allow 5–6 months for the entire PCT. No more, thanks to ultralight backpacking espoused by Ray and Jenny Jardine. In 1991 this couple completed the entire trail (their second thru-hike) in only three months and three weeks, and Ray subsequently wrote a how-to book (see the next chapter) based on this accomplishment. This was comparable to the length of time taken by Bob Holtel (in his mid-50s), who over the summers of 1985, '86, and '87 ran the PCT at the pace of a marathon a day, and he also wrote a book about it.

A few thru-hikers not only did the PCT, but also did the two other major north–south national scenic trails, the CDT (Continental Divide Trail) and the AT

(Appalachian Trail). The first person to have accomplished this task may have been Jim Podlesay, hiking the AT in 1973, the PCT in 1975, and the CDT in 1979. Back in 1975 many new stretches of the PCT had yet to be built, and in 1979 the CDT's route was still largely a matter of whatever you chose it to be. By 1980 the PCT was essentially complete, except for gaps between the Mexican border and the southern Sierra and the initial southern Washington stretch, which would become an annoying, out-of-the-way ascent and descent to the level, direct, temporary route. And with the PCT mostly complete, the first person who hiked it plus the AT and CDT may have been Lawrence Budd, who did all three in the late 1980s. Starting earlier but finishing later was Steve Queen, who hiked the PCT in 1981, the AT in 1983, and the CDT in 1991. The first woman may have been Alice Gmuer, who hiked the PCT in 1987 and '88, the AT in 1990, and the CDT in 1993. Close behind was Brice Hammack, who over eight summers completed the last of the three trails in 1994—at a very respectable age of 74.

While there have been hundreds of successful thru-hikers on the PCT, very few equestrians have matched this feat. Perhaps the first equestrians to do the trail were Barry Murray and his family, who rode it in two summers in the early 1970s. Much later, in 1988, Jim McCrea became the first "thru-equestrian," completing the entire trail in just under five months. Very few thru-hikers actually do every foot of the trail, and for thru-equestrians this feat so far has proved to be unfeasible, due to icy snowfields impassable to stock.

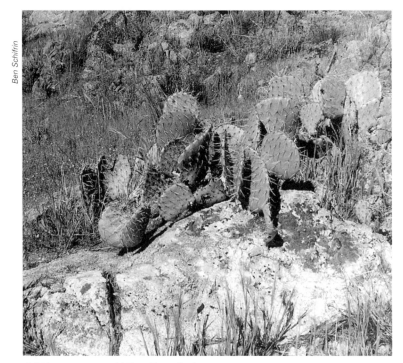

*Prickly pear cactus, Yellow Rose Spring*

## Chapter 2

# Planning Your PCT Hike

## Trekking Days or Weeks versus Trekking Months

On the basis of our limited research we have concluded that approximately 90 percent (or more) of those who buy this book will do parts of the trail as a series of short excursions, each lasting about two weeks or less. For those people, little planning is necessary; you should be able to carry enough food in your pack. You need not worry about mailing supplies to post offices along or near the trail. Furthermore, you can hike the desired stretch in its optimal season, and not need the additional clothing and gear that thru-hikers must carry for the times they may have to traverse miles of snow and confront many cold-weather storms. If you prefer to dayhike along the PCT, consider obtaining a two-volume set, *Day Hikes on the Pacific Crest Trail* (California and Oregon & Washington) by George and Patricia Semb. (For books on or related to the PCT, see the section "Pacific Crest Trail" under "Recommended Reading and Source Books." For books on general hiking or riding, see the section "Backpacking, Packing, and Mountaineering.")

At the other end of the spectrum of PCT trekkers are 200-300 or so each year who start at the Mexican border and attempt to do the entire trail in one multi-month Herculean effort. Before the early 1990s there was a rather high attrition rate among these thru-hikers—typically 50+ percent don't complete it. This need not be so. Today there are great books out there to prepare you—mentally, physically, and logistically—for the grand odyssey. Ray and Jenny Jardine were instrumental in a long-distance backpacking revolution with their 1992 how-to book, *The PCT Hiker's Handbook*, published by AdventureLore Press (unfortunately, out of print since the late 1990s). The Jardines' book advocated ultralight backpacking. If you have only 20 pounds on your back, you'll be able to traverse more miles per day than if you have 60. No longer do you have to take 5½-6 months for a thru-hike; traveling light, you can do it in 4½-5 months or less (the Jardines did it in under 4 months). Fortunately, *Beyond Backpacking: Ray Jardine's Guide to Lightweight Hiking* is available, cov-

Jeffrey P. Schsffer

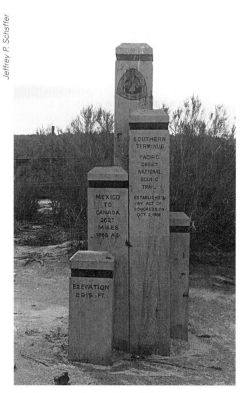

*Southern Terminus of the PCT*

ering this material and other useful tips, with sections also tailored to the "casual" backpacker.

There are several advantages to ultra-light backpacking. A lighter pack is easier on your joints and muscles, making the excursion more pleasurable. Furthermore, by traveling light you are less likely to have an injury because: 1) your body isn't overly stressed; 2) you're less likely to fall; 3) and if you do, the impact isn't as great. Traveling light, you'll perspire less, which is a plus on the long dry stretches. Additionally, you'll burn fewer calories, getting by with less food and, hence, less weight. By reducing your pack's weight to less than 20% of your body weight (that is, about 25-35 pounds for most hikers), you probably can get by with lightweight running or walking shoes, or even high-quality hiking sandals, making you less prone to those painful blisters

synonymous with almost all boots. Both lighter packs and lighter footgear increase your daily mileage, providing an advantage other than comfort. You can start later and finish earlier, thereby encountering less storm-and-snow problems in the High Sierra early in your trek, and less storm-and-snow problems in Washington near completion.

However, there is a drawback to ultra-light backpacking. If you're caught in a blizzard or some other adverse condition, you may not have sufficient gear to survive; indeed, some ultralighters on long-distance trails have died. Also—and this applies to everyone, whether they take 4 or 6 months for a thru-hike—foremost on your mind will be keeping to your schedule, but because unexpected events or trail conditions can delay you and force you to make up for lost time, you likely won't have the time or energy to "stop and smell the flowers." For this reason alone we suggest to those intent on doing the entire trail, to do it in two to five or more hiking seasons, each one to three months long, taking sufficient time to enjoy your trek. To most hikers 10 miles per day under optimal trail and weather conditions is far more pleasurable than 20 miles per day under hell-or-high-water conditions.

Perhaps the best book in print on thru-hiking the PCT is Karen Berger's *Hiking the Triple Crown: How to Hike America's Longest Trails: Appalachian Trail, Pacific Crest Trail, Continental Divide Trail.* Where Ray Jardine's books advocate ultralight backpacking, Karen Berger offers you a smorgasbord of choices since each successful thru-hiker has his or her own preferences. The first third of her book is a how-to on long-distance backpacking, while the remainder addresses specific issues on the AT, PCT, and CDT. If you plan to be on the PCT for more than a month, then by all means read Berger's book.

There are other books for the long-distance backpacker to consider, especially two inexpensive ones published by the Pacific Crest Trail Association. The first is Leslie C. Croot's *Pacific Crest Trail Town Guide,* which has detailed accounts of supplies and services available for most PCT towns or resorts, each complete with a detailed map. This is great for planning and, at only 5 ounces, is easily carried. The second PCTA book is Benedict Go's *Pacific Crest Trail Data Book.* Although the guidebook in your hand has all the necessary mileages (state mileages, section mileages, point-to-point mileages), some trekkers want more when planning their hike, and Ben delivers. The bulk of his book is a synopsis of the Wilderness Press PCT guidebooks' point-to-point mileages, each named, and each accompanied by overall mileage from Mexico, plus elevation, and what water and/or services are available.

How-to books and reference books certainly are useful for preparing and planning a thru-hike, but so too are personal accounts, and several (both in-print and out-of-print) are listed under "Recommended Reading and Source Books." Larger libraries may have copies of out-of-print books. There's nothing like first-hand accounts to give you a feel for the thru-hike and its challenges. And don't forget to subscribe to the outstanding Internet mail list, "PCT-L." To join the verbal give-and-take, and to learn about the most up-to-date trail conditions, send an e-mail to *pct-l@mailman.backcountry.net,* with no subject and a message that reads, "subscribe pct-l [your e-mail address]."

Given that few equestrians attempt most or all of the PCT, it is not surprising that a how-to book for them does not exist. However, Ben and Adeline York have self-published their notes on the whole trail, which are quite useful for potential PCT equestrians. To obtain a copy of their publication, *PCT by 2 in 1992,* write them at 1363 Peaceful Place, Alpine, CA 91901. For horse use in the mountains, they recommend you obtain the packers' Bible, *Horses,*

*Hitches and Rocky Trails,* by Joe Back (Johnson Books, Boulder, CO). You will encounter more problems than do backpackers, and so the following caution is even more important: a short horseback trip does *not* qualify you for a lengthy excursion on the PCT.

Halfway between hikers and equestrians are those who walk the trail but pack with llamas. Like horses, llamas were native to western North America before going extinct there. Unlike horses, llamas are native to *high mountains,* and on erodible tread their foot pads have less impact than horses' hooves. They are also much less damaging to mountain meadows, and do not spread exotic grass seed there. David Harmon and Amy S. Rubin have written a llama-packer's guide, which stresses minimum-impact in the wilderness. Unfortunately, it's now out of print.

# Organizations Relevant to the Pacific Crest Trail

The previously mentioned books should answer most of your questions about hiking or riding the PCT. But if questions linger, they may be answered by contacting one or more of the following organizations.

## Pacific Crest Trail Association (PCTA)

Those planning a long trek can write or phone this organization for advice that is either timely (e.g., current snowpack conditions) or expert (e.g., providing specific answers tailored to each individual). If those in the office cannot answer your questions, they will attempt to find one of their directors or members who can. Since this organization has both hikers and equestrians as members, they should be able to answer questions for either type of travel.

The organization is part of the legacy of Warren Rogers (the PCT itself is the other part). After the demise of the Pacific Crest

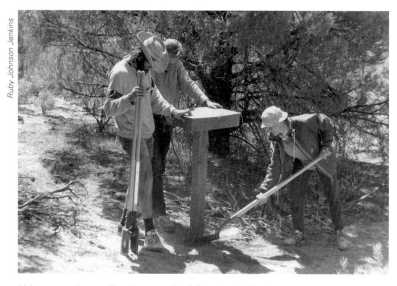

*Volunteers place trail registry north of Canebrake Road*

Trail System Conference with the death of Clinton Clarke, Rogers in 1971 formed the Pacific Crest Club to be a "world-wide fellowship of persons interested in the PCT," as his son, Don, put it. Then in 1977 he founded the Pacific Crest Trail Conference, which addressed the needs of both the trail and its users. But old age eventually interfered with running these organizations, so in 1987 the club was merged with the conference, and for several years Larry Cash was its chief officer. The conference campaigned against trailside clearcutting and against mountain bikes, and for additional water sources along the drier stretches and for volunteer trail maintenance. In 1992 the organization changed its name to the Pacific Crest Trail Association. The mailing address is 5325 Elkhorn Blvd., PMB 256, Sacramento, CA 95842-2526; phone is (916) 349-2109; e-mail is *info@pcta.org*; and Web is *www.pcta.org*. Increasingly, this organization has become active in coordinating volunteer trail maintenance. For example, in 2000 the PCTA coordinated trail crews that donated more than 20,000 hours of their time. For this reason alone the organi-

zation deserves support, and you should consider becoming a member. Most hikers and equestrians on any trail give little thought to trail maintenance. Indeed, many PCT trekkers complain about sections being not up to snuff. Without the volunteers, though, there would be far more to complain about, since, in these years of tight government budgets, trail maintenance is one of the lowest priorities. (Trail maintenance is ongoing locally, where erosion damages parts of the trail, fallen trees and rolling boulders obstruct it, and shrubs continually encroach upon it.)

What services does the PCTA provide the potential trekker? In addition to answering your PCT letters, phone calls, and faxes, it publishes a bimonthly newsletter, *The Communicator*. While addressing general issues and timely matters, it provides informative accounts by those who have hiked or ridden much or all of the PCT. *The Communicator* also has a section on trip partners where people can post their background, experience, and what kind of partner they'd like. Through an agreement with the Forest Service, Park Service, Bureau of

Land Management, and other agencies, the PCTA also provides wilderness permits for trips of 500 miles or more on the PCT. The association's Web site contains hundreds of pages of information, including trip planning, current trail conditions, trip calculators, and more (including permit applications and links to other useful sites). Additionally, the PCTA maintains registers (see below) along or near the trail. These provide the organization with a list of who did what, relative degree of trail use, and annually and seasonally changing trail conditions and special problems. By signing these registers the backpacker over time develops a camaraderie with other trekkers. Although you may never catch up to those ahead of you, by trail's end you may feel that you've come to know them. Finally, the PCTA has been making a concerted effort to

lobby Congress for funds ($4.5 million by early 2001) to help acquire nearly 300 miles of private land, ensuring future generations of PCT users a protected corridor. Related to this are suggestions to government agencies on future reroutes to make the trail safer, more practical, or more scenic.

## American Long Distance Hikers Association-West (ALDHA-West)

In 1993 Ray Jardine founded the Western States Chapter and also began publishing *The Distance Hiker's Gazette*, a quarterly newsletter. After a couple of years, Ray left his organization, and a few of its members took it over and reorganized it. Its mission is to promote fellowship and communication among long-distance hikers, and those who support (but don't necessar-

## Pacific Crest Trail Association Registers in California, South to North

Because the locations of PCTA registers are not always obvious, a list of them is presented below. These locations are subject to change, although most are quite stable, especially the sites that are post offices. Unless otherwise designated, the register is located in a post office, which at some places is just a tiny room in a store or a resort.

Campo
Mount Laguna
Julian, Banner Store
Warner Springs
Anza
Idyllwild
Cabazon
Big Bear City
Fawnskin
Wrightwood, Mountain Hardware
Agua Dulce, Agua Dulce Hardware
Tehachapi
Mojave
Onyx
Kennedy Meadows,
    Kennedy Meadows Store
Lone Pine
Independence
Vermilion Valley Resort, store

Mammoth Lakes
Tuolumne Meadows,
    concessionaire's store
Lee Vining
Bridgeport
Markleeville
Soda Springs
Sierra City
Belden Town Resort, store
Old Station
Cassel
McArthur-Burney Falls State Park,
    camper store
Castella
Seiad Valley, Seiad Valley Store
Ashland (southern Oregon),
    Youth Hostel

ily do) long-distance hiking. As the association's name implies, it is aimed at long-distance *backpackers* only (i.e., not dayhikers and equestrians). Although the association's emphasis is on the Pacific Crest Trail, it also addresses relevant backpacking matters on other long trails or treks, not only in the western United States, but even overseas, and members hail from around the country, not just from the west. If you're a long-distance hiker, there are at least two reasons to join the association: first, in *The Distance Hiker's Gazette* there are good descriptions of various trails and routes, plus backpacking advice; and second, each fall they have the ALDHA-West Gathering,

where one can find lots of camaraderie among distance hikers. To join the organization, write to ALDHA-West, Box 5286, Eugene, OR 97405, or visit its Web page at *www.aldhawest.org*.

The vast majority of PCT trekkers are hikers, but there is fair use from equestrians on certain stretches. Occasionally an equestrian party will attempt to do the whole trail. This is more difficult than hiking, since horses don't wear crampons and don't cross logs over deep, raging streams. Consequently, it's virtually impossible to do the whole trek in one long season without making serious diversions, such as skipping the High Sierra entirely or doing it

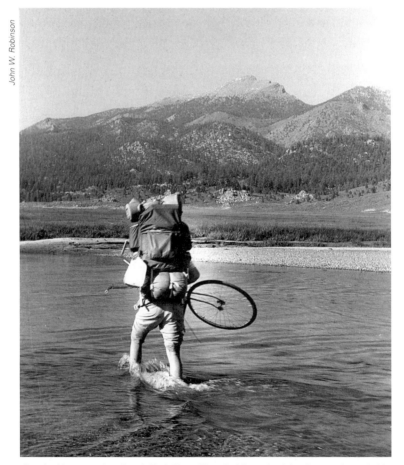

John W. Robinson

*Jim Jenkins crossing South Fork Kern River in Monache Meadows prior to bridge*

later, after the snow has melted and streams are safe. Should you want to ride the entire trail without any diversions or leapfrogging, then do it over two or more summers, making sure you do the High Sierra between mid-July and mid-September (and Washington during August— before then there is too much snow, after then, too much chance of snowstorms). For help on planning your trip through California, contact the Backcountry Horsemen of California; for Oregon and Washington, start with the Backcountry Horsemen of America.

Equestrians, you might do it while you can. Although the PCT is solely for hikers and equestrians, pressure is underway to ban equestrians from overnight stays in the backcountry, as in Yosemite National Park. (For years they've been banned overnight in the backcountry of Lassen Volcanic National Park.) What logistics could you devise if ultimately you were banned from overnight camping in wildernesses and national parks? In effect, you would only be able to do those parts you could do as day rides.

### Backcountry Horsemen of California

This organization (which, despite its name, is open to horse*women*) was created in 1981. Though its mailing address has shifted in the past, in 2001 you could reach it at Box 40007, Bakersfield, CA 93384-0007, or by phone at (888) 302-BCHC (information and fax line) and, in the 209 area code, 530-0662, or at its Web site at *www.bchc.com*. BCHC is dedicated to conserving backcountry wilderness and protecting stock users' historic use of wilderness trails. Among other things, the organization offers clinics that show you how to pack with a horse and/or mule in the mountains. Besides teaching the fundamentals of packing, it stresses low-impact use, courtesy, and common sense. Available from the organization, directly off its Web site, is "Gentle Use: A Pocket Guide to Backcountry Stock Users." *Much of their good advice also applies to backpackers.* The BCHC is a member organization of the Backcountry Horsemen of America (BCHA).

### Backcountry Horsemen of America

Like the previous organization, BCHA also includes horse*women*, but it does not include all of the United States, but only 11 western states plus several others of the conterminous 48 states. If you plan to continue riding north beyond California, into Oregon and/or Washington, you might start with this organization. It publishes a quarterly newsletter plus a book—very relevant for California equestrians—*Back Country Horsemen Guidebook* (see "Recommended Reading and Source Materials: Backpacking, Packing, and Mountaineering").

## Mailing Tips

As was stated in the beginning of this chapter, the great majority of PCT hikers will not be on the trail long enough to bother with resupply points, which are mostly post offices. Those who will be on the trail for, say, one to several hiking sections can use the following table. The minority who attempt to do all of California also should consider obtaining Leslie C. Croot's *Pacific Crest Trail Town Guide*, mentioned early in this chapter, since she gives post office hours as well as some of their phone numbers. (Be aware that this kind of information has changed in the past, and likely will do so in the future.)

You can mail yourself almost any food, clothing or equipment. Before you leave home, you should have a good idea of your consumption rate of food, clothing, and fuel for your stove. You can arrange for mailings of quantities of these things, purchased at home, where they are probably cheaper than in the towns along the way. Address your package to:

[Your Name]General Delivery
[Post Office, State Abbr. Zip Code]
Hold Until [Date]

## Post Offices Along or Near the Route, South to North

\* = recommended for use

Some stations are seasonal. The best pickup time is weekdays 1–4 P.M. Hours of most are 9–12 and 1–5 or longer. Some are open Saturday mornings. Plan your trip schedule accordingly in order to avoid waiting two or three days in town because a post office was closed for the weekend (don't forget about the three-day weekends: Memorial Day, Fourth of July, Labor Day). Additionally, some resorts or concessionaires may accept mailed or UPS parcels so check the introductory section in each of the trail-description chapters (Sections A–H).

Campo 92006
*Mount Laguna 91948
Julian 92036
Borrego Springs 92004
*Warner Springs 92086
Anza 92539
*Idyllwild 92549
Cabazon 92230
Palm Springs 92262
*Big Bear City 92314
Fawnskin 92333
*Cedar Glen 92321
Lake Arrowhead 92352
Hesperia 92340
*Wrightwood 92397
Acton 93510
Palmdale 93590
Santa Clarita 91380
*Lake Hughes 93532
Lancaster 93534

*Tehachapi 93561
Mohave 93501
Onyx 93255
Kernville 93238
*Kennedy Mdws. Gen. Store
    Box 3A-5
    Inyokern, 93427
Lone Pine 93545
Independence 93526
Bishop 93514
*Lake Edison:
    Vermilion Valley Resort
    c/o Rancheria Garage
    Huntington Lake Road
    Lakeshore, CA 93634
*Mammoth Lakes 93546
June Lake 93529
*Tuolumne Meadows 95389
Lee Vining 93541 (Use this when
    Tuolumne Meadows is
    closed)

# Federal Government Agencies

Most of the Pacific Crest Trail through California is on federal government lands and, while all have similar regulations, each may have specific requirements. For example, some of the federal government's wildernesses do not require a wilderness permit for entry while others do, and for some there may be campfire, campsite, and/or food-storage restrictions, while some will have none. As stated earlier, the Pacific Crest Trail Association provides wilderness permits for trips of 500 miles or more on the PCT. However, most of this book's users will do less than 500 miles, and may need to apply directly to a federal government agency for a permit; they may contact it for some other reason, such as to query trailhead parking fees or check for temporary road or trail closures. Therefore, the appropriate Bureau of Land Management, National Forest, and National Park offices are presented in the following table. While you can write or phone each, you may find it easier to check its Web site first for all pertinent information. If you need a wilderness permit, obtaining it through a Web site is perhaps the most painless way of getting it.

## Federal Government Agencies, South to North

\* = wildernesses and national parks that require a wilderness permit for an overnight stay

BLM-El Centro Field Office
    1661 South Fourth Street
    El Centro, CA 92243
    (760) 337-4400
    *www.ca.blm.gov/elcentro*

Cleveland National Forest
    10845 Rancho Bernardo Road
    Rancho Bernardo
    CA 92127-2107
    (858) 674-2109
    *www.r5.fs.fed.us/cleveland*

Hauser Wilderness
    contact: Cleveland NF

Sawtooth Mountains Wilderness
    contact: BLM-El Centro

BLM-Palm Springs Field Office
    690 West Garnet Avenue
    Box 1260
    North Palm Springs
    CA 92258-1260
    (760) 251-4800
    *www.ca.blm.gov/palmsprings*

Santa Rosa and San Jacinto
Mountains National Monument\*
    contact: BLM-Palm Springs

San Bernardino National Forest
    1824 Commercenter Circle
    San Bernardino, CA 92408-3430
    (909) 884-6634
    *www.r5.fs.fed.us/sanbernardino*

San Gorgonio Wilderness
    contact: San Bernardino NF &
    BLM-Palm Springs

Angeles National Forest
    701 North Santa Anita Avenue
    Arcadia, CA 91006
    (626) 574-1613
    *www.r5.fs.fed.us/angeles*

Sheep Mountain Wilderness\*
    contact: Angeles NF

BLM - Bakersfield Field Office
   3801 Pegasus Drive
   Bakersfield, CA 93308
   (661) 391-6000
   *www.ca.blm.gov/bakersfield*

Owens Peak, Chimney Peak, Dome
Land (east) wildernesses
   contact: BLM-Bakersfield

Sequoia National Forest
   900 West Grand Avenue
   Porterville, CA 93257
   (559) 784-1500
   *www.r5.fs.fed.us/sequoia*

Kiavah Dome Land (west),
South Sierra, and Golden Trout*
wildernesses
   contact: Sequoia NF

Sequoia and Kings Canyon
National Parks*
   47050 Generals Highway
   Three Rivers, CA 93271
   (559) 565-3341
   *www.nps.gov/seki*

Inyo National Forest
   873 North Main Street
   Bishop, CA 93514
   (760) 873-2400
   *www.r5.fs.fed.us/inyo*

John Muir Wilderness*
   contact: Inyo NF

Sierra National Forest
   900 W. Grand Avenue
   Porterville, CA 93257
   (559) 784-1500
   *www.r5.fs.fed.us/sierra*

Ansel Adams Wilderness*
   contact: Mammoth Ranger Station
   and Visitor Center
   Box 148
   Mammoth Lakes, CA 93546
   (760) 873-2500, 924-5500

Yosemite National Park*
Wilderness Center
   Box 545
   Yosemite, CA 95389
   (209) 372-0740
   *www.nps.gov/yose/wilderness*

Humboldt-Toiyabe National Forest
   2035 Last Chance Road
   Elko, NV 89801-4938
   (775) 738-5171
   *www.fs.fed.us/r4/htnf*

Stanislaus National Forest
   19777 Greenley Road
   Sonora, CA 95370
   (209) 532-3671
   *www.r5.fs.fed.us/stanislaus*

Emigrant Wilderness* and
Carson-Iceberg Wilderness*
Sonora Pass trailhead
   contact: Summit Ranger District
   #1 Pinecrest Lake Road
   Pinecrest, CA 95364
   (209) 965-3434

Carson-Iceberg Wilderness*
Ebbetts Pass trailhead
   contact: Carson Ranger District
   1536 S. Carson Street
   Carson City, NV 89701
   (775) 882-2766

Mokelumne Wilderness*
   contact: Carson Ranger District
   (above)

Eldorado National Forest
   100 Forni Road
   Placerville, CA 95667
   (530) 622-5061
   *www.r5.fs.fed.us/eldorado*

also:

Eldorado Information Center
   3070 Camino Heights Drive
   Camino, CA 95709
   (530) 644-6048

## Federal Government Agencies, South to North

\* = wildernesses and national parks that require a wilderness permit for an overnight stay

Desolation Wilderness*
Lake Tahoe Basin Management Unit
   870 Emerald Bay Rd., Suite 1
   S. Lake Tahoe, CA 96150
   (530) 573-2600
   *www.r5.fs.fed.us/ltbmu*

Tahoe National Forest
   Highway 49 & Coyote St.
   Nevada City, CA 95959
   (530) 265-4531
   *www.r5.fs.fed.us/tahoe*

Granite Chief Wilderness
   contact: Tahoe NF

Plumas National Forest
   Box 11500
   159 Lawrence Street
   Quincy, CA 95971
   (530) 283-2050
   *www.r5.fs.fed.us/plumas*

Bucks Lake Wilderness
   contact: Plumas NF

Lassen National Forest
   2550 Riverside Drive
   Susanville, CA 96130
   (530) 257-2151
   *www.r5.fs.fed.us/lassen*

Lassen Volcanic National Park*
   Box 100
   Mineral, CA 96063
   (530) 595-4444
   *www.nps.gov/lavo*

Shasta-Trinity National Forest
   2400 Washington Avenue
   Redding, CA 96001
   (530) 244-2978
   *www.r5.fs.fed.us/shastatrinity*

Castle Crags and Trinity Alps* wildernesses
   contact: Shasta-Trinity NF

Klamath National Forest
   1312 Fairlane Road
   Yreka, CA 96097
   (530) 842-6131
   *www.r5.fs.fed.us/klamath*

Russian and Marble Mountain wildernesses
   contact: Klamath NF

Rogue River National Forest
   Box 520
   333 West 8th Street
   Medford, OR 97501
   (541) 858-2200
   *www.fs.fed.us/r6/rogue*

Red Buttes Wilderness
   contact: Rogue River NF

## Hiking the Pacific Crest Trail

### Dayhiking

Roughly 86 percent of the PCT in California can be dayhiked, averaging about 15 miles a day, though over some sections you'll do less than 5 miles, while over others more than 25 (but less than 30). As mentioned early in this chapter, George and Patricia Semb have a two-volume set, *Day Hikes on the Pacific Crest Trail,* and their California volume presents 124 dayhikes for the California PCT (this two-volume guidebook's sections A-R). According to the authors, the only hiking sections that cannot be entirely dayhiked in the *Pacific Crest Trail: Southern California* are: (with their total inaccessible mileages) are: F (17.3 miles), G (41.7 miles), and H (110.9 miles).

Should you dayhike the trail? Maybe not, but perhaps most of those on the trail are just doing a dayhike. There are at least five advantages to dayhiking. First, the national parks and the popular wildernesses require wilderness permits for overnight stays, and some popular PCT stretches even have trailhead quotas for overnighters, yet there are no permits or quotas for dayhikers. Second, dayhiking requires very little planning or preparation. Third, because your pack is lighter, you may enjoy the hike more, since you'll expend less effort with less wear and tear on your body, especially your feet. Dayhikers can usually get by with running shoes or cross-training boots, which, though still likely to furnish blisters during the break-in period, are much lighter than hiking boots. Fourth, you can easily carry a day's supply of water. This is an advantage, for some lakes, streams, and springs contain harmful microorganisms. You can leave water-treatment chemicals or water filters behind. And finally, dayhikers have less impact on the environment. For one thing, dayhikers usually use toilets near trailheads rather than along the trail. Particularly around a popular lake, excrement can affect the water quality and lead to an increase in microorganisms. Excrement from humans infected with harmful intestinal microorganisms, such as *Giardia lamblia,* discussed under "Drinking water," can lead to the establishment of these microorganisms in a previously untainted lake or stream.

### Backpacking

If you are a typical backpacker, you may hike for two days—usually over a weekend—up to two weeks. For hikes of such length, you won't need to resupply. (Those doing considerably longer hikes with a number of resupply points might consult the books mentioned early in this chapter.) What follows is a checklist to help with your packing. You may want to carry more or less, but regardless of your preferences, be prepared for potentially bad weather. Without food, your backpack should weigh only about 15-20 pounds; with food, an additional 2 pounds per person per day. If you are out for a week, your pack initially should be 40 pounds or less (some get by on 30). Too often you see backpackers in massive boots, using trekking poles, and needlessly suffering under their 60+ pound packs. If your pack weighs less than 25% of your body weight, you probably can get by just fine without poles or boots.

## Trail Advice

Once you have your wilderness permit (if required) and a full pack, you are ready to start hiking. The following advice, most of it from the Park Service and Forest Service, is provided to help make your hike more enjoyable and also safer.

1. **The wilderness permit does not serve as a registration system for hikers.** Leave an itinerary, a route description,

## Items to consider for your backpack

waist or fanny pack
your keys
watch
wilderness permit
guidebook(s)
additional maps (e.g., USFS)
compass
first-aid book
nature books, novels
camera, film, and accessories
binoculars
fishing gear
California fishing license
trekking poles
ice ax
other special gear
sleeping bag
pad or air mattress
ground cloth
tent or ground cloth large enough to
    serve as emergency rain shelter
raingear or poncho (the latter can
    double as a ground cloth)
windbreaker and/or sweatshirt
vest or parka (down, wool, or other)
hiking shoes or boots
lightweight camp shoes (e.g., gym-
    nastics slippers) or sandals
socks (preferably polypropylene and/
    or wool)
shorts
pants
T-shirt or short-sleeved shirt
long-sleeved shirt
underwear (incl. thermal)
handkerchiefs and/or bandana

cap or hat
dark glasses (preferably polarized)
gloves
swim suit
towel and/or washcloth
toilet paper
plastic bag for used toilet paper
trowel
personal-hygiene items
contraceptives
first-aid kit
molefoam
mosquito repellent
bear repellent (pepper spray)
lip balm (with sunscreen)
sunblock
prescription medicine
pocket knife
flashlight or headlamp
extra bulb and batteries
cigarette lighter or matches in water-
    proof container
stove & fuel
cooking and eating utensils
Sierra cup or coffee cup
water bottle(s)
water filter or purifying chemicals
food and drink
several trash bags
salt, pepper, spices
2 or more stuff sacks for bearbagging
50' of parachute cord for bearbagging
50' of parachute cord for emergencies
bearproof food container
duct tape for emergencies (broken
    pack, bone, etc.)

and expected time of return with friends or relatives, or inquire at the nearest ranger station about hiker sign-out procedures.

2. **Stay on maintained trails unless you are good at using a compass and topographic maps.** When off the trail, you can easily lose your sense of direction, especially in a viewless forest or in bad weather.

3. **Solo hiking can be dangerous, particularly if you have large streams to ford.** If you do set out alone, stick to frequently used trails so that you can get help if you become sick or injured.

4. **Watch your step on trails; the mountains are no place to get a sprained ankle.** Don't shortcut across switchbacks, for this leads to trail erosion.

5. **When you meet pack stock on the trail, remain quiet and in plain view.** Allow them to pass by stepping off the trail on the downslope side; equestrians have the right-of-way.

6. **Close all gates.** They prevent stock from wandering up and down the trail.

7. **If you want to wear hiking boots, make sure they are well broken-in to avoid blisters.** Wear at least two pairs of socks and carry molefoam just in case.

8. **If you bring children along, be sure they have some personal identification on them at all times.** Tell them what to do if they get lost (they should stay put) and give them a whistle or other means of signaling for help. Don't leave them alone; there are mountain lions out there.

9. **Confusion about which trail to take at trail junctions frequently results in spread-out parties becoming separated.** To avoid confusion and the possibility of

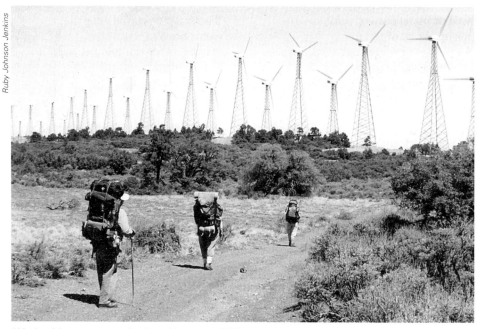

*Wind-turbine towers perched on ridges near PCT*

Ruby Johnson Jenkins

someone getting lost, faster party members should wait for slower members at all trail junctions. If your party has members who want to travel at different paces, then be sure enough of them have a marked map that shows the party's route and campsite for each night.

10. **Be prepared for rain or snow any time of the year above 7000 feet.** Learn survival techniques, especially how to stay warm and dry in inclement weather. Above 9000 feet, wear dark glasses and/or a hat, for the dangerous ultraviolet radiation up there is very intense, and prolonged exposure increases your risk of skin cancer and damage to your eyes. On exposed skin, use a strong lip balm and a strong sunscreen (30+).

11. **Don't underestimate the power of moving water, particularly since streambeds tend to be quite slippery.** One of the greatest dangers to backcountry travelers is crossing streams. White water and areas above cascades and waterfalls are especially dangerous. A rope is useful in crossing swift streams, but hang on to it rather than tie into it. Hikers tied in have drowned before they could untie the rope after slipping, because their taut rope forced them underwater.

12. **Lightning is a hazard in the mountains.** You can gauge how far away a lightning strike is by counting the seconds it takes for thunder to arrive after you see a lightning flash. A 5-second delay means the strike was about a mile away. A 1-second delay means that it was about 1000 feet away, and you are too close for comfort—absolutely seek shelter. Do not continue upward into a thunderstorm. Get off ridges and peaks. Stay away from meadows and lakes and also avoid exposed lone objects such as large rocks, isolated trees, railing, cable, and

sizable objects. Find shelter in forested areas. Your vehicle is a safe place to wait out a storm.

13. **If the trail's tread is vague, if it is under snow, or if there are multiple paths due to cycles or cattle, then look for blazes or ducks.** A blaze is a place on a tree trunk where someone has carved away a patch of bark to leave a conspicuous scar. A duck is one or several small rocks placed upon a larger rock in such a way that the placement is obviously human-made. Where a trail crosses bedrock, it is often bordered by large rocks placed there by trail crews. Occasionally a large human-made rock pile, or cairn, will be found, usually marking a route.

14. **Pets aren't allowed on national park trails.** Elsewhere, you still shouldn't take your pets on the trail. Dogs in particular annoy other hikers, spook stock, harass wildlife, pollute campsites, and sometimes import diseases harmful to other mammals. Furthermore, dogs do get lost, contrary to what many people believe. Finally, rocky trail treads can badly cut a dog's feet. Carry bandages or duct tape if you do bring your dog.

15. When John Muir roamed through the Sierra during the 19th Century, he cut branches to sleep on and built a bonfire to warm himself through the night. Muir made very little impact on the environment, but due to the great number of backpackers today, each of us must treat the environment with a great deal of care. One consideration is where to camp. **Set up camp at least 100 feet away from lakes and streams (200+ feet is better) to prevent water contamination and damage to protective shore and bank vegetation.** Also, try to camp at least 100 feet or more from trails. Avoid the fragile sod of meadows, lake

shores, and stream banks. You'll sleep better on a forest floor: it tends to harbor fewer mosquitoes than found in wet areas, and you will stay warmer and drier if you sleep under the trees rather than in the open. The forest retains heat better, tends to have drier ground, and certainly has less nighttime condensation. Once you have selected your campsite, minimize your impact on it. Don't clear away brush, level the ground, cut trenches, or build a fire ring. Don't destroy, deface, or carve up trees, shrubs, or any other natural or cultural features.

**16. Litter and food scraps not only are unsightly intrusions on a wilderness experience, but also are an unnatural food source that attracts animals— bears and rodents in particular.** Your food source in the long run is detrimental to the well-being of these animals. All trash, including cans, bottles, metal foil, tampons, disposable diapers, toilet paper, orange peels, apple cores, etc. must be packed out. Do not burn or bury trash or scatter organic wastes. Carry plastic bags for trash. An old cliché is still true: If you can pack it in, you can pack it out.

**17. Chemicals found in both biodegradable and nonbiodegradable soaps and detergents pollute backcountry lakes and streams.** Pollution by organic wastes has led to bacteria spreading through many lakes and streams, so you should bring your water to a boil, or treat it with chemicals, or—most conveniently— purify it with a water filter. Unfortunately, our own bodies, as carriers of bacteria, contribute to the bacterial population. Keep the bacterial count low by cleaning pots, washing clothes, and bathing yourself—at least 100 feet away from any body of water. On the trail, soap is unnecessary and is best left at home. You can let the toughest of the baked-on food accumulate and then clean your

pots thoroughly when you get home. To eliminate the need for pot scrubbing, as well as the weight of pots, a stove, and fuel, you could eat cold meals, and indeed, many trekkers have hiked the entire PCT this way.

**18. Proper disposal of human waste is another serious environmental consideration.** Pick a spot at least 50 yards away from any trail, camping area, meadow, stream, or lake. Dig a hole about 6-8 inches deep and 8-10 inches across. After use, put the toilet paper in a plastic bag; don't bury it. Cover the hole with the soil and duff you removed, and make the site blend in with the surroundings. Women should not burn or bury tampons or sanitary napkins, and parents should not burn or bury disposable diapers. They are difficult to burn and require years to decompose. Pack them out in a plastic bag. If you have a large group, make a latrine site, then thoroughly cover it when you leave.

**19. Wildfires are caused by lightning strikes and human stupidity.** The first is not anything you can prevent; the second is completely under your control. If you must build a fire, use only dead wood lying on the ground, and build a fire no larger than you actually need, in an already existing fire ring. Put it out at least ½ hour before you are ready to leave, adding water to it and stirring the ashes. In the High Sierra, fires usually are banned at elevations above 9000 feet. At a few popular backcountry lakes camping and/or campfires are banned, and these are mentioned in the text.

# Animal and Plant Problems on the PCT

If you hike the entire California PCT, you'll see dozens of bird species. You'll also pass by dozens of mammal species, but will *see* very few, except for deer, marmots, pikas, and squirrels, particularly the nearly ubiquitous California ground squirrel. However, the animals are around; just camp near a spring in Southern California, and you'll hear quite a flurry of activity during the night. Without a tent, you may hear or feel toads and mice traversing around or over you, and a scorpion or two may get under or, worse, into your sleeping bag. The rodents are harmless, although they can carry fleas that transmit diseases. What follows is a brief synopsis of animal and plant problems you can face on the PCT.

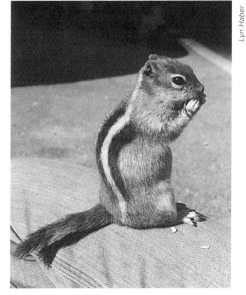

*Golden-mantled ground squirrel*

### Poison Oak

Some botanists have claimed that there are places in the chaparral belt, stretching from Southern California's coastal plains north through Sierran foothills, where poison oak is the single most common plant! In some locations, optimal conditions allow the waist-high shrub to assume the proportions of a small tree, or a thick, climbing vine. Certainly, many PCT travelers would agree that, with the possible exceptions of flies or mosquitos, poison oak is the most consistent nuisance along the trail in California. The allergic rash it causes in most people leads, at worst, to a few days of insane itching and irritation. It may, however, completely incapacitate a luckless few.

Poison-oak dermatitis is best managed by avoidance, and avoidance is best accomplished by recognition of the plant, in all phases of its life cycle: In spring and summer, it puts forth shiny green leaves, each divided into three oval, lobed leaflets, which, even on the same plant, exhibit an unusual variety of sizes. Toward fall, the

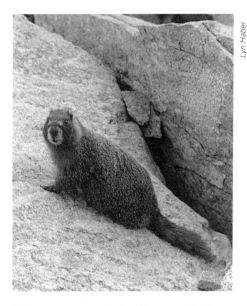

*Marmots are most likely to be seen at higher elevations*

leaves and stems turn reddish, and the small whitish flowers become smooth berries. In winter and early spring, when its leaves are gone, identification is most difficult: look for gray-dusty bark on stems, with smooth green, red-tipped new growth, and possibly some white-green berries left over from the previous season.

Avoid touching any part of the plant in any season—all parts contain an oily toxin that will, in a few days, lead to an allergic reaction where it has penetrated the skin. If you do brush against the shrub, wash the area immediately. Water helps to inactivate the toxin, and alcohol helps to extract the oil from skin, as does soap. Try to avoid spreading the oil by rubbing, however, since it takes a few minutes to an hour to fully penetrate the skin, and so one might actually spread the dermatitis by rubbing the oil around, without washing. Better yet, avoid exposure entirely by wearing loose, long-sleeved clothing, tucked into boot tops. But beware—poison-oak oil on clothing can, hours later, be wiped onto the skin, with toxic results. If you must wear shorts, try applying a commercial barrier cream, which catches the oil before it can reach your skin. Above all, avoid smoke from burning poison oak, and never eat any of the plant—fatal internal reactions have occurred.

If you do develop the itchy, red, blistering, weeping rash of poison-oak dermatitis, console yourself with the knowledge that it will be gone in a week or so. In the meantime, try not to scratch it—infection is the biggest hazard. Use calamine lotion, topical hydrocortisone cream and oral benadryl for itch relief. Severe allergic reactions, characterized by trouble breathing, dizziness, or swelling around the eyes or mouth, should be treated as soon as possible by a doctor.

### Waterborne Microscopic Organisms

Many of the PCT's springs, streams, and lakes have clear water, but what you can't see might make you ill. The microscopic organisms probably are far more threatening than virtually any black bear you'll meet on the trail. One microscopic organism is *Giardia lamblia*, which causes giardiasis (jee-ar-dye-a-sis). Although giardiasis can be incapacitating, it is not usually life-threatening. After ingestion by humans, *Giardia* organisms normally attach themselves to the small intestine, and disease symptoms usually include diarrhea, increased foul-smelling gas, loss of appetite, abdominal cramps, and bloating. Weight loss may occur from nausea and loss of appetite. These discomforts may last up to six weeks. Most people are unaware that they have been infected and return home from trips before the onset of symptoms. If not treated, the symptoms may disappear on their own, only to recur intermittently over a period of many months. Other diseases may have similar symptoms, but if you drank untreated water, you should suspect giardiasis and so inform your doctor. If properly diagnosed, the disease is curable with prescribed medication.

There are several ways for you to treat raw water to make it relatively safe to drink. The treatment most certain to destroy *Giardia* is to bring your water up to a boil. Chemical disinfectants such as iodine tablets or chlorine drops may not be as reliable, although they work well against most waterborne bacteria and viruses that cause disease. However, they are not effective against a certain intestinal parasite, *Cryptosporidium*, which can occur at water holes fouled by cattle. The most convenient safeguard is to use a portable water purifier. While relatively expensive and somewhat bulky, it gives you safe water in a minute or two—no chemical taste and no waiting for chemicals to act or for boiled water to cool.

### Mosquitoes and Other Invertebrates

"Truth bids me to say that mosquitoes swarmed in myriads, with not one tenth the fear but with twice the ferocity of a southern Secessionist." So wrote William H. Brewer about his evening in Yosemite National Park's upper Lyell Canyon on July 1, 1863. This statement is still very true for most of the High Sierra, for Lassen Volcanic National Park, and for the Klamath Mountains. Still, trekkers may encounter mosquitoes even in Southern California, and wherever there is a water source suitable for their breeding. They can be quite abundant along the Sacramento River, which you encounter at a low elevation in Northern California's Castle Crags State Park. Mosquitoes occur near water from sea level up to around 11,000 feet, that is, near treeline. All mosquitoes can transmit various diseases, but those found along the PCT rarely do. Only females ingest blood, and their biting and buzzing are more of a nuisance than a health hazard. By late July the mosquito populations wane in the high mountains, as snow melts and meadows dry out (although they can still be abundant lower down, where water is available). Until then, you'll probably want to carry a tent with mosquito netting just to get a good night's sleep. This is especially true in June. From midmorning until late afternoon, when you are likely to be on the trail, a wind usually keeps their numbers down. Of course, you can postpone your hike until August, but this is not an option for thru-hikers. Mosquitoes are pollinators, which explains why they are near their maximum numbers when wildflowers are so profuse. Without them, perhaps mountain wildflower gardens would be less glorious.

Flies can be a problem at lower elevations. Small black flies typically become numerous in warm weather, that is, from about June through early October. One favored habitat is among shady canyon live oaks, which can be locally common in Southern California. They are attracted to sweat from your face and body, but if you clean up, the flies generally cease to bother you. Occasionally at low to mid elevations you'll meet large, biting flies, usually deer

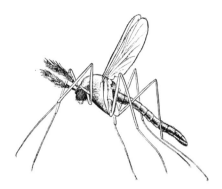

*Potentially hungry mosquito*

flies, but they don't attack in numbers. Furthermore, when one is preoccupied biting into your skin, it is easy to swat.

Another problem is the yellowjacket, a wasp that occasionally builds a ground nest under or beside a trail; if you trample on it, the yellowjackets will swarm you. You are very unlikely to meet them, though your chances increase if you ride a horse, for it tramples the ground far more than a hiker does. Their stings are multiple and painful, but not dangerous unless you happen to be allergic to bee stings. (More people in the US die from bee stings than from rattlesnake bites.)

One of the best arguments for avoiding squirrels, which frequent popular campsites looking for food, is that they may be rabid or their fleas may carry the plague. This is extremely unlikely, but small areas of plague-infested rodents are occasionally found in the mountains. Avoid fleas by avoiding rodents.

Ticks, the slow-moving relatives of spiders, are another potential carrier of disease. These blood-sucking arachnids are usually found in brushy areas below 6000 feet in Southern California and below 4000 feet in Northern California. Check your clothing and skin for them after you hike through brush at low elevations.

And finally there are scorpions, which are not merely desert creatures. You may find them in Southern California up to about 7000 feet and in Northern California up to about 5000 feet. These creatures, active at night, can give you a painful sting, although the species found along the PCT are not life-threatening.

### Rattlesnakes

Few animals are more unjustly maligned in legend and in life than the western rattlesnake, and no other animal, with the possible exception of the American black bear, causes more concern among walkers and riders along the California PCT. Indeed, most thru-hikers will have 5-6 encounters with these common reptiles by the time they reach the High Sierra! Even so, the authors know of only one PCT hiker who was ever bitten.

Frequenting warmer climes generally below the red-fir belt (although they have been seen much higher), rattlers will most often be encountered basking on a warm rock, trail or pavement, resting from their task of keeping the rodent population in check. Like other reptiles, rattlesnakes are unable to control their internal body temperature (they are "cold blooded"), and therefore can venture from their underground burrows only when conditions are suitable. Just as rattlers won't usually be seen in freezing weather, it is also no surprise that they are rarely seen in the heat of day, when ground temperatures may easily exceed 150°—enough to cook a snake (or blister human feet, as many will learn). One usually will see rattlers toward evening, when the air is cool but the earth still holds enough heat to stir them from their lethargy for a night of hunting. They naturally frequent those areas where rodents feed—under brush, in rock piles, and at streamsides.

It is their nocturnal hunting equipment that has inspired most of the legends and fears concerning rattlesnakes. Rattlers have heat-sensitive pits, resembling nostrils, in their wedge-shaped heads that can sense nearby changes in temperature as subtle as 1°F. Rattlers use these pits to locate prey at night, since they do not have well-developed night vision. More important perhaps is their sensitivity to vibrations, which can alert a rattler to footfalls over 50 feet away. With such acute organs, useful for sensing either a meal or danger, a rattler will usually begin to hurry away long before a hiker spots it. Furthermore, if you do catch one of these reptiles unawares, these gentlemen among poisonous snakes will usually warn you away with buzzing tail rattles if you get too close for comfort.

Like many of man's pest-control projects, efforts to quell rattlesnake populations have been to our detriment—rattlers are invaluable controllers of agricultural pests, and fewer people are hurt each year by rattlers than by household pets. One unsuccessful program carried out in the 1960s eliminated the conspicuous, noisy rattlers and left the silent ones to breed. A population developed in which the snakes would strike without buzzing. Luckily, most rattlers encountered along your PCT way will gladly move aside without incident.

The easiest way to avoid a snake bite is to avoid snakes. Over 75 percent of rattler bites are in people who are handling a snake, and over 80 percent of all bites are on the hand. The lessons: don't catch snakes, and look before you put your hands under rocks or logs, or into tall grass. Snakes will usually graciously depart as you approach, if you make enough noise—a good reason to carry a walking stick.

If bitten, get help immediately. The only truly useful treatment for rattlesnake bite is intravenous antivenin, which can be administered in most emergency departments in Southern California. The sooner it is given, the better, even if you must hike a distance for help. Walk out immediately. Because antiquated first-aid measures such as cold packs, tourniquets, and incision and suction devices are dangerous, they should never be used. There is no substitute for rapid evacuation to a hospital.

Finally, some special mention should be made of one of the West's most feared vipers, the uncommon Mojave "Green" Rattlesnake. This desert denizen may be encountered along the Southern California PCT. Thankfully, it, like other rattlers, is not aggressive. Its real danger is the lack of early symptoms of envenomation in its victims. These are delayed for the first 6–12 hours after a strike. This quiescent period may be followed by severe neurologic symptoms and shock, too late for treatment. Hence, all victims of rattler bite are urged to get immediate medical attention. No special treatment is needed for a Mojave Rattler bite—one type of antivenin treats all North American pit viper cases.

## Cougars

These large cats, also called pumas or mountain lions (but they also live in lowlands), range up to about 200 pounds for males, about half that for females, and they strike fear in many hikers. There seem to be two views about how threatening they are to humans. One is that they are merely curious, and that is why they track you. The other is that they are hungry, and that is why they stalk you. In California, it is a rare occurrence that a cougar would attack a human. Certainly if they wanted to, a cougar could easily kill you, best while you're asleep, tent or no tent. So far this has not happened, but in March 2001 a cougar attacked a hiker on the Mt. San Jacinto section of the PCT.

Before the mid-1990s, cougars were hunted throughout the state, which kept their numbers down and gave them a fear of humans. With the hunting ban, their numbers are increasing and they may lose this fear. As urban areas sprawl into their territory, they sometimes take pet dogs (just as coyotes take pet cats). You are not likely to have a close encounter with a cougar, although one may get close to you. If the

trail tread is soft, look for its tracks: paw prints about 3 inches across, like those left by a large dog, but without claw marks, since cats walk with retracted claws.

Since 1993, the Park Service in Yosemite has been warning visitors of increased lion sightings, and rarely, dogs, left alone in the park's campgrounds, have been attacked. For hikers, here is amended advice offered by the Park Service. Foremost, avoid hiking alone; there is safety in numbers. If you hike alone, you may be safer with a backpack than a day pack because with the latter, more of your body, especially your neck, is exposed. Second, if you bring children, watch them closely; they are easy prey. Should you see a cougar, don't approach it. Hopefully it, like you, will try to avoid a confrontation (also true for bears and rattlesnakes). Prey such as deer run, so don't act like prey and excite its killing instinct. Stay calm, not fearful (easier said than done). Hold your ground, or back away slowly. Face the cougar and do all you can to appear larger and more threatening. Grab a stick; raise your arms. If you have small children with you, pick them up. If the cougar behaves aggressively, wave your arms, shout, and throw sticks and/or stones at it. Convince the cougar that you may be dangerous. Finally, if attacked, fight back. To flee is to die.

## Bears

Black bears, which can come in a variety of colors and hues, are almost as far-ranging as cougars, and may now even occur south of San Gorgonio Pass, that is, in Sections A and B. You will not see them as you traverse dry lands, as in Sections E and F. Elsewhere they are present, although generally not seen, except in the High Sierra from Sequoia National Park north through Yosemite National Park (and in the future they may also become a problem in Desolation Wilderness, west of Lake Tahoe). In the High Sierra they can be found well above their normal range, taking the PCT over alpine passes, such as Glen and Dono-hue, despite these being, respectively, about 12,000 and 11,000 feet in elevation. Up here there's little for them, except for what trekkers have brought along. If a bear does go after your food, and if you try to stop it, especially if you try to retrieve your food once it has taken it, you could end up in the hospital.

Novice backpackers dread the thought of meeting one of these incredibly strong, 300-400+ pound adults who can out-run, out-swim, and out-climb you. Waking up in the dark of night to have one sniffing your head certainly gets your adrenaline rushing. However, although bears are carni-vores by structure, in California they are mostly herbivores by habit, only about 10 percent of their diet being animal matter, and that is mostly insects. Humans are not a part of their diet. For example, in Yose-mite National Park's history not even one visitor has been killed by any of these usu-ally gentle creatures (unlike grizzlies, which once ranged over much of California, but went extinct there in the 1920s). It is best for both you and the bears that they not get your food in the first place (problem bears are killed). Bears are boldest in Sequoia and Yosemite national parks, so the park personnel there have installed anti-bear food-storage devices, mostly bearproof metal boxes (see "Bears" in the Section H).

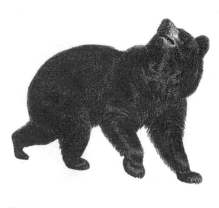

*Black bear*

### Safeguarding Your Food

There are several strategies you can use to safeguard your food. First, in the national parks use the food-storage boxes, vertical metal posts, or horizontal wire cables where available. Black bears are incredibly good tree climbers and are very intelligent, so suspending your food in trees, or "bearbagging," is not always secure. You can store food inside deep cracks found either in the bedrock or in oversized, cracked boulders. If the crack is at least 3 feet deep and less than 6 inches wide, then neither adult nor cub can reach food placed

in it. Before you store your food in one or more of these deep cracks, first place it in a stuff sack and then push it into the crack with a stick. Alternatively, if you are a good rock climber, you can climb up to a small ledge at least 15 feet off the ground and leave your stuff sack atop it. Bears are poor rock climbers. Many camping areas have adequate rock cracks and/or ledges within a few minutes' walking distance. Be aware that rodents may eat through your stuff sack to get at your food, although this is very unlikely. Finally, you can carry your food in bearproof canisters. These are heavy and expensive (you can rent them), but are okay if you will be out for only a few days. A prime advantage of them is that you have quick access to your food.

Bearbagging is time consuming, both getting the food sacks hung and then get-ting them down. Still, it may be an accept-able option south of Sequoia or north of Yosemite, where bears aren't likely to be as common or as savvy. You bearbag your food either on a cable (if one is available) or on a tree branch. The process is essen-tially the same for both. If you must use a branch, be sure your food is suspended at least 5 feet below it, at least 10 feet from the trunk, and at least 15 feet above the ground. Use the counterbalanced method of bear-bagging, described here for a tree branch.

Counterbalanced bearbagging is simply suspending your food sack at one end of a rope and another weight (which may also be a food sack) at the other end, so carry two stuff sacks. When you set up camp, set aside your dinner food and put the rest in your two stuff sacks. To bearbag, you then:

1. Tie a rock or other object to the end of your 50+ feet of parachute cord and toss it over an appropriate branch.

2. Remove the rock and tie on your heavier stuff sack (one should be noticeably heavier than the other).

3. Hoist that stuff sack up to the branch and then tie your other stuff sack (or counterweight) to the cord you are holding. Tie it on as high as you can reach.

4. You will have some cord left over. Stuff all of it in the stuff sack except for the end. Tie a small loop on this end.

5. With a stick or similar object, push your smaller stuff sack up until it is the same height as your larger one, hopefully 15 or more feet above the ground, though this is often hard to do. If these two sacks are equal in weight, you'll have difficulty pushing your second sack up due to friction. (Because a tree branch creates more friction than a cable, in trees the first stuff sack should be perhaps twice as heavy as the second.)

6. To retrieve your food, snag the small loop at the end of the parachute cord with your stick. Without a stick or similar object, adequate bearbagging is almost impossible. Unfortunately, sticks left by knowledgeable backpackers too often end up in someone's campfire.

# Weather

If you adequately prepare for bad weather, your backpack trip won't be all that bad even if such weather occurs. Storms come in two categories: frontal storms and thunderstorms. The farther north you are on the PCT the more likely you are to get caught in a frontal storm moving east across the state, since the storm season is several months longer than in Southern California. In Northern California frontal storms may come in mid- or late August, but they don't get serious until sometime in September. By October you'll generally want to be out of the highlands, which likely will become snow-covered before month's end and stay that way into early July. When you're in the Klamath Mountains you can get snow any time of the year, although in July and August the storms are infrequent and may dump only a few inches, which is no real impediment if you're prepared. In the High Sierra, from about the Lake Tahoe environs south to Sequoia National Park, the storm season is shorter. In average years these lands are not closed by snowfall until late October or early November; you can still have frontal storms in August or September, but the snow usually melts in several days. In Southern California frontal storms may occur in November, but the serious ones will more likely be from January through March. Still, thru-hikers starting in April from the Mexican border can get snowed on anywhere en route.

Contrasting with winter-centered frontal storms, thunderstorms are centered around summer and move north up the state. If you're caught in one, you can get a real drenching from copious rain or a beating from hard-hitting hail. This can occur in the San Jacintos and the San Bernardinos (the San Gabriels are less likely), and in the southern and central Sierra Nevada. Especially in the high lands of Sequoia and Kings Canyon National Parks, these storms are likely, particularly in July. They are less frequent in Yosemite National Park, and once you're north of the Lake Tahoe area they are rare events. The cumulonimbus clouds that create these storms build in the afternoon, and the storms themselves typically occur from midafternoon into early evening, that is, from about 2 or 3 P.M. until about 7 or 8 P.M. Therefore, if you have an exposed alpine pass to cross, try to do it before midafternoon. As mentioned under item 12 of "Trail Advice" earlier in this chapter, if you see the clouds looming and hear distant thunder, be prepared to seek shelter. Exposed high lands are no place to be dodging lightning strikes.

To minimize any storm encounter, hike during an optimal time. For Southern California lowlands this can be March or April, when frontal storms are less likely, temperatures are neither too cold nor too hot, there is still enough groundwater for springs to be reliable, and even some seasonal streams may still be flowing. The higher elevations in the San Jacinto, San Bernardino, and San Gabriel mountains will still be under snow (as may the Laguna Rim), and are best left for June. In July and August they can be quite hot and, as summer progresses, flowing water becomes increasingly sparse. Temperatures become optimal by October, but the water situation is at about its worst, unless a major storm has recently moved through.

Beyond the San Gabriels and before the High Sierra is a land of transition, essentially Sections E and F, which traverse partly through the desert lands of Antelope Valley and the dry lands of the Tehachapi Mountains. Like Southern California lowlands, they are very hot and dry in the summer, so it's best to do them in March or April. May is pushing it, at least through the desert.

From Section G north to the Oregon border (midway through Section R) constitutes two thirds of the California PCT, and most of this is relatively high lands, above 6000 feet. In Northern California such high lands can remain largely snowbound through June, while in Section G, which is farther south, snow is not a likely problem in June until you reach elevations of around 10,000 feet, which are quite common in Golden Trout Wilderness. Immediately north of it is Sequoia National Park where much of the trail is above 11,000 feet; the snowpack is serious, even though the snow is melting fast. Snowmelt presents another problem—swollen streams you have to ford. These can be just as life-threatening as icy passes. Therefore, generally don't hike there before mid-July in a year with average precipitation. August is better, but it also will be the most crowded, especially in Sections G and H further north. September usually has fair weather and after Labor Day it lacks the crowds, although this month is best from the Lake Tahoe area south. In Lassen Volcanic National Park and certainly the lands north of it, September weather can be chancy.

Choosing an optimal hiking month is not an option with thru-hikers bound for the Canadian border. They must start at the Mexican border by mid-April through early May, when there are still enough springs flowing and not too much snow in higher elevations. The hike through Antelope Valley (the western part of the Mojave Desert) can be grueling, usually too hot and always too dry. But a couple of weeks later they will be entering the High Sierra, which will be too snowy. Not until early July, when hopefully they've reached Interstate 80 at Donner Pass, will their problems be over—temporarily: snow storms await them in Washington in September.

If you plan to thru-hike and can choose the year to do it, then pick one in which the south half of the Sierra and all lands south of it (Sections A-H) are having a relatively dry year. Though springs will dry up earlier in Southern California, with a light Sierra snowpack you can start a month sooner, in early April rather than in early May. When central and Southern California are having relatively low precipitation in fall, winter, and spring, Oregon and Washington usually are having relatively high precipitation, which means a thick, long-lasting snowpack. However, by the time you reach Oregon, perhaps in early July, the snow problems won't be that bad and the snow will continue to melt as you advance northward to the really snowy country. Another bonus of hiking in such a year is that you can finish by early or mid-September, before the frontal storms start coming in thick and fast, besieging you with one snow dusting after another.

Perhaps the worst kind of year is one with heavy precipitation both in the central and southern Sierra Nevada and in Southern California. On the plus side (which does not approach the heavy minus side), springs and seasonal streams will be flowing in Southern California. On the minus side, snowpacks can slow you down in Southern California's mountains, and especially so in the Sierra. Hiking slower than average, you could run out of time, for Washington's North Cascades can be snowbound and that section can be indecipherable when you reach it. If you don't have access to information about the water situation in California, contact the Pacific Crest Trail Association (PCTA), mentioned early in this chapter. They keep track of trail conditions, including drinking-water availability, snow problems, and other issues pertinent to the PCT trekker.

## Hypothermia

Hypothermia is the rapid and progressive mental and physical collapse that accompanies chilling of the human body's inner core. It is caused by exposure to cold, and is intensified by wetness, wind, and exhaustion. Therefore, it's always a good idea to carry raingear. An unexpected storm could otherwise soak you to the bone.

Hypothermia almost always occurs at temperatures *well above freezing.* Anyone who becomes fatigued in wet and windy conditions is a potential victim. If you experience a bout of uncontrolled shivering, you should seriously consider yourself a candidate for hypothermia and take appropriate measures.

The best defense against hypothermia is to avoid exposure. Stay dry. When clothing is wet, it can lose as much as 90 percent of its insulating value, draining heat from the body. Unlike cotton, down and some synthetics, wool and polypropylene retain most of their insulating value when wet. If you can afford them, buy waterproof-breathable garments, which are made by a number of manufacturers. Be aware of the wind. Even a slight breeze carries heat away from your body, and forces cold air under as well as through clothing. Wind intensifies cold by evaporating moisture from the skin's surface. Put on raingear immediately, not after you are fairly soaked. Add a layer of clothing under your raingear before shivering occurs. A hat or ski cap, preferably made of wool or polypropylene, should be worn to protect and help retain body heat.

If your party fails to take these precautionary steps, a hiker with hypothermia may progress to more advanced symptoms, which include slurred speech, drowsiness, amnesia, frequent stumbling, a decrease in shivering, hallucinations and, finally, stupor, coma, and death. The victim may strongly deny he or she is in trouble. Believe the symptoms, not the patient.

It is far more dangerous to hike alone than in a group. You may not recognize the signs of hypothermia by yourself and, if you do, you may have a harder time restoring your body heat than if you have others to help you. In the mountains it is extremely important to keep your sleeping bag and a set of clothes dry. If they get wet, and threatening weather prevails, try to get out of the mountains as quickly as possible. But, don't abandon your pack and make a

dash for the trailhead, which can be tanta-
mount to suicide. If weather gets too bad,
stay put in a sheltered area and keep warm
and dry. Unless you are a very seasoned
mountaineer, you should not attempt to
continue hiking in bad weather.

# High Altitude Problems

### Altitude Sickness

Altitude sickness may occur at elevations of about 8000 feet or more. Symptoms include fatigue, weakness, headache,
loss of appetite, nausea, vomiting, and
shortness of breath on exertion. Sleep may
be difficult for the first night and, if you are
above 10,000 feet, perhaps even for one or
more additional nights. Regular periods of
heavy breathing separated by periods of no
breathing at all may awaken the sleeper
with a sense of suffocation. Hyperventil-
ation may also occur, causing lightheaded-
ness, dizziness, and tingling of the hands,
feet, and mouth. Altitude sickness results
from exposure to the oxygen-deficient
atmosphere of high elevations. It is aggra-
vated by fatigue and cold. Some people are
more susceptible to it than others. As the
body adjusts to the lower oxygen pressure,
symptoms usually disappear. Resting and
drinking extra liquids are recommended. If
symptoms persist, descend to lower altitudes.

### High-Altitude Pulmonary Edema

However rare, this is a serious and
potentially fatal condition. Cases have been
reported at altitudes of 8500 feet, but usually it occurs considerably higher. The basic
problem, as with altitude sickness, is a
reduction of oxygen, and early symptoms
are often unrecognized or else confused
with altitude sickness. However, in the case
of pulmonary edema, reduced oxygen initi-
ates blood diversion from the body shell to
the core, causing congestion of the lungs,
brain, and other vital organs. Besides exhib-
iting symptoms similar to those of altitude
sickness, the victim is restless, coughs, and
eventually brings up frothy, blood-tinged
sputum. The only treatment is immediate
descent to at least 2000 feet lower and, if
available, administration of oxygen. You
should secure medical help as soon as possible.

### Blood in Urine

If you are at high elevations and exercising to the point of dehydration, you can,
like serious long-distance runners, have
reddish urine. You are not dying, but this is
a good sign that you are overexerting yourself. Slow down.

### Ultraviolet Radiation

Above 9000 feet, wear UV-absorbing
or reflecting glasses and a hat to protect
your eyes, for the dangerous ultraviolet
radiation at these elevations is very intense.
You can get quite a splitting headache if
your eyes get too much radiation. Prolonged exposure to ultraviolet radiation
increases your risk of skin cancer, so be liberal with sunscreen on all your exposed
skin.

*Chapter 3*

# PCT Natural History

## Geology

It is very likely that the California section of the Pacific Crest Trail is unequaled in its diversity of geology. Many mountain trails cross glacial and subglacial landscapes, but which ones also cross arid and semi-arid landscapes? Some parts of your trail will have perennial snow; others are usually dry. Precipitation may be more than 80 inches per year in places, less than 5 inches in others. In each of the three major rock classes—igneous, sedimentary, and metamorphic—you'll encounter dozens of rock types. Because the PCT provides such a good introduction to a wide spectrum of geology, we have added a liberal dose of geologic description to the basic text. You start among granitic rocks at the Mexican border, and then we inform you of almost every new major rock outcrop you'll encounter along your trek northward. We hope that by the end of your journey you'll have developed a keen eye for rocks and that you'll understand the relations between the different rock types. Since we assume that many hikers will have only a minimal background in geology and its terminology,

we'll try to cover this broad subject for them in the next few pages. Those wishing to pursue the subject further should consult the list of references at the end of this book.

## Rocks

First, you should get acquainted with the three major rock classes: igneous, sedimentary, and metamorphic.

### Igneous rocks

Igneous rocks came into being when liquid (molten) rock material (*magma*) solidified. If the material solidified beneath the earth's surface, the rock is called *intrusive*, or plutonic, and a body of it is a *pluton*. If the material reached the surface and erupted as *lava* or *ash*, the rock is called *extrusive*, or volcanic.

**Intrusive rocks:** The classification of an igneous rock is based on its texture, what minerals are in it, and the relative amount of each mineral present. Since intrusive rocks cool more slowly than extrusive rocks, their crystals have a longer time to grow. If, in a rock, you can see an abundance of individual crystals, odds are that it is an intrusive rock. These rocks may be classified by crystal size: fine, medium, or coarse-grained, to correspond to average diameters of less than 1 millimeter, 1–5, and greater than 5.

Some igneous rocks are composed of large crystals (*phenocrysts*) in a matrix of small crystals (*groundmass*). Such a rock is said to have a *porphyritic* texture. The Cathedral Peak pluton, which is well exposed on Lembert Dome at the east end of Tuolumne Meadows in Yosemite National Park, has some feldspar phenocrysts over four inches long. High up on the dome these phenocrysts protrude from the less resistant groundmass and provide rock climbers with the holds necessary to ascend the dome.

The common minerals in igneous rocks are quartz, feldspar, biotite, hornblende, pyroxene, and olivine. The first two are light-colored minerals; the rest are dark. Not all are likely to be present in a piece of rock; indeed, quartz and olivine are never found together. Intrusive rocks are grouped according to the percentages of minerals in them. The three common igneous groups are *granite, diorite,* and *gabbro.* Granite is rich in quartz and potassium feldspar and usually has only small amounts of biotite.

Diorite is poor in quartz and rich in sodium feldspar, and may have three dark minerals. Gabbro, a *mafic* rock (rich in magnesium and iron), lacks quartz, but is rich in calcium feldspar, pyroxene, and may have some olivine. You can subdivide the granite–diorite continuum into granite, quartz monzonite, granodiorite, quartz diorite and diorite. These rocks, which are usually called "granitic rocks" or just plain "granite," are common in the Sierra Nevada and in most of the other ranges to the south. If you start your hike at the Mexican border, you'll begin among granitic rock known as Bonsall tonalite. *Bonsall* refers to the location where this rock is well exposed. *Tonalite* is the name given to diorite with quartz, or quartz diorite. In PCT Section D you'll encounter another intrusive rock with an unusual name: anorthosite. This rock, usually found with gabbro, is overwhelmingly composed of calcium-rich feldspar crystals.

Since it is unlikely that you'll be carrying a polarizing microscope in your backpack, let alone a great deal of mineralogical expertise in your head, your best chance of identifying these granitic rocks lies in making educated guesses based upon the following table.

At first you'll probably estimate too high a percentage of dark minerals, partly because they are more eye-catching and partly because they show through the glassy light minerals. If the intrusive rock is com-

| Rock | Color | % Dark Minerals |
|------|-------|-----------------|
| Granite | Creamy white | 5 |
| Quartz monzonite | Very light gray | 10 |
| Granodiorite | Light gray | 20 |
| Quartz diorite | Medium gray | 30 |
| Diorite | Dark gray | 40 |
| Gabbro | Black | 60 |

posed entirely of dark minerals (no quartz or feldspar), then it is an ultramafic rock. This rock type, which can be subdivided further, is common along the trail from Interstate 5 at Castle Crags State Park northwest to the Oregon border.

**Extrusive rocks:** Extrusive, or volcanic, rocks are composed of about the same minerals as intrusive rocks. *Rhyolite, andesite,* and *basalt* have approximately the same chemical compositions as granite, diorite, and gabbro, respectively. As with the intrusive rocks, the three volcanics can be subdivided into many groups, so it is possible to find ordinary rocks with intimidating names like "quartz latite porphyry"—which is just a volcanic rock with quartz phenocrysts and a composition in between rhyolite and andesite.

Texture is the key feature distinguishing volcanic from plutonic rocks. Whereas you can see the individual crystals in a plutonic rock, you'll have a hard time finding them in a volcanic one. They may be entirely lacking, or so small, weathered and scarce that they'll just frustrate your attempts to identify them. If you can't recognize the crystals, then how can you identify the type of volcanic rock? Color is a poor indicator at best, for although rhyolites tend to be light gray, andesites dark gray, and basalts black, there is so much variation that each can be found in any shade of red, brown or gray.

One aid to identifying volcanic rock types is the landforms composed of them. For example the high silica ($SiO_2$) content of rhyolite makes it very viscous, and hence the hot gases in rhyolite magma cause violent explosions when the magma nears the surface, forming *explosion pits* and associated rings of erupted material (*ejecta*). For the same reason, a rhyolite lava flow (degassed magma) is thick, short, and steep-sided and may not even flow down a moderately steep slope. The Mono and Inyo craters, north of Devils Postpile National Monu-

ment, are perhaps the best examples of this volcanic rock in California. You will find very little of it along the trail.

The landform characteristically associated with andesite is the *composite cone*, or stratovolcano. Mt. Shasta and some of the peaks in the Lassen area, including Brokeoff Mountain, are examples. These mountains are built up by alternating flows and ejecta. In time *parasitic* vents may develop, such as the cone called Shastina on Mt. Shasta; and the composition of the volcano may shift to more silica-rich *dacite* rock, an intermediate between rhyolite and andesite, which, like rhyolite, gives rise to tremendous eruptions, but also can produce lava domes such as Lassen Peak.

The least siliceous and also the least explosive of volcanic rocks is basalt. A basaltic eruption typically produces a very fluid, thin flow and a cinder cone, usually less than 1000 feet high. When in Lassen Volcanic National Park, take the alternate route up to the rim of the Cinder Cone. From this vantage point you can see what an extensive, relatively flat area its thin flows covered. Contrast this with Lassen Peak, to the west, California's largest dacite dome.

## Sedimentary rocks

We often think of rocks as being eternal—indeed, they do last a long time. But even the most resistant polished granite eventually succumbs to the effects of weathering, although on broad, unglaciated ridges and gentle slopes the rate of removal (denudation) is about a foot or less per million years. Granite rocks solidified under high pressures and rather high temperatures within the earth. At the surface, pressure and temperature are lower and the rock's chemical environment is different, and in this environment it is unstable. The rock weathers, and the pieces are gradually transported to a place of deposition. This place may be a lake in the High Sierra, a closed basin with no outlet such as the Mono Lake basin, an open structure such as the great Central Valley, or even the continental shelf of the Pacific Ocean. The rocks formed of the sediment that collects in these basins are called sedimentary rocks.

Most sedimentary rocks are classified by the size of their particles: clay that has been compacted and cemented forms *shale*; silt forms *siltstone*, and sand forms *sandstone*. Sandstone derived from granitic rock superficially resembles its parent rock, but if you look closely you'll notice that the grains are somewhat rounded and that the spaces between the grains are usually filled with a cement, usually calcite. Pebbles, cobbles and boulders may be cemented in a sand or gravel matrix to form a *conglomerate*. If these particles are deposited on an *alluvial fan* and then gradually cemented together to form a hard rock, collectively they become *fanglomerate*. Alluvial fans are usually formed where a stream debouches from the mouth of a canyon and drops its sedimentary load, or alluvium, over a fan-shaped area. Alluvial fans are seen along the south edge of the Mojave Desert, where it abuts the north base of the San Bernardino and the San Gabriel mountains. If the larger particles in a conglomerate or fanglomerate are angular rather than rounded, the sedimentary rock is called a *breccia*.

*Limestone*, another type of sedimentary rock, is formed in some marine environments as a chemical precipitate of dissolved calcium carbonate or as cemented fragments of shells, corals and foraminifers. The individual grains are usually microscopic. If the calcium in limestone is partly replaced by magnesium, the result is *dolomite*.

Since the PCT attempts to follow a crest, you'll usually find yourself in an area being eroded, rather than in a basin of deposition, so you'll find very ephemeral sediments or very old ones. The young ones may be in the form of alluvium, talus slopes, glacial moraines, or lake sediments. The old ones are usually resistant sediments that the intruding granitic plutons bent (*folded*), broke (*faulted*) and changed (*metamorphosed*).

## Metamorphic rocks

A volcanic or a sedimentary rock can undergo enough alteration (metamorphism) due to heat, pressure, and superhot, corrosive fluids that it loses its original characteristics and becomes a *metavolcanic* or a *metasedimentary* rock. Metamorphism may be slight or it may be complete. A shale undergoing progressive metamorphism becomes first a *slate*, second a *phyllite*, then a *schist*, and finally a *gneiss*. The slate resembles the shale but is noticeably harder. The schist bears little resemblance and is well-foliated, with flaky minerals such as biotite or other micas clearly visible. The gneiss resembles granite, but has alternating layers of light and dark minerals.

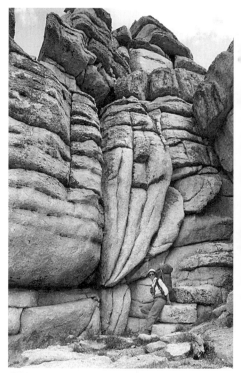

*"Fang-toothed" granitic rock formation prior to Sequoia National Park entrance*

*Hornfels* is a hard, massive rock, common in parts of the High Sierra, formed by contact of an ascending pluton with the overlying sediments. It can take on a variety of forms. You might find one that looks and feels like a slate, but differs in that it breaks across the sediment layers rather than between them.

*Quartzite* is a metamorphosed sandstone and resembles the parent rock. The spaces between the grains have become filled with silica, so that now if the rock is broken, the fracture passes through the quartz grains rather than between them as in sandstone. Metamorphism of limestone or dolomite yields *marble*, which is just a crystalline form of the parent rock. Check out Marble Mountain, in Northern California, when you reach it.

## Geologic Time

You cannot develop a feeling for geology unless you appreciate the great span of time that geologic processes have had to operate over. A few million years' duration is little more than an instant on the vast geologic time scale (see the following Geologic Time Scale). Within this duration a volcano may be born, die and erode away, and dozens of major "ice ages" may have come and gone.

A mountain range takes longer to form. Granitic plutons of the Sierra Nevada first came into being about 240 million years ago, and intrusion of them continued until about 80 million years ago, a span of 160 million years. Usually there is a considerable gap in the geologic record between the granitic rocks and the older sediments and volcanics that they intrude and metamorphose—often more than 100 million years.

## Geologic History

With the aid of a geologic section, like the one that follows, we can reconstruct in part the geologic history of an area. Our geologic section represents an idealized slice across the Sierra Nevada to reveal the rocks and their relations.

Through dating methods that use radioactive materials, geologists can obtain the absolute ages of the two granitic plutons, the andesite flow, and the basalt flow, which respectively would likely be Cretaceous, Pliocene, and Holocene. The overlying, folded sediments intruded by the plutons would have to be pre-Cretaceous. The metabasalt could be dated, but the age arrived at may be for the time of its metamorphism rather than for its formation. A paleontologist examining fossils from the marble and slate might conclude that these rocks are from the Paleozoic era.

Before metamorphism the Paleozoic slate, quartzite, metabasalt, and marble would have been shale, sandstone, basalt, and limestone respectively. The shale–sandstone sequence might indicate marine sediments being deposited on a continental shelf, then on a coastal plain. Lack of transitional rocks between the shale and the sandstone leads us to conclude that they were eroded away, creating a gap in the geologic record. We then have an *unconformity* between the two *strata* (layers), the upper resting on the *erosional surface* of the lower. The basalt, shale, and limestone sequence indicates first a localized volcanism, followed by a marine and then a shallow-water environment.

These Paleozoic rocks remained buried and protected from erosion for millions of years until the intrusion of granitic plutons and associated regional volcanism. Radiometric dating would show that the quartz-monzonite pluton was emplaced before the granodiorite pluton. Field observations would verify this sequence because the latter intrudes the former as well as the overlying sediments. During the Mesozoic period, plutonism and volcanism were at times accompanied by mountain building. This occurred when large pieces of continental crust, which were riding atop a plate

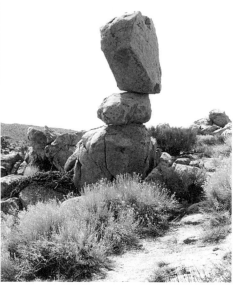

*Trail passes east of precariously balanced crest-line boulders*

that generally was diving eastward beneath the edge of the continent, were transported toward the range. Being relatively low in density, this continental crust did not descend with the rest of the plate, and so was forced against the range. The resulting compression caused uplift, and the Paleozoic rocks became folded, metamorphosed, and often faulted. Until plutonism ceased about 80 million years ago, the Mesozoic Sierra Nevada was just a small part of a much longer range that extended continuously along the western coasts of North America and South America. The climate was mostly tropical, and both weathering and erosion were intense; so as uplift occurred, these processes removed much of the Paleozoic rocks.

After plutonism ceased in California, late Cretaceous through early Tertiary faulting broke up the longer range and the Sierra Nevada became separated from the Klamath Mountains on the north, and the Coast, Transverse, and Peninsular ranges on the south. (This, and much that follows, cannot be deduced from the geologic section.) Before the breakup, the longer range was high, similar to today's Andes, but with the faulting into smaller blocks there also was *detachment faulting*—the separation of upper crust from lower crust. This occurred when the lower continental crust, under tremendous pressure from the thick, overlying upper crust and from high heat flow below, started to flow laterally. The upper continental crust lacked sufficient heat and pressure to flow. Rather, this brittle layer detached at its base and was transported laterally, atop the flowing lower continental crust. Where the upper several miles of Sierran proper crust went is not yet known. However, in the southern Sierra, (PCT Sections E, north part, and F and G), most of the upper crust was transported westward. Then, when the San Andreas fault system developed, it was transported northwest, slivering into linear blocks in the process.

With the upper crust removed—more than 65 million years ago for most of the Sierra—the unburdened lower crust rose to heights that probably were a bit higher than today's. In the ensuing millions of years, broad summits such as Mt. Whitney's have been reduced through weathering and erosion by only a few hundred feet, if that. Back in those early days following detachment, the range already had achieved a largely granitic landscape, since most of the exposed lower crust was granitic. Because stepped topography develops in granitic rocks, it would have begun generating cliffs and benches as well as streams, almost level reaches alternating with rapids, cascades, and even falls. Also in this early time there existed shallow forms of Owens Valley and Kern Canyon (which developed along a late Cretaceous fault). Like the Sierra Nevada, the Peninsular Ranges (Sections A-B) and the Klamath Mountains in the northernmost sections of the California PCT had also experienced a similar postplutonic history of uplift and erosion to expose their lower continental crusts. This also may have been true for the eastern and central

# Geologic Time Scale

| Era | Period | Epoch | Began (years ago) | Duration (years) |
|-----|--------|-------|-------------------|------------------|
| Cenozoic | Quaternary | Holocene | 10,000 | 10,000 |
|  |  | Pleistocene | 2,480,000 | 2,470,000 |
|  | Tertiary | Pliocene | 5,200,000 | 2,720,000 |
|  |  | Miocene | 22,900,000 | 20,420,000 |
|  |  | Oligocene | 33,400,000 | 10,500,000 |
|  |  | Eocene | 56,500,000 | 23,100,000 |
|  |  | Paleocene | 65,000,000 | 8,500,000 |
|  |  |  |  |  |
| Mesozoic | Cretaceous | *Numerous* | 145,000,000 | 80,000,000 |
|  | Jurassic | *epochs* | 200,000,000 | 55,000,000 |
|  | Triassic | *recognized* | 251,000,000 | 51,000,000 |
|  |  |  |  |  |
| Paleozoic | Permian |  | 302,000,000 | 51,000,000 |
|  | Carboniferous |  | 360,000,000 | 58,000,000 |
|  | Devonian | *Numerous* | 408,000,000 | 48,000,000 |
|  | Silurian | *epochs* | 438,000,000 | 30,000,000 |
|  | Ordovician | *recognized* | 490,000,000 | 52,000,000 |
|  | Cambrian |  | 543,000,000 | 53,000,000 |
|  |  |  |  |  |
|  | Precambrian |  | No defined periods or epochs; oldest known rocks are about 4.2 billion years old; Earth's crust solidified about 4.6 billion years ago. | |

These dates are derived from latest sources available in the early 2000s, but as in the past, they are bound to be slightly revised in the future. Most earth scientists still recognize the Tertiary–Quaternary boundary at 1,800,000 years, which is a poor choice except in Italy (where the boundary was so defined). The 2,480,000-year date is that of the Gauss-Matuyama reversal of the earth's magnetic poles, and this date is virtually synonymous with the commencement of the dozens of cycles of major glaciations in the northern hemisphere; and it also marks the approximate date of earliest man (origin of genus *Homo*[1]). Thus it accommodates the two classic concepts of the Quaternary, this period originally being the Ice Age and the Age of Man.

[1] The line of humans (*Homo* species) goes back about 2½ million years. Before then the *Australopithicus* species existed, and although they lasted longer they eventually became extinct.

parts of the Transverse Ranges (Sections C, D, and half of E), but they have been so disrupted by faulting, especially over the last 30 million years, that some additional uplift probably has occurred.

Thirty-three million years ago was an important time. Roughly about then the climate began changing from one that was somewhat tropical to one that was drier and more seasonal. In the northern half of the Sierra Nevada the range was in part buried by extensive rhyolite-ash deposits. Furthermore, the San Andreas fault system was born 33 million years ago, west of the modern coast of Southern California. By 15 million years ago, California had acquired an essentially modern summer-dry climate; the northern half of the Sierra Nevada was buried under even larger amounts of andesitic deposits (burying the old, granitic river canyons); and the fault system was beginning to migrate eastward onto existing lands, thereby disrupting them. As today, lands west of any fault segment moved northward with respect to those on the east (*right-lateral* faulting). Also by 15 million years ago, the composite Sierra Nevada–Central Valley block had begun migrating from its location near the southwestern Nevada border, first west, then northwest, some 150-180 miles to its present location. Today on a very clear day, from Mt. Whitney's summit you can see granitic Junipero Serra Peak, highest summit of central California's outer coast ranges, about 170 miles west. Likewise, back then from the same summit, on a very clear day you could have seen the Grand Canyon plateau (no canyon yet), a similar distance east.

Most of the volcanic deposits in the northern Sierra Nevada were readily eroded, but the new canyons cut in such deposits were inundated by additional sediments. About 10–9 million years ago several massive outpourings of lava flowed westward from faults near the present Sierran crest. These faults were created by extension of the Great Basin lands, which before widespread down-faulting had been a rugged, mountainous highland. The floor of the Owens Valley sank, but the already high Sierra Nevada did *not* rise; the opposite-direction arrows along the fault in the idealized geologic section indicate only relative movement, not absolute up or down. Note that the fault cuts the bedrock but not the *lateral moraine* (an accumulation of debris dropped off the side of a glacier), and this indicates that no faulting has occurred since the moraine was deposited (or else it too would have been disrupted).

Significant parts of these lava flows still remain, and the remnants best preserved are those that lie directly atop old bedrock, as does the remnant of an *andesite*

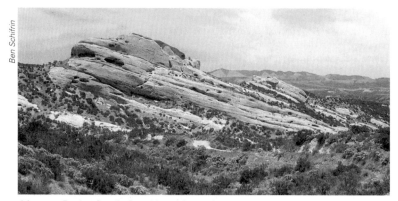

*Mormon Rocks, Devils Punchbowl formation*

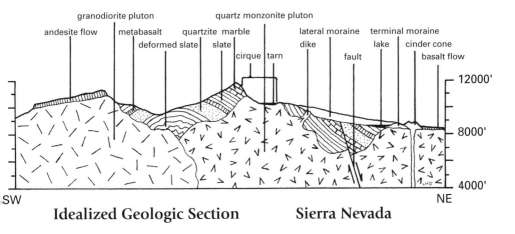

## Idealized Geologic Section    Sierra Nevada

*flow* in the idealized geologic section. Such remnants stand high above the floor of today's granite-walled canyons, which had been mostly exhumed of volcanic deposits before glaciation commenced. From this relation, geologists have concluded—incorrectly according to Schaffer—that major postflow uplift raised the flows to their present high positions, and that the steepened rivers then cut through thousands of feet of granite to their present low positions. According to this view, glaciers aided in the excavation, but misinterpretation of the field evidence has led geologists to infer major glacial erosion in some canyons, such as Yosemite Valley, and very little in others, such as the Grand Canyon of the Tuolumne River—two adjacent drainages both in Yosemite National Park.

The Sierra Nevada first experienced major glaciation about two million years ago, although it could have had episodes of minor glaciation long before that. These first large glaciers eroded the layer of rough, fractured, weathered bedrock, then retreated to leave behind much smoother surfaces. Where the bedrock floor was highly fractured and/or deeply weathered (in Yosemite Valley, the most extreme example, tropical weathering had penetrated some 2000 feet down), glaciers could excavate quite effec-

tively, leaving behind bedrock basins that quickly filled with water each time the glaciers retreated, creating a bedrock lake, or *tarn*. (In some canyons a lake formed behind a *terminal moraine*, although such a lake exists not so much because of a moraine dam, but rather because of impervious bedrock that is buried by the moraine.) On the resistant, smoothed and polished bedrock, succeeding glaciers could do very little, despite a century of claims by glaciologists.

Some of the evidence for lack of major glacial erosion lies along or close to the PCT. In Section G you reach the South Fork Kern River in Rockhouse Basin (Map G6). This basin and lands around it have changed so little in the last 15 million years—only a few feet of erosion—that back then you could have used today's topo maps. The ridge separating the basin from Tibbets Creek canyon (Section 15, Map G6) provides a particularly instructive view. From it you can look west across the canyon and see a splendid glacial landscape: straight, hanging tributary canyons that are U-shaped in cross section. The only problem is that there was no glaciation! This is a relict tropical landscape. Farther north, in the Sonora Pass to the Echo Lake Resort section of the PCT (described in *Pacific Crest Trail:*

*Northern California*), a descent from the Wolf Creek Lake saddle north takes you into the deep, glaciated East Fork Carson River canyon. After about two trail miles from there, and before you cross the river's second tributary, there are remnants of volcanic deposits on the west slopes that descend to within 200 feet of the canyon floor. These remnants are dated at about 20 million years old, indicating that back then—before any supposed uplift and before any glaciation—the canyon was about as wide as it is today and almost as deep.

Returning to the idealized geologic section, we see both a lateral and a terminal moraine on the east side of the crest, these usually being massive deposits left by a former glacier. (However, some lateral moraines are thin, merely a veneer atop an underlying bedrock ridge.) If glaciers do not erode, then why are moraines so large? Rockfall is the answer. It can occur at any time, but it is especially prevalent in late winter and early spring (due to cycles of freeze and thaw that pry off slabs and blocks). During and after a major earthquake, a tremendous amount of rockfall occurs, as noted in the 1980 Mammoth Lakes earthquake swarm, which was centered near the town along the east base of the range. Rockfall was greatest along and east of the crest, and so perhaps it is good that the PCT lies a few miles west of it. The greatest amount of local rockfall along the PCT route was from the ragged southeast face of Peak 11787, north of Purple Lake (Map H16). What glaciers do best is haul out a lot of rockfall, from which moraines are constructed and with which rivers are choked. Over the last two million years there were 2–4 dozen cycles of major glacier growth and retreat, and the glaciers transported a lot of rockfall. At the head of each canyon, where physical weathering was extremely pronounced, there usually developed a steep-walled half-bowl called a *cirque*. Before glaciation these already exist-

ed in a less dramatic form, as can be seen in the unglaciated lands west of Rockhouse Basin.

In the idealized geologic section, the last significant change was the eruption of lava to produce a *cinder cone*, which partly overlapped the terminal moraine, thereby indicating that it is younger. A *basalt flow* emanated from the cinder cone during or immediately after its formation. A carbon-14 date on wood buried by the flow would verify the youthfulness of the flow. Weathering and erosion are oh-so-slowly attacking the range today, at a rate much slower than in its tropical past, but nevertheless they are seeking to reduce the landscape to sea level. This will not occur. Future PCT hikers in the distant geologic future can expect a higher range, for eventually the Coast Ranges of central California should be thrust across the Great Central Valley and onto the Sierra Nevada, the crust-crust compression generating a new round of mountain building.

For now, PCT hikers can study the existing landscape. When you encounter a contact between two rocks along the trail, you might ask yourself: Which rock is younger? Which older? Has faulting, folding, or metamorphism occurred? Is there a gap in the geologic record?

# Biology

One's first guess about hiking the Pacific Crest Trail—a high adventure rich in magnificent alpine scenery and sweeping panoramas—turns out to be incorrect along some parts of the trail. The real-life trail hike will sometimes seem to consist of enduring many repetitive miles of hot, dusty tread, battling hordes of mosquitoes, or slogging up seemingly endless switchbacks. If you find yourself bogged down in such unpleasant impressions, it may be because you haven't developed an appreciation of the natural history of this remarkable route. As there is a great variety of minerals, rocks, landscapes and climates along the PCT, so also is there a great variety of plants and animals.

Even if you don't know much about basic ecology, you can't help noticing that the natural scene along the Pacific Crest Trail changes with elevation. The most obvious changes are in the trees, just because trees are the most obvious—the largest—organisms. Furthermore, they don't move around, hike, or migrate in their lifetimes, as do animals. When you pay close attention, you notice that not only the trees but the shrubs and wildflowers also change with elevation. Then you begin to find latitudinal differences in the animal populations. In other words, there are different *life zones.*

## Life zones

In 1894 C. Hart Merriam divided North America into seven broad ecosystems, which he called "life zones." These zones were originally based primarily on temperature, though today they are based on the distribution of plants and animals. The zones correspond roughly with latitude, from the Tropical Zone, which stretches from Florida across Mexico, to the Arctic Zone, which includes the polar regions. Between these two are found, south to north, the Lower Sonoran, Upper Sonoran, Transition, Canadian and Hudsonian zones. All but the Tropical Zone are encountered along the California PCT.

Just as temperature decreases as you move toward the earth's poles, so too does it decrease as you climb upward—between 3° and 5.5°F for every 1000-foot elevation gain. Thus, if you were to climb from broad San Gorgonio Pass for 10,000 feet up to the summit of San Gorgonio Peak, you would pass through all the same zones that you would if you walked from Southern California north all the way to Alaska. It turns out that 1000 feet of elevation are

about equivalent to 170 miles of latitude. Although the California PCT is about 1600 miles long, the net northward gain in latitude is only about 650 miles—you have to hike 2.5 route-miles to get one mile north. This 650-mile change in latitude should bring about the same temperature change as climbing 3800 feet up a mountain. On the PCT you enter Oregon at a 6000-foot elevation, finding yourself in a dense, Canadian Zone pine-and-fir forest. Doing your arithmetic, you would expect to find an equally dense fir forest at the Mexican border 3800 feet higher—at a 9800-foot elevation. Unfortunately, no such elevation exists along the border to test this prediction. However, if we head 85 miles north from the border to the Mt. San Jacinto environs, and subtract 500 feet in elevation to compensate for this new latitude, what do we find at the 9300-foot elevation? You guessed it, a Canadian Zone pine-and-fir forest. Ah, but nature is not quite that simple, for the two forests are unmistakably different.

## Plant geography

Every plant (and every animal) has its own *range, habitat* and *niche.* Some species have a very restricted range; others, a very widespread one. The sequoia, for example, occurs only in about 75 groves at mid-elevations in the western Sierra Nevada. It flourishes in a habitat of tall conifers growing on shaded, gentle, well-drained slopes. Its niche—its role in the community—consists of its complex interaction with its environment and every other species in its environment. Dozens of insects utilize the sequoia's needles and cones, and additional organisms thrive in its surrounding soil. The woolly sunflower, on the other hand, has a tremendous range: from California north to British Columbia and east to the Rocky Mountains. It can be found in brushy habitats from near sea level up to 10,000 feet.

Some species, evidently, can adapt to environments and competitors better than others. Nevertheless, each is restricted by a complex interplay of *climatic, physiographic* (topography), *edaphic* (soil) and *biotic* influences.

### Climatic influences

Of all climatic influences, temperature and precipitation are probably the most important. Although the mean temperature tends to increase toward the equator, this pattern is camouflaged in California by the dominating effect of the state's highly varied topography. As was mentioned earlier, the temperature decreases between 3° and 5.5°F for every 1000-foot gain in elevation. The vegetational changes reflect this cooling trend. For example, the vegetation along San Gorgonio Pass in Southern California is adapted to its desert environment. Annuals are very ephemeral; after heavy rains, they quickly grow, blossom and die. Perennials are succulent or woody, have deep roots, and have small, hard or waxy leaves—or no leaves at all. Only the lush cottonwoods and other associated species along the dry streambeds hint at a source of water.

As you climb north up the slopes of San Gorgonio Mountain, not only does the temperature drop, but the annual precipitation increases. On the gravelly desert floor below, only a sparse, drought-adapted vegetation survives the searing summer temperatures and the miserly 10 inches of precipitation. A doubled precipitation on the mountainside allows growth of chaparral, here a thick stand of ocean spray, birchleaf mountain mahogany, Gregg's ceanothus and great-berried manzanita. By 7000 feet the precipitation has increased to 40 inches, and the moisture-loving conifers—first Jeffrey pine, then lodgepole pine and white fir—predominate. As the temperature steadily decreases with elevation, evaporation of soil water and transpiration of moisture from plant needles and leaves are both reduced. Furthermore, up here the precipitation may be in the form of snow, which is preserved for months by the shade of the forest, and even when it melts is retained by the highly absorbent humus (decayed organic matter) of the forest soil. Consequently, an inch of precipitation on the higher slopes is far more effective than an inch on the exposed, gravelly desert floor. Similar vegetation changes can be found wherever you make dramatic ascents or descents. In Northern California significant elevation and vegetation changes occur as you descend to and then ascend from Highway 70 at Belden, Interstate 5 at Castle Crags State Park, and Highway 96 at Seiad Valley.

### Physiographic influences

As we have seen, the elevation largely governs the regime of temperature and precipitation. For a *given* elevation, the mean maximum temperature in Northern California is about 10°F less than that of the San Bernardino area. Annual precipitation, however, is considerably more; it ranges from about 20 inches in the Sacramento Valley to 80 inches along the higher slopes, where the snowpack may last well into summer. When you climb out of a canyon in the Feather River country, you start among live oak, poison oak and California laurel, and ascend through successive stands of Douglas-fir and black oak, incense cedar and ponderosa pine, white fir and sugar pine, then finally red fir, lodgepole, and western white pine.

The country near the Oregon border is one of lower elevations and greater precipitation, which produces a wetter-but-milder climate that is reflected in the distribution of plant species. Seiad Valley is hemmed in by forests of Douglas-fir, tanbark-oak, madrone, and canyon live oak. When you reach Cook and Green Pass (4750′) you reach a forest of white fir and noble fir. To the east, at higher elevations, you encounter weeping spruce.

A low minimum temperature, like a high maximum one, can determine where a plant species lives, since freezing temperatures can kill poorly adapted plants by causing ice crystals to form in their cells. At high elevations, the gnarled, grotesque trunks of the whitebark, limber, and foxtail pines give stark testimony to their battle against the elements. The wind-cropped, short-needled foliage is sparse at best, for the growing season lasts but two months, and a killing frost is possible in every month. Samples of this subalpine forest are found on the upper slopes of the higher peaks in the San Jacinto, San Bernardino, and San Gabriel mountains and along much of the John Muir Trail. Along or near the High Sierra crest and on the highest Southern California summits, all vestiges of forest surrender to rocky, barren slopes pioneered only by the most stalwart perennials, such as alpine willow and alpine buttercup.

Other physiographic influences are the *location, steepness, orientation,* and *shape of slopes.* North-facing slopes are cooler and tend to be wetter than south-facing slopes. Hence on north-facing slopes, you'll encounter red-fir forests which at the ridgeline abruptly give way to a dense cover of manzanita and ceanothus on south-facing slopes. Extremely steep slopes may never develop a deep soil or support a coniferous forest, and of course cliffs will be devoid of vegetation other than crustose lichens, secluded mosses, scattered annuals, and a few drought-resistant shrubs and trees.

## Edaphic influences

Along the northern part of your trek, at the headwaters of the Trinity River and just below Seiad Valley, you'll encounter outcrops of serpentine, California's official state rock. (Technically, the rock is serpentinite, and it is composed almost entirely of the mineral serpentine, but even geologists use "serpentine" for the rock.) This rock weathers to form a soil poor in some vital plant nutrients but rich in certain undesirable heavy metals. Nevertheless, there are numerous species, such as leather oak, that are specifically or generally associated with serpentine-derived soils. There is a species of streptanthus (mustard family) found only on this soil, even though it could grow

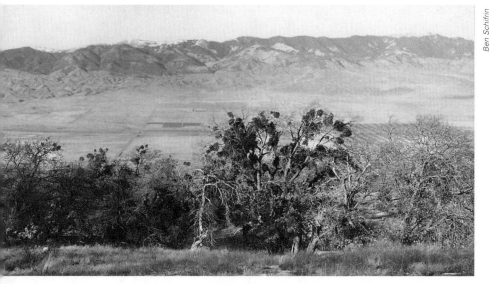

Ben Schifrin

*North over Antelope Valley to Tehachapis from Liebre Mountain*

better on other soils. Experiments demonstrate that it cannot withstand the competition of other plants growing on these soils. It therefore struggles, yet propagates, within its protected environment. Another example is at Marble Mountain, also in Northern California, which has a local assemblage of plants that have adapted to the mountain's limey soil.

A soil can change over time and with it, the vegetation. An illuminating example is found in formerly glaciated Sierran lands, where young soils today are thin and poor in both nutrients and humus. However, with passing millennia they will evolve into more-mature soils, and eventually could, given enough time, support sequoias up in the red-fir zone. These trees likely grew mostly in that zone, but glaciers removed the soils, so the trees that manage to survive today do so in the lower, unglaciated lands, that is, mostly down with the white firs and sugar pines. Once glaciation ceases in the Sierra Nevada, which could be a few mil-

lion years away, the sequoias could recolonize the lands they lost some two or more million years ago.

## Biotic influences

In an arid environment, plants competing for water may evolve special mechanisms besides their water-retaining mechanisms. The creosote bush, for example, in an effort to preserve its limited supply of water, secretes toxins which prevent nearby seeds from germinating. The result is an economical spacing of bushes along the desert floor.

Competition is manifold everywhere. On a descending trek past a string of alpine lakes, you might see several stages of plant succession. The highest lake may be pristine, bordered only by tufts of sedges between the lichen-crusted rocks. A lower lake may exhibit an invasion of grasses, sedges and pondweeds thriving on the sediments deposited at its inlet. Corn lilies

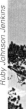

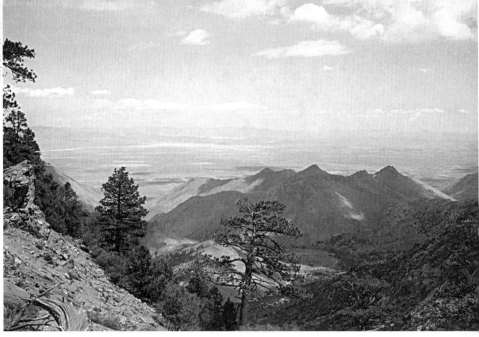

*Expansive eastern views in Owens Peak Wilderness from the Sierra crest of Sand Canyon and desert below*

and Lemmon's willows border its edge. Farther down, a wet meadow may be the remnant of a former shallow lake. Water birch and lodgepole pine then make their debut. Finally, you reach the last lake bed, recognized only by the flatness of the forest floor and a few boulders of a recessional moraine (glacial deposit) that dammed the lake. In this location, a thick stand of white fir has overshadowed and eliminated much of the underlying lodgepole. Be aware, however, that lake-meadow-forest succession is very slow, the lakes being filled with sediments at an average rate of about one foot per thousand years. At this rate, about 20–30,000 years will be required to fill in most of the lakes, and Tenaya Lake, between Tuolumne Meadows and Yosemite Valley, will take over 100,000 years. However, barring significant man-induced atmospheric warming, California's climate should cool in a few thousand years, and another round of glaciation should commence.

When a species becomes too extensive, it invites attack. The large, pure stand of lodgepole pine near Tuolumne Meadows has for years been under an unrelenting attack by a moth known as the lodgepole needle-miner. One of the hazards of a pure stand of one species is the inherent instability of the system. Within well-mixed forest, lodgepoles are scattered and the needle-miner is not much of a problem. But species need not always compete. Sometime two species cooperate for the mutual benefit, if not the actual existence, of both. That is true of the Joshua tree and its associated yucca moth, which are discussed in the Antelope Valley portion of PCT Section E. Another most important association goes unseen. Nearly all the plants you'll encounter have roots that form a symbiotic relationship with fungi. These mycorrhizal fungi greatly increase the roots' efficiency of water and nutrient uptake, and the roots provide the fungi with some of the plants' photosynthesized simple sugars.

Unquestionably, the greatest biotic agent is people. (They are also the greatest geomorphic agent, directly or indirectly causing more erosion—and therefore more habitat degradation—than any natural process.) For example, people have supplanted native species with introduced species. Most of California's native bunchgrass is gone, together with the animals that grazed upon it, replaced by thousands of acres of one-crop fields and by suburban sprawl. Forests near some mining towns have been virtually eliminated. Others have been subjected to ravenous scars inflicted by people-caused fires and by clearcutting logging practices. The Los Angeles basin's smog production has already begun to take its toll of mountain conifers, and Sierra forests may experience a similar fate. Wide-scale use of pesticides has not eliminated the pests, but it has greatly reduced the pests' natural predators. Through forestry, agriculture and urban practices, people have attempted to simplify nature, and by upsetting its checks and balances have made many ecosystems unstable. Along the Pacific Crest Trail, you'll see areas virtually unaffected by people as well as areas greatly affected by them. When you notice the difference, you'll have something to ponder as you stride along the quiet trail.

## The role of fire

Fires were once thought to be detrimental to the overall well-being of the ecosystem, and early foresters attempted to prevent or subdue all fires. This policy led to the accumulation of thick litter, dense brush and overmature trees—all of them prime fuel for a holocaust when a fire inevitably sparked to life. Human-made fires can be prevented, but how does one prevent a lightning fire, so common in the Sierra?

The answer is that fires should not be prevented, but only regulated. Natural fires, if left unchecked, burn stands of mixed conifers about once every 10 years. At this frequency, brush and litter do not accumulate sufficiently to result in a damaging forest fire; only the ground cover is burned over, while the trees remain intact. Hence, through small burns, the forest is protected from flaming catastrophes.

Some pines are adapted to fire. Indeed, the relatively uncommon knobcone pine, growing in scattered localities particularly in the Klamath Mountains of Northern California, requires fire to survive: the short-lived tree must be consumed by fire in order for its seeds be released. The lodgepole pine also will release its seeds after a fire, although a fire is not necessary. Particularly adapted to fires, if not dependent on them, are plants of Southern California's chaparral community, which is discussed in the introductory matter of PCT Section B. But in the Sierra and other high ranges, fire is important, too. For example, seeds of the genus *Ceanothus* are quick to germinate in burned-over ground, and some plants of this genus are among the primary foods of deer. Hence, periodic burns will keep a deer population at its maximum. With too few burns, shrubs become too woody and unproductive for a deer herd. In like manner, gooseberries and other berry plants sprout after fires and help support several different bird populations.

Without fires, a plant community evolves toward a *climax*, or end stage of plant succession. Red fir is the main species in the climax vegetation characteristic of higher forests in California's mountains. A pure stand of any species, as mentioned earlier, invites epidemic attacks and is therefore unstable. But even climax vegetation does not last forever. Typically the climax vegetation is a dense forest, and eventually the trees mature, die, and topple over. Logs and litter accumulate to such a degree that when a fire does start, the abundant fuel causes a crown fire, not a ground fire, and the forest burns down. Succession over time will result in an even-age stand of trees, and the cycle will repeat itself. In the

past, ecologists believed that stable climax vegetation was the rule, but we now know that unstable, changing vegetation is more common, even where man is not involved.

Fire also unlocks nutrients that are stored in living matter, topsoil, and rocks. Vital compounds are released in the form of ash when a fire burns plants and forest litter. Fires also can heat granitic rocks enough to cause them to break up and release their minerals. Even in a coniferous forest the weathering of granitic rock often is due primarily to periodic fires. This may be true even in the high desert. For example, in Anza-Borrego Desert State Park a large fire ravaged many of its granitic slopes, and a post-fire inspection revealed that the fire was intense enough to cause thin sheets of granite to exfoliate, or sheet off, from granitic boulders.

Natural, periodic fires, then, can be very beneficial for a forest ecosystem, and they should be thought of as an integral process in the plant community. They have, after all, been around as long as terrestrial life has, and for millions of years have been a common event in California plant communities.

## Plant communities and their animal associates

Plant communities are quite complex, and the general Life Zone system fails to take into account California's diverse climates and landscapes. Consequently, we'll elaborate on the biological scenario by looking at California's plant communities. Philip Munz, in his day, one of California's leading native-plant authorities, used the term *plant community* "for each regional element of the vegetation that is characterized by the presence of certain dominant species." Using this criterion, we devised our own list of California plant communities, which differs somewhat from the list proposed by Munz. We found that for the PCT, the division between Red Fir Forest and Lodgepole Pine

Forest was an artificial one. True, you can find large, pure stands of either tree, but very often they are found together and each has extremely similar associated plant and animal species. For the same reason we grouped Douglas-Fir Forest with Mixed Evergreen Forest. Finally, we've added two new communities that were not recognized by Munz, though they are recognized by other biologists: Mountain Chaparral and Mountain Meadow, each being significantly different from its lowland counterpart. Certainly, there is overlapping of species between adjacent communities, and any classification system can be quite arbitrary. Regardless of how you devise a California plant community table, you'll discover that along the PCT you'll encounter over half of the state's total number of communities—only the coast-range and eastern-desert communities are not seen. The California PCT guidebook is divided into two separate books, Southern and Northern California, (hiking sections A-H and I-R). The PCT through Southern California passes through 15 of the 16 following plant communities, the only one not seen being 10. Seven occur exclusively along the Southern California PCT: 1, 2, 3, 5, 6, 7, and 9. In contrast, the PCT through Northern California, lacking lands of Mediterranean and desert climates, passes through only nine plant communities and has only one exclusive plant community, 10. Eight plant communities are shared, found along the PCT in both parts of the state: 4, 8, 11, 12, 13, 14, 15, and 16.

As mentioned earlier, each species has its own range, which can be very restricted or very widespread. Birds typically have a wide—usually seasonal—range, and therefore may be found in many plant communities. In the following table we've listed only the plants and animals that have restricted ranges; that is, they generally occur in only one-to-several communities. Of the thousands of plant species we reviewed for this table, we found most of

them failed to serve as indicator species since they either inhabited too many plant communities or they grew in too small a geographic area. Terrestrial vertebrates pose a similar classification problem. For example, in the majority of the PCT plant communities you can find the dark-eyed junco, robin, raven, mule deer, coyote, badger and Pacific treefrog, so we didn't include them in the table.

The following table of plant communities will be useless if you can't recognize the plants and animals you see along the trail. Our trail description suggests plant communities, such as "you hike through a ponderosa-pine forest." This would clue you into plant community #11, and by referring to it, you could get an idea of what plants and animals you'll see in it. But then you'll need a guidebook or two to identify the various plants and animals. We have a few suggestions. If you can spare the luxury of carrying 12 extra ounces in your pack, then obtain a copy of Storer's *Sierra Nevada Natural History*, which identifies over 270 plants and 480 animals. Although it is dated and long overdue for revision, it is the only general book on the subject. Not only does it provide identifying characteristics of plant and animal species, but also it describes their habits and gives other interesting facts. Its title is misleading, for it is generally applicable to about three-fourths of the California PCT route: Mt. Laguna, the San Jacinto, San Bernardino, and San Gabriel mountains, and from the Sierra Nevada north almost continuously to the Oregon border. To better appreciate Southern California, read Bill Havert and Gary Gray's *Nature Guide to the Mountains of Southern California, by Car and on Foot*. For a 4-ounce pocket book, take Keator's *Sierra Flower Finder*. Finally, if you're doing all three states, bring Niehaus and Ripper's *Pacific States Wildflowers*, which has almost 1500 species. This certainly beats carrying the 4-pound authoritative reference, *The Jepson Manual*.

# Plant Communities of California's Pacific Crest Trail

### 1. Creosote Bush Scrub

**Shrubs:** creosote bush, bladderpod, brittle bush, burroweed, catclaw, indigo bush, mesquite
**Cacti:** Bigelow's cholla, silver cholla, calico cactus, beavertail cactus, Banning prickly pear, desert barrel cactus
**Wildflowers:** desert mariposa, prickly poppy, peppergrass, desert primrose, spotted langloisia, desert aster, Mojave buckwheat
**Mammals:** kit fox, black-tailed jackrabbit, antelope ground squirrel, Mojave ground squirrel, desert kangaroo rat, Merriam's kangaroo rat, cactus mouse, little pocket mouse
**Birds:** roadrunner, Gambel's quail, Le Conte's thrasher, cactus wren, phainopepla, Say's phoebe, black-throated sparrow, Costa's hummingbird
**Reptiles:** spotted leaf-nosed snake, coachwhip, western blind snake, Mojave rattlesnake, western diamondback rattlesnake, chuckwalla, desert iguana, collared lizard, zebra-tailed lizard, long-tailed brush lizard, desert tortoise
**Amphibian:** red-spotted toad
**Where seen along PCT:** base of Granite Mountains, southern San Felipe Valley, San Gorgonio Pass, lower Whitewater Canyon, Cajon Canyon, L.A. Aqueduct in Antelope Valley, lower Tehachapi Mountains

### 2. Shadscale Scrub

**Shrubs:** shadscale, blackbush, hop sage, winter fat, bud sagebrush, spiny menodora, cheese bush
**Mammals:** kit fox, black-tailed jackrabbit, antelope ground squirrel, desert wood rat, desert kangaroo rat, Merriam's kangaroo rat
**Bird:** black-throated sparrow
**Reptiles:** gopher snake, Mojave rattlesnake, zebra-tailed lizard
**Where seen along PCT:** L.A. Aqueduct in Antelope Valley

### 3. Sagebrush Scrub

**Shrubs:** basin sagebrush, blackbush, rabbit brush, antelope brush (bitterbrush), purple sage, Mojave yucca
**Mammals:** kit fox, white-tailed hare, pigmy rabbit, least chipmunk, Merriam's kangaroo rat, Great Basin pocket mouse
**Birds:** green-tailed towhee, black-chinned sparrow, sage sparrow, Brewer's sparrow
**Reptiles:** side-blotched lizard, desert horned lizard, leopard lizard
**Where seen along PCT:** Doble Road, Soledad Canyon, southern Antelope Valley, terrain near Pinyon Mountain

### 4. Valley Grassland

**Grasses, native:** bunchgrass, needle grass, three-awn grass
**Grasses, introduced:** brome grass, fescue, wild oats, foxtail
**Wildflowers:** California poppy, common muilla, California golden violet, Douglas meadow foam, Douglas locoweed, whitewhorl lupine, Kellogg's tarweed, redstem storksbill (filaree), roundleaf storksbill

**Mammals:** kit fox, Heermann's kangaroo rat, California meadow mouse

**Birds:** horned lark, western meadowlark, burrowing owl, Brewer's blackbird, savannah sparrow

**Reptiles:** racer

**Amphibians:** western spade-foot toad, tiger salamander

**Where seen along PCT:** Buena Vista Creek area, Big Tree Trail near Sierra Pelona Ridge, Dowd Canyon, Seiad Valley (human-made grassland)

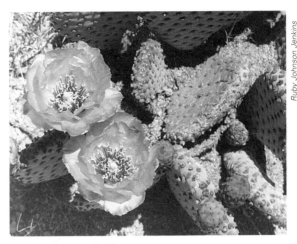

*Beavertail cactus in bloom*

Ruby Johnson Jenkins

## 5. Chaparral

**Trees:** big-cone Douglas-fir, gray (digger) pine, interior live oak

**Shrubs:** chamise, scrub oak, birch-leaved mountain mahogany, chaparral whitethorn, Gregg's ceanothus, bigpod ceanothus, hoaryleaf ceanothus, bigberry manzanita, Eastwood's manzanita, Mexican manzanita, Parry's manzanita, pink-bracted manzanita, toyon, ocean spray, holly-leaf cherry, California coffeeberry, redberry, coyote brush (chaparral broom), poison oak

**Wildflowers:** California poppy, fire poppy, Parish's tauschia, charming centaury, Cleveland's monkey flower, Fremont's monkey flower, scarlet bugler, Martin's paintbrush, foothill penstemon, Coulter's lupine, buckwheat spp.

**Mammals:** gray fox, brush rabbit, Merriam's chipmunk, dusky-footed wood rat, nimble kangaroo rat, California mouse, California pocket mouse

**Birds:** turkey vulture, California quail, scrub jay, California thrasher, green-tailed towhee, brown towhee, rufous-sided towhee, orange-crowned warbler, Lazuli bunting, blue-gray gnatcatcher, wrentit, bushtit

**Reptiles:** striped racer, western rattlesnake, western fence lizard, southern alligator lizard, coast horned lizard

**Where seen along PCT:** Mexican border, Hauser Mountain, Fred Canyon, Monument Peak, Chariot Canyon, Agua Caliente Creek, Combs Peak, Table Mountain, upper Penrod Canyon, middle Whitewater Canyon, Crab Flats Road, west slopes above Silverwood Lake, west of Pinyon Flats, Fountainhead Spring, North Fork Saddle, Soledad Canyon, Leona Divide, Spunky Canyon, Sawmill and Liebre mountains, Lamont Canyon to north of Kennedy Meadows

## 6. Joshua Tree Woodland

**Trees:** Joshua tree (tree-like stature, but really a yucca), California juniper, single-leaved pinyon pine

**Shrubs:** Mojave yucca, Utah juniper, box thorn, bladder sage, saltbush

**Wildflowers:** wild buckwheat, rock echeveria, rock five-finger, heart-leaved jewel flower, coiled locoweed, pigmy-leaved lupine, Parish's monkey flower, mouse-tail, Mojave pennyroyal, two-colored phacelia, tetradymia

**Mammals:** kit fox, antelope ground squirrel, desert wood rat, Merriam's kangaroo rat, white-eared pocket mouse

**Birds:** pinyon jay, loggerhead shrike, Scott's oriole, Bendire's thrasher

**Reptiles:** Mojave rattlesnake, California lyre snake, desert night lizard, desert spiny lizard, desert tortoise

**Amphibian:** red-spotted toad

**Where seen along PCT:** middle Whitewater Canyon, Nelson Ridge, Antelope Valley, western Mojave Desert, Walker Pass

### 7. Pinyon-Juniper Woodland

**Trees:** single-leaved pinyon pine, California juniper

**Shrubs:** Utah juniper, scrub oak, Mojave yucca, basin sagebrush, blackbush, box thorn, curl-leaved mountain mahogany, antelope brush, ephedra

**Wildflowers:** rock buckwheat, Wright's buckwheat, golden forget-me-not, adonis lupine, yellow paintbrush, Hall's phacelia

**Mammals:** black-tailed jackrabbit, California ground squirrel, Merriam's chipmunk, southern pocket gopher, pinyon mouse

**Birds:** pinyon jay, rock wren, poorwill, California thrasher, gray vireo, black-throated gray warbler, ladder-backed woodpecker

**Reptiles:** speckled rattlesnake, Mojave rattlesnake, leopard lizard, sagebrush lizard, western fence lizard, desert spiny lizard, coast horned lizard, Gilbert's skink

**Amphibian:** red-spotted toad

**Where seen along PCT:** just south of Burnt Rancheria Campground, Onyx Summit, Camp Oakes, Van Dusen Canyon, West Fork Mojave River, Highway 58 to Kennedy Meadows

### 8. Northern Juniper Woodland

**Trees:** western juniper, single-leaved pinyon pine, Jeffrey pine

**Shrubs:** basin sagebrush, antelope brush, rabbit brush, curl-leaved mountain mahogany

**Wildflowers:** sagebrush buttercup, ballhead ipomopsis, three-leaved locoweed, Humboldt's milkweed, western puccoon, sagebrush Mariposa tulip

**Mammals:** least chipmunk, Great Basin kangaroo rat, sagebrush vole

**Birds:** sage grouse, pinyon jay, sage thrasher, northern shrike, gray flycatcher, sage sparrow

**Reptiles:** striped whipsnake, sagebrush lizard, short-horned lizard

**Amphibian:** Great Basin spadefoot toad

**Where seen along PCT:** Kennedy Meadows, Little Pete and Big Pete meadows, upper Noble Canyon, much of the volcanic landscape between Highways 108 and 50, Hat Creek Rim, Buckhorn Mountain

### 9. Southern Oak Woodland

**Trees:** coast live oak, Englemann oak, interior live oak, California juniper, Coulter pine, digger pine, big-cone Douglas-fir, California black walnut

**Shrubs:** sugar bush, lemonade-berry, gooseberry, bigberry manzanita, fremontia, squaw bush, poison oak

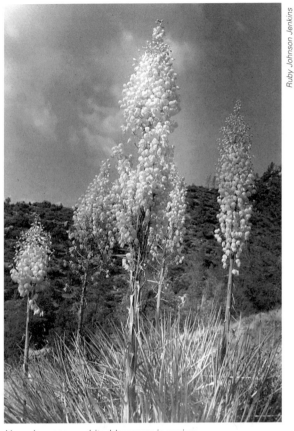

Ruby Johnson Jenkins

*Yucca's creamy white blossoms in spring*

**Wildflowers:** elegant clarkia, slender eriogonum, wild oats, California Indian pink, golden stars, wild mountain sunflower, Kellogg's tarweed, Douglas loco-weed, Douglas violet

**Mammals:** gray fox, raccoon, western gray squirrel, dusky-footed wood rat, brush mouse, California mouse

**Birds:** California quail, acorn woodpecker, scrub jay, mourning dove, Lawrence's goldfinch, common bushtit, black-headed grosbeak, plain titmouse, Nuttall's woodpecker, western wood-peewee, band-tailed pigeon, red-shouldered hawk

**Reptiles:** California mountain kingsnake, Gilbert's skink, western fence lizard, southern alligator lizard

**Amphibians:** California newt, California slender salamander, arboreal salamander

**Where seen along PCT:** Lake Morena County Park, Cottonwood Valley, Flathead Flats, Barrel Spring, Cañada Verde, Warner Springs, Tunnel Spring, Vincent Gap, Three Points, upper Tie Canyon, Mt. Gleason, Big Oak Spring, San Francisquito Canyon

### 10. Douglas-Fir/Mixed Evergreen forest

**Trees:** Douglas-fir, tanbark-oak, madrone, bay tree, big-leaf maple, canyon oak, black oak, yew, golden chinquapin

**Shrubs:** Pacific blackberry, California coffeeberry, Oregon grape, poison oak, wood rose, salal, Fremont's silk-tassel

**Wildflowers:** California pitcher plant, Indian pipe, striped coralroot, American pine sap, sugar stick, giant trillium, long-tailed ginger, one-sided wintergreen, wedge-leaved violet, California skullcap, grand hounds-tongue, Bolander's hawkweed

**Mammals:** black bear, porcupine, long-eared chipmunk, Townsend's chipmunk, red tree mouse

**Birds:** winter wren, hermit thrush, golden-crowned kinglet, purple finch, brown creeper, chestnut-backed chickadee

**Reptiles:** rubber boa, northern alligator lizard, western pond turtle

**Amphibians:** northwestern salamander, rough-skinned newt

**Where seen along PCT:** Middle Fork Feather River canyon, North Fork Feather River canyon, Pit River canyon, Sacramento River canyon, lower Grider Creek canyon, lower slopes around Seiad Valley, Cook and Green Pass, Mt. Ashland Road 20

### 11. Ponderosa Pine Forest

**Trees:** ponderosa pine, sugar pine, Jeffrey pine, incense-cedar, white fir, Douglas-fir, black oak, mountain dogwood, grand fir

**Shrubs:** deer brush, greenleaf manzanita, Mariposa manzanita, mountain misery, western azalea, Scouler's willow, spice bush

**Wildflowers:** elegant brodiaea, spotted coralroot, draperia, rigid hedge nettle, Indian hemp, slender iris, leopard lily, grand lotus, dwarf lousewort, Sierra onion, Yosemite rock cress, shy Mariposa tulip

**Mammals:** black bear, mountain lion, mountain beaver, porcupine, western gray squirrel, golden-mantled ground squirrel, yellow-pine chipmunk, mountain pocket gopher

**Birds:** Steller's jay, hairy woodpecker, white-headed woodpecker, western tanager, band-tailed pigeon, pigmy nuthatch, western bluebird, flammulated owl

**Reptiles:** rubber boa, California mountain kingsnake, western rattlesnake, western fence lizard

**Amphibians:** foothill yellow-legged frog, ensatina

**Where seen along PCT:** Laguna Mountains, upper West Fork Palm Canyon, Apache Spring, upper Whitewater Canyon, much of the Big Bear Lake area, most of the San Gabriel Mountains, Piute Mountain, Haypress Creek, Chimney Rock, Burney Falls, lower Rock Creek, Castle Crags, lower slopes of Lower Devils Peak

### 12. Mountain Chaparral

**Trees:** Jeffrey pine, sugar pine, western juniper

**Shrubs:** huckleberry oak, snow bush, tobacco brush, greenleaf manzanita, bush chinquapin

**Wildflowers:** showy penstemon, dwarf monkey flower, hounds-tongue hawkweed, pussy paws, mountain jewel flower, golden brodiaea

**Mammals:** bushy-tailed wood rat, brush mouse

**Birds:** mountain quail, dusky flycatcher, fox sparrow, green-tailed towhee
**Reptiles:** western rattlesnake, sagebrush lizard
**Where seen along PCT:** near Tahquitz Peak, near Strawberry Cienaga, in small
    areas from north of Walker Pass to Cow Canyon, above Blaney Hot Springs,
    slopes north of Benson Lake, upper North Fork American River canyon,
    Sierra Buttes, Bucks Summit, slopes west of Three Lakes, lower Emigrant
    Trail, upper Hat Creek Valley, Pigeon Hill, above Seven Lakes Basin, slopes
    south of Kangaroo Lake, South Russian Creek canyon, upper Right Hand
    Fork canyon, south slopes of Lower Devils Peak and Middle Devils Peak,
    between Lily Pad Lake and Cook and Green Pass, Mt. Ashland Road 20

### 13. Mountain Meadow

**Shrubs:** arroyo willow, yellow willow, mountain alder
**Wildflowers:** California corn lily, wandering daisy, elephant's head, tufted gen-
    tian, Douglas knotweed, monkshood, swamp onion, Lemmon's paintbrush,
    meadow arnica, mountain carpet clover, California cone flower, Gray's
    lovage, Kellogg's lupine, meadow monkey flower, tall phacelia, Jeffrey's
    shooting star, Bigelow's sneezeweed
**Mammals:** Belding's ground squirrel, California meadow mouse, long-tailed
    meadow mouse, deer mouse, ornate shrew
**Birds:** northern harrier, Lincoln's sparrow, white-crowned sparrow, Brewer's
    blackbird
**Amphibians:** mountain yellow-legged frog, Yosemite toad
**Where seen along PCT:** Little Tahquitz Valley, Vidette Meadow, Grouse Meadows,
    Evolution Valley, Tully Hole, Tuolumne Meadows, Grace Meadow, upper
    Truckee River canyon, Benwood Meadow, Haypress Meadows, Corral
    Meadow, Badger Flat, Shelly Meadows, Donomore Meadows, Sheep Camp
    Spring area, Grouse Gap

### 14. Red Fir/Lodgepole Pine Forest

**Trees:** red fir, Shasta red fir, noble fir, lodgepole pine, western white pine, Jeffrey
    pine, aspen, mountain hemlock, weeping spruce
**Shrubs:** pinemat manzanita, bush chinquapin, snow bush, red heather, Labrador
    tea, mountain spiraea, caudate willow, MacKenzie's willow, Scouler's willow,
    black elderberry, thimbleberry
**Wildflowers:** snow plant, pine drops, nodding microseris, broadleaf lupine, west-
    ern spring beauty
**Mammals:** black bear, red fox, mountain beaver, porcupine, yellow-bellied mar-
    mot, golden-mantled ground squirrel, lodgepole chipmunk, mountain pock-
    et gopher
**Birds:** blue grouse, great gray owl, mountain chickadee, red-breasted nuthatch,
    dusky flycatcher, olive-sided flycatcher, Williamson's sapsucker, three-toed
    woodpecker, ruby-crowned kinglet, Cassin's finch
**Where seen along PCT:** upper Little Tahquitz Valley, upper San Bernardino
    Mountains, Mt. Baden–Powell, Kern Plateau, lower portions of John Muir
    Trail, much of northern Yosemite, most of the stretch from Yosemite to cen-
    tral Lassen Volcanic National Park, Bartle Gap, Grizzly Peak, most of the trail
    from Seven Lakes Basin to Mt. Ashland

### 15. Subalpine Forest

**Trees:** whitebark pine, foxtail pine, limber pine, lodgepole pine, mountain hemlock

**Shrubs:** Sierra willow, Eastwood's willow, white heather, bush cinquefoil

**Wildflowers:** Eschscholtz's buttercup, Coville's columbine, mountain monkey flower, Suksdorf's monkey flower, Sierra penstemon, Sierra primrose, mountain sorrel, cut-leaved daisy, silky raillardella, rock fringe

**Mammals:** red fox, yellow-bellied marmot, pika, Douglas squirrel (chickaree), alpine chipmunk, heather vole, water shrew

**Birds:** Clark's nutcracker, mountain bluebird, mountain chickadee, Williamson's sapsucker

**Amphibian:** Mt. Lyell salamander

**Where seen along PCT:** Mt. Baden–Powell summit, much of the Sierra Nevada (above 10,000 feet in the southern part, above 8,000 feet in the northern part), higher elevations in Marble Mountain Wilderness

### 16. Alpine Fell-Fields

**Shrubs:** alpine willow, snow willow

**Wildflowers:** alpine gold, Sierra pilot, alpine paintbrush, alpine sandwort, ruby sandwort, dwarf lewisia, dwarf ivesia, Muir's ivesia, Brewer's draba, feeble saxifrage, Sierra primrose

**Mammals:** pika, alpine chipmunk

**Birds:** rosy finch, mountain bluebird, rock wren

**Where seen along PCT:** at and just below the following passes: Forester Pass, Glen Pass, Pinchot Pass, Mather Pass, Selden Pass, Silver Pass, Donohue Pass; high traverse along Leavitt Peak ridge

### A final word

Plant communities aren't the final word in plant-animal classification, since each community could be further subdivided. For example, Edmund Jaeger divides the desert environment into even more compartments than Munz does, including Desert Sand Dunes, Desert Wash, Salt Water Lake (Salton Sea), Desert Canal, Colorado River Bottom, Desert Urban, and Desert Rural. Farther north, in a glaciated basin near Yosemite's Tioga Pass, Lionel Klikoff has identified eight vegetational patterns within the subalpine forest plant community, each distribution pattern the result of a different set of microenvironmental influences. Once you start looking and thinking about organisms and their environments, you'll begin to see that all is not a group of random species. There is continual interaction between similar organisms, between different organisms, and between organisms and their environment. They are there because they fit into the dynamic ecosystem; they currently are adapted to it; they belong.

# Chapter 4

# Using This Guide

## Our Route Description

*Pacific Crest Trail: Southern California* is composed of route description and original, detailed topographic maps of the Pacific Crest Trail. In eight section chapters this guide covers the California PCT from the Mexican border north as far as Tuolumne Meadows in Yosemite National Park. The route description is divided into sections A through H because most PCT hikers will be hiking only a part of the trail, not all of it. In this book's companion volume, *Pacific Crest Trail: Northern California* by Jeffrey P. Schaffer, the PCT description picks up from Tuolumne Meadows and ends at the Oregon border (Sections I through R).

Each section starts at or near a highway and/or supply center (town, resort, park) and ends at another similar point. The one exception is the end of Section G and start of Section H, which occurs where the Pacific Crest Trail joins the John Muir Trail near Crabtree Meadows. From this point most PCT hikers will go east to climb Mt. Whitney and perhaps descend to Lone Pine to resupply. We also chose this break point because many hikers skip Southern California and start their PCT hiking on the John Muir Trail—this guide's Section H. This section is the only one that is too long for *most* hikers to do without resupplying. All of the other sections are short enough to make comfortable backpack trips ranging from 3 to 10 days. Even so, most of these have resupply points along or close to the actual route, thereby allowing you to carry a little less food.

At the beginning of each section is an introduction that mentions:

1. the attractions and natural features of that section,

2. the 7½′ topographic maps that cover the trail in the chapter, arranged south to north,

3. the declination setting, for your compass,

4. a mileage table between points on route,

5. weather and best times to go,

6. supply points on or near the route,

7. water availability or scarcity,

8. wilderness permits (if required), and

9. special problems (such as presence of rattlesnakes, snow, difficult-to-ford rivers and creeks, etc.).

(Maps can be ordered from The Map Center, 2440 Bancroft Way, Berkeley, CA 94704; phone: (510) 841-MAPS, or The Map Centre, Inc., 2611 University Avenue, San Diego, CA 92104-3830, (619) 291-3830.) Attractions and natural features will help you decide what part of the trail you'll want to hike—very few hikers do all of California. The declination setting for your compass is important if you have to get a true reading. The declinations vary from 14½°E near the Mexican border to 20°E in southern Oregon. If your compass does not correct for declination, you'll have to add the appropriate declination to get the true bearing. For example, if your compass indicates that a prominent hill lies along a bearing of 75°, and if the section you're hiking in has a declination of 15°E, then you should add 15°, getting 90° (due east) as the true bearing of that hill. If you can identify that hill on a map, then you can find where you are on the PCT by adding 180°, getting 270° (due west) in this example. Be aware that this procedure is correct for only true-bearing (true field-sighting) compasses, which list degrees from 0° to 360° in a counterclockwise direction. Most hikers, however, use the generally less expensive reverse-bearing compasses, which are harder to use. (Indeed, a whole book has been written on using them for map-orienteering purposes.) Reverse-bearing, or backsight, compasses list degrees in a clockwise direction. With these compasses, you subtract. **No one should attempt a major section of the PCT without a thorough understanding of his or her compass and of map interpretation.**

Each mileage table lists distances between major points found within its PCT section. Both distances between points and cumulative mileages at points are given. We list cumulative mileages south to north and north to south so that no matter which direction you are hiking the PCT, you can easily determine the mileages you plan to hike. Many of the points listed in the tables are at or near good campsites. If you average 22 miles a day—the on-route rate you'll need to do to complete the tri-state PCT in four months—you can determine where to camp and estimate when you'll arrive at certain supply points.

At the end of this short chapter we've included a mileage table for the entire California PCT. Any two adjacent points represent the start and end of one of this book's 8 section chapters. (We have also listed mileages for the ten sections covered in this book's companion volume, *Pacific Crest Trail Northern California*.) By scanning this table's distance between points, you can easily see how long each section is. Then you can pick one of appropriate length, turn to that section's introduction, and see if it sounds appealing. Of course, you need not start at the beginning of any section, since a number of roads cross the PCT in most sections. (Section H is an exception, having only a few access points.)

Supply points on or near the route are mentioned, as well as what you might expect to find at each. You will realize, for example, that you can't get new clothes at Old Station, but can at Burney, the next major settlement. Many supply points are just a post office and/or small store with minimal food supplies. By "minimal" we mean a few odds and ends that typically cater to passing motorists, e.g., beer and potato chips (which nevertheless are devoured by many a trail-weary trekker).

Finally, the introduction mentions special problems you might encounter in each section, such as desert thirst, snow avalanches, and early-season fords. If you are hiking all of the California PCT, you will be going through some of its sections at very inopportune times and will face many of these problems. Backpackers hiking a short stretch can pick the best time to hike it, and thereby minimize their problems.

When you start reading the text of a PCT section, you will notice that a pair of numbers follows the more important trail points. For example, at Highway 120 in Tuolumne Meadows (end of Section H) this pair is (8595-0.8), which means that you cross this highway at an elevation of 8595 *feet* and at a distance of 0.8 *mile* from your last given point. In our example this is at a junction by Tuolumne Meadows Lodge. By studying these figures along the section you are hiking, you can easily determine the distance you'll have to hike from point A to point B, and you can get a good idea of how much elevation change is involved. In the descriptions, an **Alternate route** is a trail segment that the authors think is worth considering given certain circumstances. Along this guide's **Alternate routes**, which are set aside by a shaded grey background, there are occasional second mileage figures, which represent the distance along the alternate route to that point.

**Water access** is self-explanatory, as is **Resupply access**. All these are offset with a blue shaded box.

In the trail description, numbers below the columns indicate what maps to refer to. This description of the route also tells something about the country you are walking through—the geology, the biology (plants and animals), the geography, and sometimes a bit of history. Longer highlights of interest are set aside by a shaded grey box and marked with a distinctive icon:

Camping/Permits

Geology

Fire

Historical Information

Land Management/Trail information

Plants

Views

Wildlife

## Following the Trail

The route of the PCT is mostly along trail tread, but occasionally it is along a stretch of road. Except where the trail tread may momentarily die out, there is no cross-country, although early-season hikers may go miles on snow, when accurate route finding becomes imperative. Quite naturally, you want to stay on the route. For that purpose, we recommend relying on the route description and maps in this book. To be sure, there are various markers along the route—PCT emblems and signs, California Riding and Hiking Trail posts and signs, metal in the shape of diamonds and discs nailed to tree trunks, plastic ribbons tied to branches, and blazes and ducks. (A blaze is a place on a tree trunk where bark has been removed. Typically a blaze is about 4–6 inches in its dimensions. A duck is a small rock placed on a very large boulder or a pile of several small rocks whose placement is obviously unnatural.)

Our route descriptions depend on these markers as little as possible because they are so ephemeral. They get destroyed by loggers, packers, motorbikers, hikers, wilderness purists, bears and other agents. Furthermore, the blazes or ducks you follow, not having any words or numbers, may or may not mark the trail you want to be on.

One way to find a junction is to count mileage from the previous junction. If you know the length of your stride, that will help. We have used yards for short horizontal distances because one yard approximates the length of one long stride. Alternatively, you can develop a sense of your ground speed. Then, if it is 2 miles to the next junction and your speed is 3 miles and hour, you should be there in ⅔ hour, or 40 minutes. Be suspicious if you reach an unmarked junction sooner or later than you expect. We sometimes go to great lengths to describe the terrain so that you can be alerted to upcoming junctions.

Without these clues you could easily miss the junction in early season, when snow still obscures many parts of the trail.

## The Maps

Each section contains all the topographic strip maps you'll need to hike that part of the California PCT. All these maps are at a scale of 1:50,000, or about 0.8 mile per inch, and all are aligned with north at the top. On the maps the PCT route appears as a solid black line where it exists as a trail and as a dashed black line where it exists along roads. The legend on the following page lists most of the symbols you'll see on this guide's topographic maps.

## Sample map

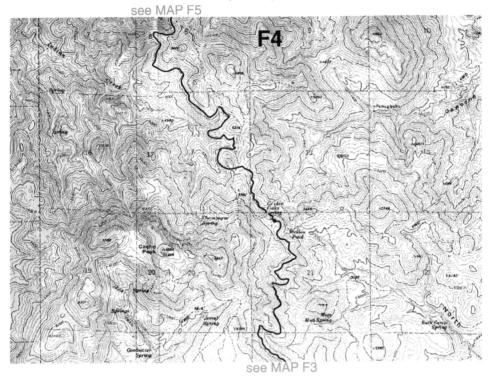

see MAP F5

F4

see MAP F3

## Southern California PCT Mileage Table

| Legend for topographic maps | | Legend for Section Maps | |
|---|---|---|---|
| Heavy-duty road | ━━━ | PCT route | ━━━ |
| Medium-duty road | ▭▭ | Other trail | ─── |
| Improved light-duty road | ═══ | Paved road | ─── |
| Unimproved dirt road | ═══ | Secondary road | ─── |
| Jeep road or trail | ─── | Park/wilderness boundary | ━━ |
| Railroad: single track | ─── | River/creek | ∼ |
| Railroad: multiple track | ═══ | Topographic map page | **H10** |
| PCT route along trails | ━━━ | Mountain peak | △ |
| PCT route along roads | ━━━ | Pass | ) ( |
| Year-round streams | ─── | Ranger station | ☗ |
| Seasonal streams | ─ ··· ─ | Spring | ●∼ |
| | | Structure | ▲ |
| | | Town | ■ |

1    0    1
Miles

Scale of maps 1:50,000

# Section

| Section/Start/End | S→N | Length | N→S |
|---|---|---|---|
| A: Mexican border near Campo | 0.0 | 1724.4 | 110.6 |
| B: Highway 79 southwest of Warner Springs | 110.6 | 1613.8 | 101.4 |
| C: near Interstate 10 in San Gorgonio Pass | 212.0 | | 1512.4 |
| | | 132.9 | |
| D: Interstate 15 near Cajon Pass | 344.9 | | 1379.5 |
| | | 112.5 | |
| E: Agua Dulce near Antelope Valley Freeway | 457.4 | | 1267.0 |
| | | 109.3 | |
| F: Highway 58 near Tehachapi Pass | 566.7 | | 1157.7 |
| | | 84.1 | |
| G: Highway 178 at Walker Pass | 650.8 | | 1073.6 |
| | | 113.5 | |
| H: John Muir Trail junction | 764.3 | | 960.1 |
| | | 175.8 | |

The mileages for the northern part of the Pacific Crest Trail are shown below for your future planning. Sections I through R are described in *The Pacific Crest Trail: Northern California.*

## Northern California PCT Mileage Table

| Section/Start/End | S→N | Section Length | N→S |
|---|---|---|---|
| I: Highway 120 in Tuolumne Meadows | 940.1 | | 784.3 |
| | | 76.4 | |
| J: Highway 108 at Sonora Pass | 1016.5 | | 707.9 |
| | | 76.2 | |
| K: Echo Lake Resort near Highway 50 | 1092.7 | | 631.7 |
| | | 64.3 | |
| L: Trailhead-parking lateral near Interstate 80 | 1157.0 | | 567.4 |
| | | 38.4 | |
| M: Highway 49 near Sierra City | 1195.4 | | 529.0 |
| | | 91.7 | |
| N: Highway 70 at Belden Town bridge | 1287.1 | | 437.3 |
| | | 134.3 | |
| O: Burney Falls in Burney Falls State Park | 1421.4 | | 303.0 |
| | | 82.9 | |
| P: Interstate 5 near Castle Crags State Park | 1504.3 | | 220.1 |
| | | 99.8 | |
| Q: Somes Bar-Etna Road at Etna Summit | 1604.1 | | 120.3 |
| | | 55.8 | |
| R: Highway 96 at Seiad Valley | 1659.9 | | 64.5 |
| | | 64.5 | |
| Interstate 5 near Mt. Ashland Road 20 | 1724.4 | | 0.0 |

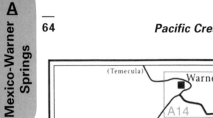

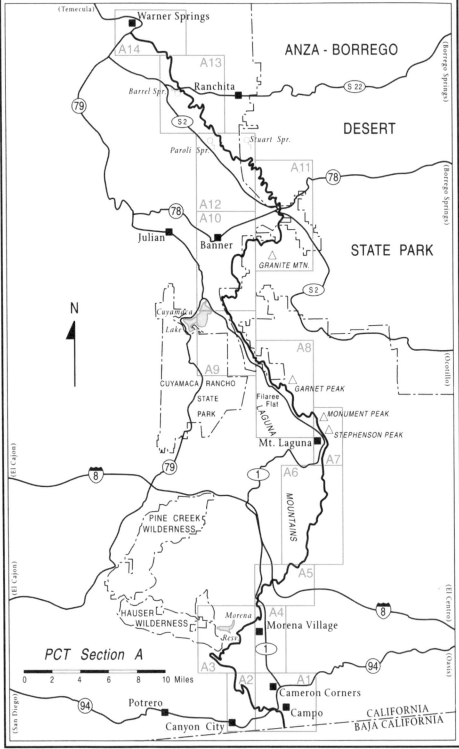

(Temecula)

Warner Springs

A14

ANZA - BORREGO

(Borrego Springs)

A13

Ranchita

S 22

*Barrel Spr.*

DESERT

S 2

*Stuart Spr.*

*Paroli Spr.*

A11

78

(Borrego Springs)

A12

A10

78

Julian

Banner

STATE PARK

△
*GRANITE MTN.*

S 2

(Ocotillo)

N

*Cuyamaca Lake*

A8

A9

△
*GARNET PEAK*

CUYAMACA  RANCHO

*Filaree Flat*

△ *MONUMENT PEAK*

STATE

△ *STEPHENSON PEAK*

PARK

LAGUNA

Mt. Laguna

A7

8

79

1

A6

PINE CREEK WILDERNESS

MOUNTAINS

A5

HAUSER WILDERNESS

*Morena Resv.*

A4

Morena Village

8

(El Centro)

PCT  Section  A

1

A3

94

A2

A1

94

(Oasis)

0   2   4   6   8   10 Miles

Cameron Corners

CALIFORNIA

94

Potrero

Campo

BAJA CALIFORNIA

(San Diego)

Canyon City

*Section A:*

# Mexican Border to Warner Springs

This southernmost section of the Pacific Crest Trail is among the most varied of all. It traces a fine line between scorching desert and dense, rolling brushlands, occasionally in fine mid-mountain forest. Although cacti and sand are encountered often, and late-spring and summer temperatures frequently rise above 100°, the PCT in this section does not traverse true desert, but rather keeps just west of the searing Colorado Desert—which you often glimpse—passing through a transitional area influenced by moist Pacific Ocean air. At the time when most long-distance hikers will be traversing the southernmost part of the PCT, in April and May, they are quite likely to encounter late-season snowstorms as they climb into the Laguna Mountains.

The Lagunas are a fault-block range of granitic rock closely related to the Sierra Nevada geologically. Here, walkers might forget sun and thirst while walking beneath shady oaks and pines also similar to those found in the Sierra. But the next day, as they swoop down to San Felipe Valley, the stifling heat returns as the route enters Anza-Borrego Desert State Park and the Colorado Desert. The furnace breath of this arid land above the Salton Sea follows you from the San Felipe Hills to Warner Springs.

*Racer*

*Ben Schifrin*

# Maps

Campo
Potrero
Morena Reseroir
Cameron Corners
Mount Laguna
Monument Peak
Cuyamaca Peak

Julian
Earthquake Valley
Tubb Canyon
Ranchita
Hot Springs Mountain
Warner Springs

# Declination
13°E

| Points on Route | S→N | Mi. Btwn. Pts. | N→S |
|---|---|---|---|
| Mexican border | 0.0 | | 110.6 |
| | | 1.3 | |
| Campo, near Border Patrol station | 1.3 | | 109.3 |
| | | 18.9 | |
| Lake Morena County Park | 20.2 | | 90.4 |
| | | 5.9 | |
| Boulder Oaks Campground | 26.1 | | 84.5 |
| | | 6.7 | |
| Fred Canyon Road to Cibbets Flat Campground | 32.8 | | 77.8 |
| | | 4.2 | |
| Long Canyon | 37.0 | | 73.6 |
| | | 4.6 | |
| Burnt Rancheria Campground | 41.6 | | 69.0 |
| | | 1.3 | |
| Stephenson Peak Rd. to Mt. Laguna | 42.9 | | 67.7 |
| | | 4.8 | |
| Sunrise Highway near Laguna Campground | 47.7 | | 62.9 |
| | | 5.3 | |
| Pioneer Mail Picnic Area | 53.0 | | 57.6 |
| | | 8.6 | |
| jeep track to Cuyamaca Reservoir | 61.6 | | 49.0 |
| | | 2.4 | |
| detour to water in upper Chariot Canyon | 64.0 | | 46.6 |
| | | 4.9 | |
| Rodriguez Spur Truck Trail: detour to spring | 68.9 | | 41.7 |
| | | 9.2 | |
| Hwy. 78 in San Felipe Valley, near Sentenac Cienaga | 78.1 | | 32.5 |
| | | 23.8 | |
| Barrel Spring | 101.9 | | 8.7 |
| | | 8.7 | |
| Highway 79 southwest of Warner Springs | 110.6 | | 0.0 |

## Weather To Go

The best time to hike is in late April and early May—biting winter winds and snow flurries in the Lagunas are usually gone, but extreme heat hasn't yet developed in the San Felipe Hills. Thankfully, this is also the optimal time window for most south-to-north thru-hikers to begin their journeys. By late May, this section's lower reaches can be uncomfortably hot.

## Supplies

Last-minute supplies may be bought in Campo, 1.2 miles along the walk. It has a small store, a laundromat, a railroad museum, and a ranch supply store (which most equestrians need). A PCTA trail register is kept at the post office. Cameron Corners, 1 mile north of Campo on Highway 94, has a hot dog stand, a convenience store, and a branch of Wells Fargo Bank. Sophisticated camping items still needed must be bought in San Diego before starting out.

As of June 2001, inbound airline passengers reach the PCT's southern terminus via the following links: Take bus Route 992 from the San Diego Airport to downtown San Diego (*www.sandag.cog.ca.us/992.htm*). Next, take the "Orange Line" trolley to the El Cajon Transit Center (*www.sandag.cog.ca.us/sdmts/trolleymap.htm*). The "Southeastern Rural Route bus" departs the center only once per day at 3:04 P.M. and arrives in Campo about 5 P.M. (*www.co.san-diego.ca.us/cts/rural/index.html*).

Morena Village, with a small store and cafe, lies 0.3 mile off route at Lake Morena County Park, 20 miles into the journey. Mount Laguna, a tiny mining community with a store, post office, restaurants and motels, is the next opportunity, about 43 miles into the hike. As of 2001, Mount Laguna Post Office has no morning service, except on Saturday.

The tourist-oriented, apple-growing ex-mining town of Julian, with stores, restaurants, lodging and post office, lies 12.5 miles west of the PCT where it strikes Highway 78 in San Felipe Valley. Julian is a welcome respite for the PCTer sporting a first set of desert-induced blisters.

Borrego Springs is a desert resort community with complete supplies, motels, laundromat, and the Anza-Borrego Desert State Park headquarters, with camping and a delightful natural history museum. It is reached from two points along the PCT. From Scissors Crossing, about 78.3 miles into your journey, find Borrego Springs by hitchhiking about 5 miles east on Highway 78 to Highway S3, then heading north about 10 miles. From Highway S22 where the PCT strikes it, just north of Barrel Springs, at the 102.2-mile point of this section, hitchhike 15 miles east on S22.

Warner Springs, at the end of this section, is the last supply point. This little resort community is clustered around a rejuvenating hot spring on the Aguanga Fault. Now a private spa, Warner Springs Ranch boasts a fine restaurant, restful bungalows, invigorating massages, and hot-spring soaks. Golf, tennis, horseback riding, and glider rides round out the experience. Contact the resort in advance: 31652 Highway 79, Warner Springs, CA 92086; (760) 792-4200; *www.warnersprings.com*. Warner Springs has a post office but no supplies.

## Water

Ground water in the dry mountains of Southern California dries up rapidly after winter snows melt. Especially from late May through summer, hikers should not count on any water away from civilization—in Section A, this could require some waterless camps and, probably, some long detours for water. Carry at least 8 liters of water per person, for each day!

In dry years, the Southern California PCT's meager accompaniment of streams and springs begins to disappear. During repeated dry years, some smaller water sources remain dry, even in spring. During drought years in Section A, expect to find water only in Campo, Lake Morena County Park, Boulder Oaks Campground, Burnt Rancheria Campground, Laguna Campground and Warner Springs. Expect Hauser Creek, Cottonwood Creek, Long Canyon Creek, Chariot Canyon, Rodriguez Spur Truck Trail well, San Felipe Creek and Barrel Spring to be dry!

Conversely, years with normal or heavy precipitation will deposit heavy snows on the San Jacintos, San Bernardinos, and San Gabriels. These often pose a problem through mid-May. The higher Tehachapis, as well, routinely have over a foot of snow on northern slopes. Hence, the springtime PCT traveler must have a flexible resupply strategy, ready to load up tents, gaiters, warm parka and ice ax when

needed, and to jettison them in favor of extra water bottles through the dry spells.

Walkers should carry lots of water from Mount Laguna, for it is a long, blistering 23.9 miles (including a 1.8-mile detour) to springs in Chariot Canyon. When the water tank at Pioneer Mail Trailhead Picnic Area is in operation, it will deduct 10.1 miles from this leg. An alternative to Chariot Canyon is the well on Rodriguez Spur Truck Trail, 28.1 miles beyond Mount Laguna (including a 1.3-mile detour). In either case, carry a big water container, since the next stretch to water at Barrel Springs is a mind-broiling 37.9 miles from Chariot Canyon, and 33.0 miles from Rodriguez Spur Truck Trail!

## Permits

Wilderness permits are usually required for both day and overnight visits to Hauser Wilderness, through which you briefly pass early in this section. PCT trekkers, however, are exempt. Still, if you'll be

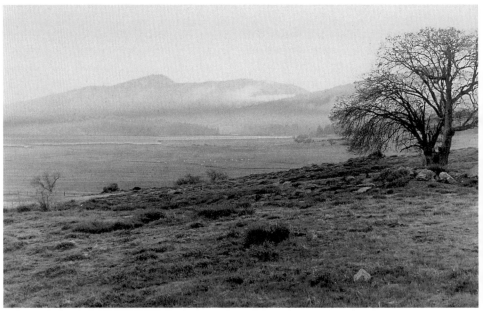

Ben Schifrin

*Cuyamaca Peak and Reservoir*

heading into future wildernesses on your northward trek, then you should get a permit at the Cleveland National Forest's office—see Chapter 2's "Federal Government Agencies."

## Special Problems

### Rattlesnakes

Refer to this section in Chapter 2.

# THE ROUTE

State Highway 94 leads 50 miles east from San Diego to Campo, where one turns south on Forrest Gate Road, which in one block passes a US Border Patrol station, where hikers should check in. The pavement ends beyond Rancho del Campo, and you continue south up the graded road. It jogs east at Castle Rock Ranch, turns south at a T-junction with a poorer road, then climbs moderately along a telephone line. After passing under a 500 KV powerline, you reach a junction with a good dirt road that parallels the Mexican border. This road is used nightly by Border Patrol officers to scout for footprints of illegal aliens. Now look uphill to the left, southeast, to see the gray PCT monument atop a low knoll at the edge of the wide, defoliated border swath. This swath has a welter of paralleling roads which run alongside the barbed-wire border fence. Walk up a short jeep road to the monument, an eight-foot-high gray wooden affair constructed of five 12x12 posts, and capped with the soon-to-be familiar delta-shaped PCT emblem. An inscription reads: SOUTHERN TERMINUS PACIFIC CREST NATIONAL SCENIC TRAIL. ESTABLISHED BY ACT OF CONGRESS ON OCTOBER 2, 1968. MEXICO TO CANADA 2627 MILES. 1988 A.D. ELEVATION 2915 FEET. Fifty feet south of the border monument, another dirt road has been bulldozed, parallel to the border. Its southern verge, the border itself, is protected from the Mexican influx by a 4-to-6-foot-high fence of metal runway-repair panels, painted olive-green. Reach across it for a feel of *tierra Mexicana*, and then return to the knoll for photos. Sign the register on the back of the monument, then turn north and start your adventure (2915-0.0).

Your first vistas north show the steep southern flanks of the Laguna Mountains on the northern horizon, while the low green dome of Hauser Mountain stands in the northwest. The prominent orange buttresses of Morena Butte overlook its northern shoulder.

To find the start of the PCT, look due north, downhill from the monument to a lone 12-foot-high scrub oak, just left (west) of the road you just came up, and immediately north of the grassy defoliated border strip. Next to it is a gray sign at the actual start of the trail tread. It announces: PACIFIC CREST TRAIL: LAKE MORENA 19.5 MILES. The PCT's obvious trail tread starts, heading north, downhill into high brush. A sandy descent curves to parallel the access road. In a few minutes, you pass under the San Diego Gas and Electric powerline and walk northeast across a poor road (2810-0.4) that subserves the line. Continue gently down, just east of the access road, in a low, arid chaparral of chamise, sagebrush, ribbonwood and yucca, which is punctuated with protruding boulders of bonsall tonalite—a light gray granitic rock—and white popcorn flowers.

A 2000-acre fire that started near Tecate in November 1995 burned eastward across the PCT's route from near the border, and north past Castle Rock Ranch. It is an early reminder of the flammability of the Southern California landscape, and just one of many "burns" crossed by the

**See Map A1**

PCT. Please be fire-safe! Thankfully, trail tread is still easily visible.

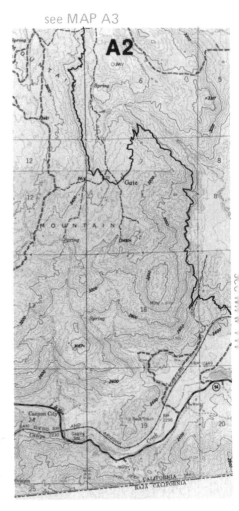

In minutes, descent ends as you cross another dirt road (2710-0.3), then, the way marked by 4x4 posts, swing west on the edge of a large dry meadow, dotted with mustard and large canyon live oaks. Look for posts to indicate the way, since the tread is poorly defined. Just west of the entrance to Castle Rock Ranch, you step across Forrest Gate Road (2710-0.1) to its west side, where you wind and undulate easily above the now-paved road through stands of feathery, stringy-barked ribbonwood and around granitic blocks. Soon, you note the buildings and exercise yards of Ranchos del Campo and del Reyo—cavalry camps in World War I but now San Diego County boys' camps. Marked by a post, the path dips to merge with the paved road shoulder across from their entrances. Walk along the road's west shoulder, going north for 250 yards, past a cluster of tan-pink bungalows. Just across from Rancho del Reyo's entrance, and just up Forrest Gate Road from the Border Patrol Station, trail tread resumes and veers left, northwest, away from the roadside (2600-0.5), via three old concrete steps.

**Resupply access:** Before heading off on the PCT, be sure you are adequately provisioned, since the next certain water is at Lake Morena County Park, 18.9 miles away. A post office and ranch-supply store are situated just 2 blocks north in sleepy, agricultural Campo. A good store lies 0.3 mile north, at the junction of Forrest Gate Road and Highway 94. The next supply point is in Mount Laguna, about 41.6 miles away.

Now turning your attention to the trail, you climb gently from the road, pass a lone live-oak tree, momentarily reach a terrace and then cut obliquely across a road serving the bungalows. Beyond, the sandy path climbs minimally across a brushy slope, then swings southwest at an overlook of Highway 94 and Campo Valley. Paralleling the highway, the PCT undulates over a string of low ridges, comes close to a descending jeep road, then descends easily to a PCT-posted crossing (2475-1.0) of two-lane Highway 94. North of it, the PCT leads counterclockwise around a low hill, then descends into a grove of cottonwoods alongside Campo Creek. Just before crossing that attractive, but seasonal, stream on a log telephone-pole bridge built in spring 1994 by PCTA volunteers, you ignore a jeep road climb-

see MAP A4

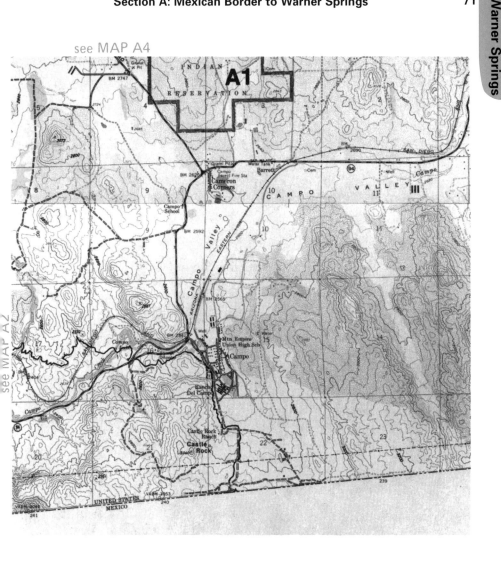

ing south. Instead, you follow PCT posts to the northwest bank, then traverse southwest on an alluvial terrace for a few minutes. Presently the route veers uphill, soon to find the abandoned San Diego & Arizona Eastern Railroad's tracks (2475-0.6). You have a gentle ascent as you continue over the tracks and wind westward over the nose of a low ridge. Now in a maze of small gullies and waist-high chamise chaparral, the tread descends gently to a larger ravine, which is just north of the tracks. Here the cool shade of willows and cottonwoods, with an under-

story of mint and cattails, makes a picturesque lunch spot. Alas, the creeklet here flows only in winter and early spring.

After momentarily coming close to the tracks again, you undertake a longer but still easy climb northwest to a low gap. A minute's walk beyond it, you strike a poor jeep road (2550-2.2), which descends in a south-trending valley. Now climbing more in earnest, you swing southwest on Hauser Mountain's broad, sunny slopes, then switchback to find a north-ascending line. The well-built, alternately sandy and rocky path soon rises high enough to afford

**See Maps A2, A3**

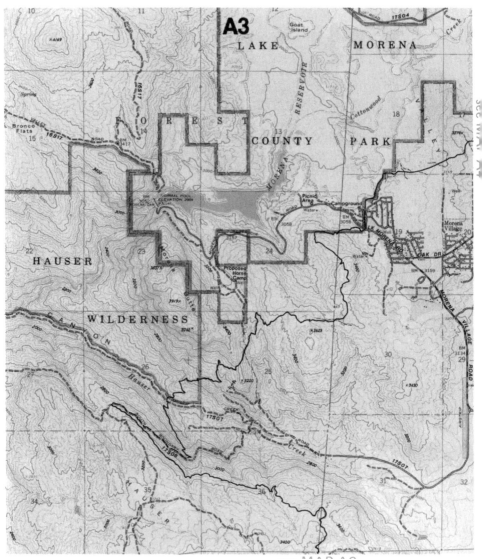

see MAP A2

fine, clear vistas southeast back to the border, and east over a lovely ranch that lies below Hauser Mountain's eastern escarpment. Pleasant walking leads northwest, more or less level, then the trail abruptly switchbacks up to the south to gain a canyon rim. Here the steep slopes yield to the chaparral-covered summit dome of Hauser Mountain. The path continues south, ascending gently and then passing through a pipe gate to a little-used road (3350-3.7). Beyond it you climb only minutes more before striking a second jeep road (3400-0.2). Next you undertake a contour north, and you can see your trail snaking ahead for over a mile. Umpteen hillside ravines later, you step across an east-descending jeep road (3345-2.0) before winding up to a viewful point (3400-0.5) low on the northeast ridge of Hauser Mountain.

**See Maps A2, A3**

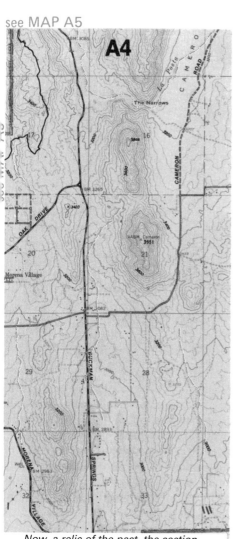

see MAP A5

A4

*Now, a relic of the past, the section shown on Map A4 is no longer in use. The map is to provide historical context and to maintain the map numbering system that PCT users have long relied on.*

To the north and west, an impressive panorama of Hauser Canyon unfolds. On the northern canyon wall stand orange granitic pillars of Morena Butte. This area now lies in one of California's smallest wilderness areas, Hauser Wilderness, created in 1984.

The trail now descends in a northwestern direction along the north face of Hauser Mountain, making a long traverse down-canyon. Presently, you note a road below you and continue out onto the nose of a low ridge to meet it—South Boundary Road 17S08 (2910-2.7). The PCT route heads southeast on this little-traveled road, first climbing gently and then descending likewise to a junction (2810-0.8) with a 1988-vintage trail segment. This branches left, east, dropping rapidly from the road where it begins to bend north on a rocky hillside. To stay on public lands, but to avoid unnecessary elevation loss, the trail makes a willy-nilly, rocky descent northwestward across the canyon wall, via five switchbacks. Finally, the grade moderates to reach a pleasant glade of live oaks and sycamores. In it, the PCT crosses Hauser Creek (2320-0.7), which is usually flowing in winter and early spring, but probably dry by April of drought years. A small flat just downstream could offer the best first night's camp north of the Mexican border for those who are disinclined to make the 1,000-foot climb to reach Lake Morena County Park. However, beware of cattle pollution of the stream and of plentiful poison oak.

Just across Hauser Creek you find Hauser Creek Road, then cross it to begin an earnest, sweaty ascent of the southern slopes of Morena Butte. The first leg of this climb lies in the southeastern corner of Hauser Wilderness, and it consists of a moderate-to-steep grade through straggly chaparral. As the climb progresses, vistas unfold down-canyon to meadows and to sky-blue Barrett Lake, which is framed by the bluffs of nearby Morena Butte. Switchbacks long and short eventually bring you to a saddle (3210-1.3) on the granitic southeastern spur of Morena Butte. Now the PCT undertakes a traversing descent north, shortly joining and then leaving a jeep trail (3150-0.2), which climbs more directly up from Hauser Canyon. Beyond

see MAP A6

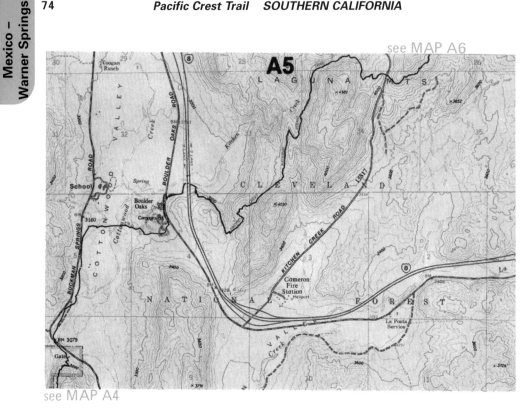

A5

see MAP A4

it, you wind for a minute or two along a dry creek bed, then step across its sandy wash to climb moderately north, then east, through lush mixed chaparral. In spring, the heavy perfume of startling lilac-blue ceanothus shrubs hangs heavy in the air, while a number of red-and-yellow-flowered globe mallows line the trailside. After reaching a low ridgecrest, you climb southeast a bit to a fair viewpoint (3495-1.0), which gives panoramas north over the southern Laguna Mountains.

Now you drop gently east to find a good jeep road in a saddle (3390-0.3). Walk right, east, on the jeep road for 50 yards, then leave it to angle first northeast and then north along a viewful, outcrop-strewn ridge. Eventually the route veers northwest down a chaparral-cloaked nose, then leaves the heights for a descending traverse east to an oak grove and a gate in a barbed-wire fence at the corner of Lake Morena Road and Lakeshore Drive (3065-1.7), at a trailhead parking area. Just north

is the entrance to John Lyons-Lake Morena Regional Park. This large facility offers, for a fee, 90 campsites with showers, water, picnic areas, and angling for bass, bluegill and catfish in Morena Reservoir. Just 0.3 mile southeast on Lake Morena Road is a malt shop and grocery store.

The PCT continues from the corner of the two paved roads, following Lakeshore Drive north 80 yards to where one steps through a fence to follow a paved road that traces the campground's perimeter. Beyond the camp area the route becomes trail and continues north to an oak-shaded overlook of Morena Reservoir and its chaparral-cloaked basin. Now walk levelly east and north around the lakeshore on trail that is often confused by a welter of use paths. PCTA volunteers have installed signs so, hopefully, the route is now more certain. Ignore intersecting paths made by local homeowners, which cross the PCT for lake access. Stay essentially level, and don't head away from the shoreline until

**See Maps A3, A4**

PCT emblems mark the way. Only 0.1 mile from the campground, ignore some prominent but rapidly fading paths that fishermen use to continue along the lakeshore. Rather, just after passing below the last house built in an adjacent cul-de-sac to the east, head right, northeast, uphill through a gated barbed-wire fence, onto a sandy rolling upland, clothed in waist-high chemise scrub. The route next crosses many jeep tracks in the open chamise chaparral as it turns east, then northeast, climbing gently to a low ridgetop (3220-1.5). Now the way drops northeast into a nearby secluded, oak-shaded canyon, hops its seasonal creek, and climbs moderately east, then southeast, to gain a 3375-foot ridge with expansive vistas west over the reservoir, Morena Butte and Hauser Mountain. The Laguna Mountains are seen on the northern skyline. You romp easily north on the spine of the ridge in mixed chaparral. After a mile the route makes a traversing descent along the ridge's west flank to a switchback, then to a gate on the ridge's northern nose. You quickly reach Buckman Springs Road S1, which you parallel briefly to its bridge over Cottonwood Creek (3065-2.6), which may be dry by April of drought years. The PCT's ford of the seasonally swollen creek may be too deep. If so, use the road's bridge and drop off its west end to find the PCT—an abandoned road. **You can camp here, although grazing cattle may have contaminated the creek.**

Continuing north, PCT trail tread soon diverges from the roadbed to wind through a pleasant mile of oak stands and dry meadows, always within earshot of Buckman Springs Road. Abruptly the route then veers east and descends to the 0.1-mile wide, sandy-gravelly bed of Cottonwood Creek (3105-1.4). Dry most of the year, the creek in winter and spring may be flowing and may be a couple of yards wide. Across it the trail heads east up a ravine, then joins a steadily improving and climb-ing jeep road that leads through a gate and over a low ridge to reach the equestrian section of **Boulder Oaks Campground** (3170-0.4). **This pleasant and little-used facility offers picnic tables, piped water, toilets and horse corrals among boulders and shady live oaks.** Marked by posts the PCT winds east across the campground, then momentarily goes north to reach paved, 2-lane Boulder Oaks Road (3165-0.1) just south of the campground's entrance. Now walk north along the road's west shoulder to the southern verge of Cottonwood Valley's grassy plain (3150-0.3), where well-signed PCT tread resumes, leading east. The Boulder Oaks Store used to stand at this intersection, and was the object of a pitched legal land-use battle for the entire past history of the PCT. A now-victorious Forest Service has erased its last vestiges.

Soon the route leads north and then east under two concrete spans of Interstate Highway 8. Just beyond the second bridge, switchbacks climb south to an ascending traverse that heads to a brushy gap. Here the route turns northeast for a long, traversing climb on open, sometimes rocky slopes, eventually finding a position some 100 feet above the cool, pooling early-season flow of Kitchen Creek. Arcing north around Peak 4382, you then switchback up, east, to find paved Kitchen Creek Road (3990-3.8) on a viewful pass.

The northbound PCT from atop the pass is found beyond a firebreak east of the pavement. Panoramas expand back to the Mexican border and to Cameron Valley as one ascends gently-to-moderately along slopes composed of foliated, red-stained gneiss, colored in season with blossoms of white forget-me-nots. After leveling off momentarily on a 4310-foot saddle, the trail drops, flanked by nodding, brown-flowered peonies and mixed chaparral, to a glade of oaks beside the usually dry creek of Fred Canyon (4205-1.9). Now on the west side of the canyon, the trail ascends to

**See Maps A5, A6**

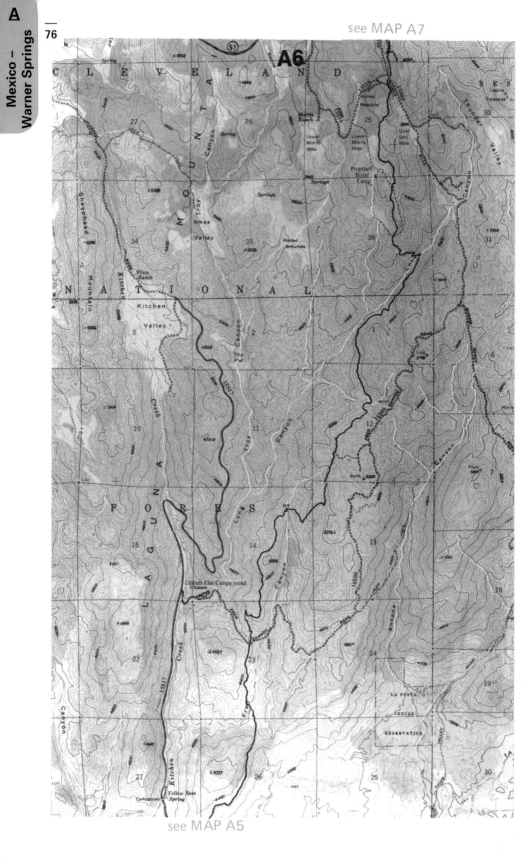

Fred Canyon Road 16S08 (4410-0.6), which descends 0.8 mile northwest to **Cibbets Flat Campground with toilets, tables and water.**

Now the path climbs moderately in heavy ceanothus/ocean spray/chamise cover, switch-backing once around a nose and then climbing to a traverse past Peak 5036 over to the dry headwaters of Fred Canyon. Next the PCT gains 500 feet, passes a jeep trail east to Fred Canyon Road, and then makes an undulating traverse and a gentle descent into Long Canyon (5230-4.2), where a camp could be made beside a seasonally trickling creek near wild roses. A gentle ascent in this pretty, meadowed canyon, dotted with black oaks, finds a ford (5435-0.8) of Long Canyon Creek, followed by switchbacks and two crossings of a jeep road from Horse Meadow. At the second crossing (5900-1.1) you could follow the jeep road northwest 0.3 mile to pretty **Lower Morris Meadow**, which has a horse-trough spring and a cozy cluster of Jeffrey pines—**the best camp so far. The USFS plans an equestrian/backpacker trail camp here in the future.**

Climbing still into the relatively cool Laguna Mountains proper, you alternate between mountain mahogany and Jeffrey-pine/black-oak forest to cross a saddle, then descend slightly to a crossing of Morris Ranch Road (6005-1.2). A few minutes north of the crossing of Morris Ranch Road, the undulating duff-treaded path intersects, then for 80 yards ambles along, a jeep road under open cover of Jeffrey pines and black oaks, before clearly branching away to descend. A few minutes' walk leads you to cross a much better road (5825-0.7) beside shaded La Posta Creek.

Here you'll see outstanding examples of acorn-woodpecker food caches—custom-built niches for individual black-oak and interior-live-oak acorns in Jeffrey pine bark. When tasty insect larvae hatch in the stored acorns, the birds return to feast!

Leaving La Posta Creek, the route contours above a pumphouse that in the future may become the site of a backpacker camp. Trekkers should be aware that in the Laguna Mountain Recreation Area camping is restricted to designated sites. The recreation area stretches from near this site north 10.4 miles to Pioneer Mail Trailhead Picnic Area.

Your trail ascends into the recreation area, passing abandoned wood-rat nests and the first pinyon pines of the trail before reaching the south boundary of **Burnt Rancheria Campground** (5950-0.8) **has toilets, water and tables.**

Cattlemen invaded the Laguna Mountains in the later 1800s, fattening their herds to the displeasure of the natives, called "Dieguenos" by the Spanish padres. The natives attested to their dislike of the white man's invasion by burning down a seasonal ranch house—whence the name "Burnt Rancheria."

**Northbound hikers should know that the next water lies in Chariot Canyon, a 1.8-mile detour from the PCT after a long, usually too warm, 22.4-mile trek. Less reliable water is found at Pioneer Mail Trailhead Picnic Area, 10.1 miles north.**

Climbing away from the campground, the PCT does double-duty as the Desert View Nature Trail, passing live-forever, pearly everlasting, thistle, yerba santa and beavertail cacti, all of them xeric (drought-tolerant) plants that reflect your proximity to the searing Colorado Desert to the east. Bending north and passing numerous, poorer side trails, your now nearly level path leads back into restful forest, joins dirt Desert View Road, and passes a dirt-road spur leading southwest to Burnt Rancheria Campground (5970-0.6). A con-

**See Maps A6, A7**

see MAP A9

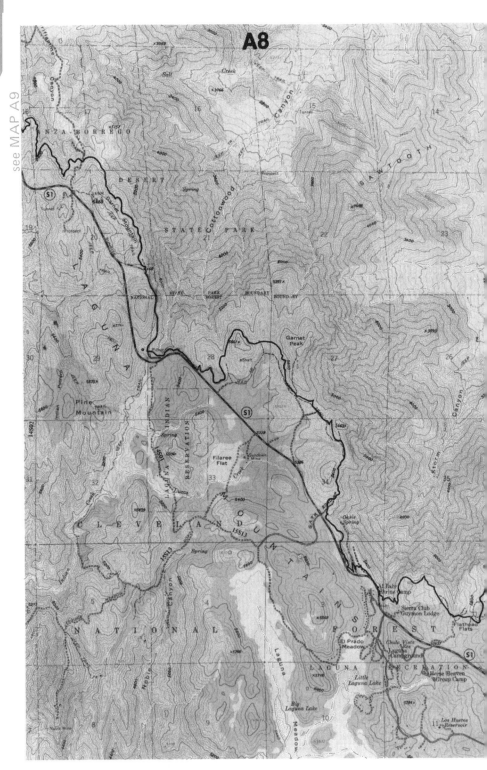

crete culvert horse trough and faucet were installed here in 1993 by a group of local PCT advocates. Travelers should rely on it only during seasons when Burnt Rancheria Campground is open, from mid-May thru late October.

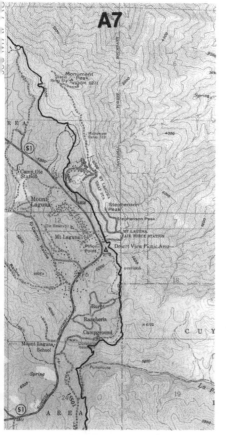

From here the PCT climbs north along the Desert View Nature Trail, reaching a spectacular overlook of arid Anza-Borrego Desert State Park, its floor—Vallecito Valley—lying 4400 feet below you in the rain shadow of the Laguna Mountains. The 35,080-acre Sawtooth Mountains Wilderness, designated in

see MAP A6

1994, lies east of and below the PCT, as it threads north around Stephenson Peak, Monument Peak, and Garnet Peak. The wilderness was designed to protect the rugged canyons that descend to the Vallecito Valley.

The rocks you stand on are now-familiar banded Mesozoic intrusive rocks: just to the east, a contact separates these from well-foliated pre-Cretaceous metasediments blotched with yellow lichens—a cliff on the east face of Stephenson Peak, to the north, is a good example. To your east Vallecito Valley is bedded in Pleistocene sediments, and beyond it the Tierra Blanca Mountains are composed of intrusive tonalite and the Vallecito Mountains of several-million-year-old nonmarine sediments.

Leaving this overlook, the PCT descends into cooler black-oak forest, passes below tables of the Desert View Picnic Area, now with toilets and a faucet, and then switchbacks up to a paved road (5980-0.7), which leads to Stephenson Peak and the abandoned Mount Laguna USAF Western Air Defense Network Station, now a Federal Aviation Administration navigation-control site.

**Resupply access:** Hikers in need of supplies can turn left on the road and walk 70 yards west to Sunrise Highway S1, and thence south 0.4 mile to Mount Laguna Post Office, a store, phones, restaurants and motels, and a Forest Service station. The next supply point along the PCT is Warner Springs, 67.7 miles away.

Continuing on the PCT, you have an easy traverse through high scrub and forest that lie below the golf-ball radar domes on Stephenson Peak. The traverse then ends at a second paved road (5895-0.6) climbing

**See Map A7**

to the summit. Iris, snowberry, yellow violets and baby blue eyes lend springtime color to the forest floor as the route skirts north around the Air Force station's boundary. Then it crosses a succession of jeep roads, and rises moderately in huckleberry-oak, manzanita and ocean-spray chaparral below Monument Peak before dropping easily to a saddle (5900-2.0) where some jeep roads terminate.

 A startling contrast of vegetation is presented when the PCT tops the next small ridge. To the east nothing but drought-tolerant, clumped shrubbery survives, while on the Laguna Mountains' summits to the west, a nearly uniform Jeffrey-pine and black-oak forest stretches from North, Cuyamaca and Stonewall peaks, in Cuyamaca Rancho State Park, over to hazy mountains above San Diego. A disparity of rainfall maintains these two different life zones, caused by the Laguna Mountains' geography. Warm, moisture-laden air sweeping inland from the Pacific Ocean cools as it rises over the obstructing Lagunas. This cooling causes moisture in the air to condense, bringing rain to nurture pine forests, and leaving parched, water-absorbing air to blast down desert slopes in the mountains' lee.

Leaving this instructional vista, the PCT descends, perhaps vaguely, through a small burn, crosses bulldozer tracks that encircle it, and then turns west, descending easily into oak-shaded Flathead Flats (5715-0.9). Here an obvious patchwork of poor roads leads west for 75 yards at the head of Storm Canyon. If the tread has been vague, it will become obvious here, as the trail ascends just under a northwest-trending road, crossing that road in a moment to emerge from shade onto a chaparral-covered nose. Merging with the road, your thoroughfare narrows as it descends viewfully northwest past rock and chaparral, then turns south to switchback down to a ravine and resume a gently undulating traverse below the Sunrise Highway. In just a moment you reach a dirt spur (5440-1.3) descending from the highway.

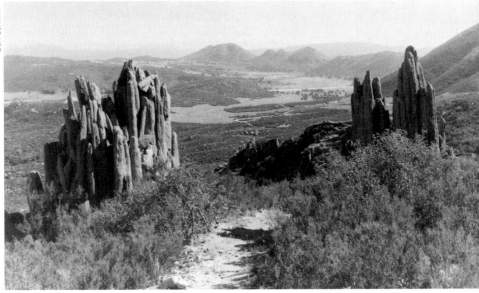

*Cameron Valley, view south from Peak 4737*

**See Map A8**

**Water access:** To get water, head west up the road to the highway and take it south 0.2 mile to Laguna/El Prado Campground.

Back on route, a few minutes' walk leads to a lone switchback that raises you to a ridgetop pole-line road, which you cross westward to descend to a quiet draw and a better dirt road (5430-0.5) that descends north to Oasis Spring. After you leave this road, live and black oaks, scattered pines and mountain mahogany line the viewful way around the spectacular furnace-breathed head of Storm Canyon to reach closed GATR Road (5440-0.9) on cooler forested land. This intersection is now trail, and marks an important detour to water.

**Water access:** Just beyond a pipe swing-gate, there is now an unmarked trail junction, where the roadbed used to be. Continuing straight ahead (northwest), a spur trail curves gently down and west, then momentarily south, to reach Sunrise Highway S1 in less than 0.1 mile. Here, a monument to the Penny Pines reforestation program stands beside a busy trailhead parking area. Directly across two-lane Highway S1 is the start of Noble Canyon Trail 5E04, which strikes west-southwest only 50 yards to a permanent water supply. Here lie a green faucet and a galvanized horse trough, in an open stand of black oaks. This level flat is quite hospitable but, unfortunately, no camping is allowed in this vicinity. A moment farther on is a junction with the southbound Big Laguna Trail, which heads back to Mount Laguna in about 3 miles.

This is the last certain water source close to your route until Cuyamaca Reservoir, 12.5 miles farther along the PCT and then 1.7 miles along a lateral. Closer but less certain water may be had during late spring and summer at Pioneer Mail Trailhead Picnic Area, in 3.9 miles. Possibly

more convenient to some northbound travelers are the year-round springs in Chariot Canyon, a 1.8-mile detour from the PCT in 14.9 miles, or the well on Rodriguez Spur Truck Trail, a 1.3-mile detour from your path in 19.8 miles.

North across the closed fire road, the PCT swings right (north), then ascends gently east, recrossing the road to climb easily under the Lagunas' steep eastern scarp to a saddle with the end of a jeep road (5540-0.5). From it the route undulates northwest on scrub-bound slopes while keeping just above the rough jeep track. Your path crosses jeep spurs to the summits of Peak 5663 and Garnet Peak and then strikes another spur at a saddle (5495-1.6) west of Garnet Peak. The PCT next traverses around Peak 5661, passing through hoary-leaved ceanothus brush and providing excellent vistas of Oriflamme Mountain to the north. Beyond, the route drops first south and then west to a sandy saddle with a grass-floored pine forest. The route then heads northwest before winding west to shaded Pioneer Mail Trailhead Picnic Area (5260-1.8), which lies at the end of a parking spur coming from Sunrise Highway. Here the PCT is signed as Laguna Rim Trail 5E08.

The massive Pines Fire of July 2002 has devastated the PCT on it's traverse from the Lagunas to Barrel Springs— much of the route surrounding the trail has burned. Be very alert for trail junctions, which may no longer be easily distinguished due to destruction of signs and markers.

**Water access:** In 1994 the USFS placed a 6-foot-diameter, 4-foot aboveground, 1000-gallon water tank in low brush just 50 feet beyond the trailhead information sign. It is filled only during

see MAP A10

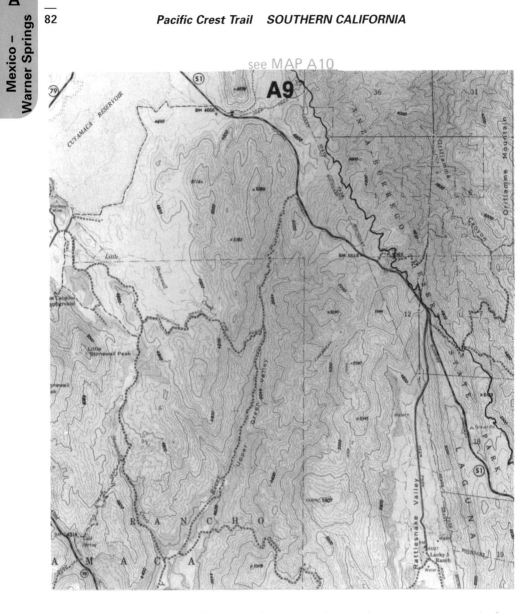

late May and summer and only with untreated water. A 4-foot-diameter concrete trough is fed by the tank. Contact Cleveland National Forest's Descanso Ranger District before leaving Mount Laguna, for the tank's status. Alternately, contact the PCTA at (888) PC-TRAIL or *www.pcta.org*. Please conserve water, and don't promote vandalism by advertising the tank's presence!

The PCT's continuation north from the picnic area follows the old, unpaved alignment of Sunrise Highway gently up across a cliff at the head of Cottonwood Canyon to meet the end of paved Kwaaymi Point Road (5450-0.7). Northbound tread recommences a few yards up this road only 40 yards south of a defunct jeep road climbing Garnet Mountain. Now you contour on the mountain's eastern declivity and enter Cuyamaca Rancho State Park. A

**See Map A8**

he mountain's north end, you drop briskly north on sunny slopes to a jeep road 5250-1.4) that descends into Oriflamme Canyon.

Oriflamme ("golden flame") Mountain, whence the canyon derives its name, received its appellation from numerous sightings, since the 1880s, of "burning balls" or "spirit lights" on the mountain's east side. These led to insistent prospecting for gold over the years, but scientists have at least one more-interesting theory—that the lights are static electricity, discharged when dry desert winds blow sand against quartz boulders on the hillside.

The next leg meanders northwestward long steep hillsides of light-colored granodiorite—weathered to futuristic knobs—nd affords excellent panoramas of seemgly sterile Vallecito Valley. But these views hardly compensate for the shadeless, monotonous trail.

Vallecito Valley was once the site of a Butterfield Overland Mail Stage station. Following an old Spanish trail from Fort Yuma, stages ran from St. Louis to California from 1858 to 1861. The first Europeans to traverse this part of the Colorado Desert, however, were Spanish forces led by Lieutenant Pedro Fages from the San Diego Presidio, who marched through in search of deserters in 1772. Two years later Captain Juan Bautista de Anza, for whom the park is named, scouted this area for a life-line trail from Mexico to impoverished Alta California settlements.

Presently the route descends to meet a second road to Oriflamme Canyon (4875-2.8). Across it you climb through brush on a trail that soon closely parallels Sunrise Highway.

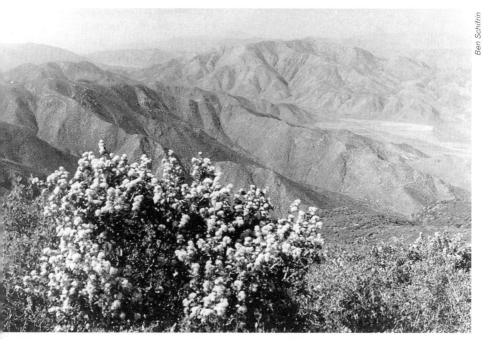

Ben Schifrin

*Oriflamme Mountain, from west of Garnet Peak*

**See Maps A8, A9**

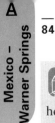

The rocks lining your route from here to Chariot Canyon are Julian schist—metasediments of Paleozoic age. This particular schist (a rock, once a shale, that now breaks along paper-thin parallel planes) shows abundant flecks of reflective, glassy mica, and it weathers to a rusty brown containing frequent mineral-stain bandings.

Presently you cross a ridgetop jeep road, and then another (5025-1.3). ADZP-CTKOP volunteers have established a **springtime water cache** in this area—look for blazes and water jugs beside the trail. Take only what you need, and don't count on these supplies!

A sweeping vista unfolds to the north; green forested Volcan Mountain stands above your unfortunate route down to arid San Felipe Valley and the brown San Felipe Hills. Beyond, Combs Mountain, Thomas Mountain and the Desert Divide rise to the rugged subalpine splendor of San Jacinto Peak. Over its west shoulder, the bald white alpine cap of San Gorgonio Peak thrusts its height—your next two weeks' work is displayed!

Continuing, the PCT undulates above Oriflamme Canyon to reach a faint jeep track (4770-2.4) at a low gap.

**Water access:** Here thirsty hikers may opt to follow that track west for 1.0 mile through a verdant meadow to Sunrise Highway. There is a horse trough at the barbwire gate here, which may afford a water gift in springtime, but must not be relied on. From the highway, follow California Riding and Hiking Trail (CRHT) posts 0.7 mile west to Cuyamaca Reservoir, where long-overdue draughts of water are available. **Los Caballos Camp-**ground, in Cuyamaca Rancho State Park, is 1.6 miles farther along the well-marked CRHT. It is reserved for equestrians only. Cuyamaca Rancho State Park (from the Native American "Ah-ha-kwe-ah-mac", meaning "the place where it rains") is a recommended layover spot, having cool forests, seasonally chortling streams, and campgrounds with showers. An excellent Native American cultural exhibit and the old Stonewall Mine could round out the visit.

Returning to your trek, you follow the PCT as it winds north along chaparral clothed summits to the Mason Valley Truck Trail (4690-1.1), just east of a locked gate. Northbound travelers here turn right and curve 100 yards east to a junction with Chariot Canyon Road, now barely distinguishable as a road. **Emergency water is sporadically available 75 yards east of this junction, where a spigot juts out of the hillside below a concrete-box water tank used by fire crews. If the spigot is locked, look 10 feet uphill in a grove of Coulter pines—the large cistern has an unlocked metal access plate. Don't count on it.** Back on route, the PCT leads north down rocky Chariot Canyon not-a-road, on a bone-jarring descent, which ends at a lupine flat holding the canyon's seasonal creek. Fair but waterless camping may be found here, by a road junction (3860-1.3).

**Water access:** If you are low on water, you should detour here, and continue north down Chariot Canyon Road in search of that precious desert commodity. But check upstream from the PCT before heading down-canyon to the springs—water is sometimes found there. Otherwise, walk north down the gently sloping sandy, sunny wash, passing, in a few yards, a set of native American mortars ground in a large boulder near the creek bed. Presently you pass in and out of stands of cottonwoods and live oaks.

and leave Anza-Borrego Desert State Park (3700-0.6). Beyond, you begin to encounter tailings, mine tunnels and shacks of some of the many gold mines that dot Chariot Canyon. One commonly finds water in the streambed in the next quarter mile, relieving the hiker of the full trek down to the main springs. If not, continue north, cross to the east bank, and presently find a short dirt spur road (3565-0.6). It branches right, east, uphill for 75 yards to an 18-foot-diameter, buried concrete water tank set in the hillside. This road is marked near its junction by a square concrete valve box. Water can be had from the tank by way of a 4′x18″ iron plate set in its top. Camping is adequate, nearby. If water or accommodations here aren't to your liking, continue down-canyon farther, recrossing Chariot Canyon Creek twice in quick succession to find permanent springs (3490-0.6), just short of dirt Ben Hur Mine Road. In severe drought years, the springs have become very close to dry.

If they are dry, continue down-canyon to one of a half-dozen active gold-mining claims, and ask for water. If that is futile, continue out to the road's end on Highway 78 at Banner (2755-3.2), a small resort with a store, restaurant, phones and camping. From there it is 7.5 miles west on Highway 78 to beautiful Julian, with complete supplies and delicious apple pie. The northbound traveler could get back on route by heading east from Banner to the PCT near Scissors Crossing, in 5 miles.

Those who return to the PCT in upper Chariot Canyon should note that their watery treasure must last a while: the well on Rodriguez Spur Truck Trail is the next near-route water for the northbound, a 1.3-mile detour from the PCT in 4.9 miles. Barrel Spring, 33.0 blistering hot miles ahead from the junction, has the next on-route water. Heading south, the next completely reliable water is at reliable water is at GATR Road, 14.9 long miles up in the Laguna Mountains.

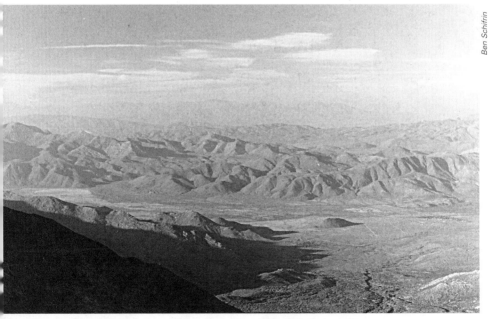

*Ben Schifrin*

*Anza-Borrego Desert State Park and Santa Rosa Mountains, from Laguna Rim*

**See Map A10**

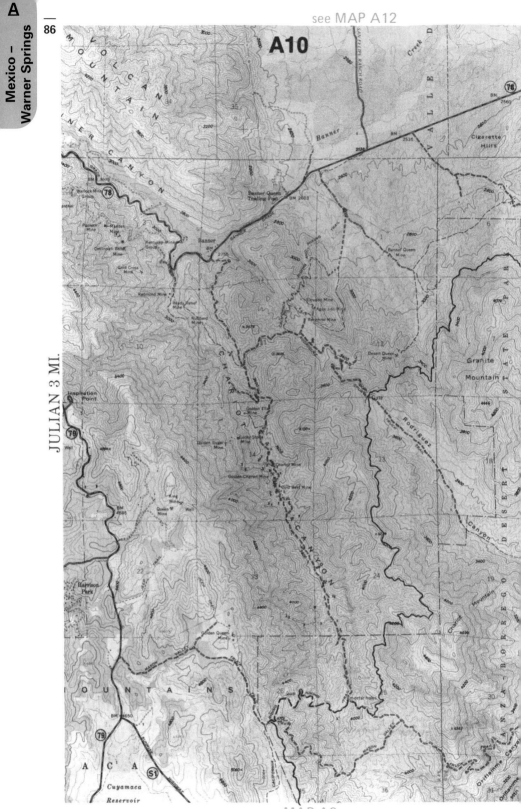

# A10

JULIAN 3 MI.

From the road junction in upper Chariot Canyon you climb steeply east up the Mason Valley cutoff road to a resumption of PCT trail tread (4075-0.3). This branches left, northeast, the junction perhaps marked with a brown and white state park sign. Now, a well-built tread snakes gently uphill around the western and northern slopes of rounded Chariot Mountain. Eventually the path skirts briefly northwest along a crest saddle, veers left, and then soon veers northeast across a gap (4240-2.6). Just beyond it you get vistas southeast, down desertlike Rodriguez Canyon and into the mirage-wavering, incandescent heart of Anza-Borrego Desert State Park. Thankfully, your way continues north and skirts the hottest regions. A businesslike descent now leads down to the head of Rodriguez Canyon, where you cross Rodriguez Spur Truck Trail (3650-2.0).

**Water access:** Here you can detour north to an important water source: Follow Rodriguez Spur Truck Trail left, west, for a brisk descent northward. Make two big switchbacks, then turn right, east, on a dirt road spur (3410-0.9) leading in just a minute to a cream-colored clapboard house in grove of poplars. Ask for water, from a small spring and pond just uphill of the house. Alternatively, one may continue down Rodriguez Spur Truck Trail for a few minutes more to find a well (3270-0.4) just 40 feet below the road. It is 12 feet high, capped with a blue plastic barrel. A circular concrete horse trough in a small patch of irrigated grass lies just to the northwest, only yards below the road. The vicinity is private property, so no camping is allowed hereabouts.

Immediately beyond good dirt Rodriguez Spur Truck Trail, you pass through a pipe gate and angle across an east-curving jeep track, then you too swing east. A graded but persistent descent next

leads northward on the steep, rocky, barren slopes of Granite Mountain, offering impressive panoramas.

North over arid San Felipe Valley, look carefully for the next leg of the PCT, which traverses along the San Felipe Hills, low on the northern horizon. In the far distance, green San Jacinto Peak and glistening, bald San Gorgonio Peak rear above 2-mile heights. Closer by, the rusty headframes of a few old gold mines—part of the once rich Julian mining complex which caused excitement in 1869-70—lie in ravines below you.

After winding down a succession of dry slopes, the PCT turns more east and almost levels just above the gentle, brushy alluvial fans at the foot of Granite Mountain. Unfortunately, a logical, direct PCT route from here—northeast to the southern San Felipe Hills—was blocked by uncooperative landowners, who denied right-of-way to trail construction. Hence your route now makes a frustrating, hot, time-consuming detour east to remain on public lands.

First you ascend to a rocky gap (3390-3.2) on Granite Mountain's north ridge. Next you descend to cross a succession of bouldery washes, then undulate east some more to a second gap (3130-1.9) behind a prominent light-colored granitic knob. A final descent is begun on four small switchbacks, followed by a descending traverse eastward. Abruptly, near the base of a cluster of pinnacles below Granite Mountain's northeast ridge, you veer north, debouching onto a sandy alluvial plain. After quickly crossing a jeep track, you proceed almost arrow-straight across northern Earthquake Valley, imperceptibly descending through an open desert association of low buckwheat, rabbitbrush and teddy-bear cholla shrubs, these sprinkled with larger junipers and graceful agave. You eventually pass

**See Maps A10, A11**

through a gate in a barbed-wire fence, then swing northeast, tracing an old jeep road that is immediately west of the fenceline. This stretch ends at busy, 2-lane Highway S2 (2245-2.9) at a spot just west of a white, wooden cattle guard.

Now locate a faint trail that turns left, west, near the south shoulder of Highway S2 just south of a 4-strand green barbed-wire fence. It winds fairly level past low shrubs, many of them equipped with murderously efficient, thigh-slashing, clothes-grabbing spines. Nearing a junction with Highway 78, find a red metal pipe gate and cross Highway S2 (2275-0.8), safe from attack by menacing vegetables, but now exposed to a considerable traffic of desert-bound vacationers. This was the route of the Butterfield Stage Line, which carried mail across the western US, passing this way in the 1850s. Now walk directly north, at first paralleling a wooden-post fence, then drifting vaguely away to the left through cat-claw shrubs, beyond which trail tread peters out as you walk down to cross a dry sandy wash. Momentarily, you emerge on a low terrace, just beneath the south shoulder of Highway 78. Now head right, northeast, along the shrubby terrace, close beside Highway 78, to find another cattle gate adjacent to the concrete bridge where the highway spans San Felipe Creek (2250-0.2).

**Water access:** San Felipe Creek stream almost always runs well into summer, even during drought years, but should not be counted upon. Even when present, it is usually heavily contaminated by cattle.

Just to the north of the bridge is a large cottonwood tree which could afford a fair camp.

Continuing, step across San Felipe Creek's sandy bed, then resume a parallel course to Highway 78, again on a low terrace, where trail tread is often overgrown by tumbleweeds, mustard and baccharis. It was cleared of brush by PCTA volunteers in late 1994, but the riparian shrubbery will no doubt grow back quickly. If it is too dense, simply step north onto the road shoulder, instead. In just a few minutes, we cross Highway 78 to find a resumption of PCT tread (2252-0.2). It climbs northwest, up from the highway at a junction that may be marked with a CHAINS REQUIRED sign.

**Water access:** Northbound hikers should be reminded that Barrel Spring, the next possible (but not certain) water-hole, is still 23.8 potentially scorching miles away. If your water reserves are low, consider walking one mile northeast on Highway 78 to Sentenac Cienaga, a marsh along San Felipe Creek. Water is usually found here all spring. Better yet, hitch-hike 5 miles southwest to Banner to refill. Southbound hikers will find water in Banner too, or near-route at Rodriguez Canyon Truck Trail, in 9.2 miles, or in Chariot Canyon, 14.1 miles hence. This is also a reasonable spot to detour for supplies as well as water—delightful and cool Julian is 12.5 miles west up Highway 78, while Borrego Spring is about 15 miles east on Highway 78.

A number of selfless volunteers have stepped in to help with the already dicey water-availability problem around the San Felipe Hills. Members of the San Diego Chapter of the Sierra Club, the PCTA, and ADZPCTKOP have repeatedly placed water bottles at Scissors Crossing, and in the San Felipe Hills, for the last three hiking seasons. Current plans call for the same effort in late April of each year. However, count on this gracious act at your peril! The best way to monitor the water situation here, as well as through-out Southern California, is to subscribe

**See Map A11**

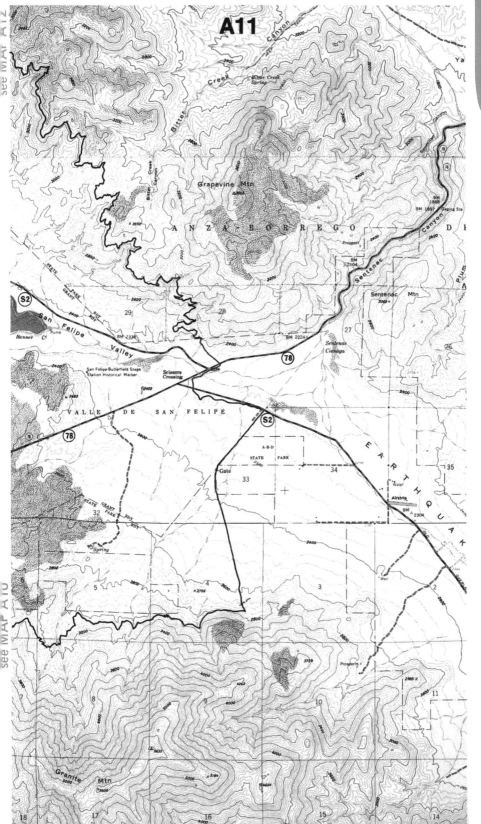

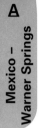
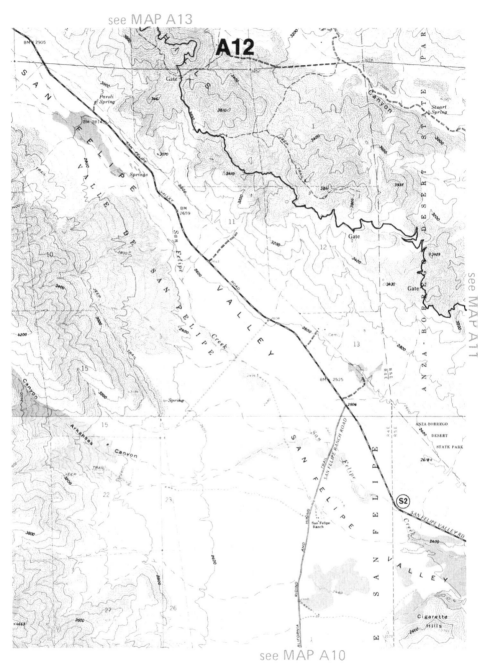

see MAP A13

**A12**

see MAP A11

see MAP A10

to the outstanding Internet mail list, "PCT-L." To join the verbal give-and-take, and to learn about the most up-to-date trail conditions, send an e-mail to *pct-l@ mailman.backcountry.net*, with no subject and a message that reads, "subscribe pct-l [your e-mail address]."

An alternative way to water from the Scissors Crossing environs would be to hop on a bus and retreat west up to the cool green haven of Julian. (See "Supplies," page 67). A San Diego County bus stops at Scissors Crossing each morning at about 8:30 A.M., and returns by 5:30 P.M. Contact San Diego County for an up-to-date schedule.

Commencing a long, exposed traverse of the San Felipe Hills, the PCT ascends briefly across a cobbly alluvial fan to the southern foot of Grapevine Mountain. Here you cross into Anza-Borrego Desert State Park and, now on rotten granite footing, begin to climb Grapevine Mountain's truly desertlike southwestern flanks. Even in springtime PCT hikers would do well to attack this ascent in the very early morning, since temperatures over 100° are commonplace, and most of the next 24 miles are virtually shadeless. Hikers trying to walk the length of the San Felipe Hills in one hot day will be either gratified or frustrated by the extraordinarily gentle grade of the route, which adds many extra switchbacks and a few unnecessary miles to the task.

Early on the walk, however, the easy grade allows one to marvel at the "forest" of bizarre ocotillo shrubs. Standing 10–15 feet tall and resembling nothing more than a bundle of giant, green pipe cleaners, ocotillos are perfectly adapted to their searing desert environment. Much of the year, ocotillos' branches look like spiny, lifeless stalks. But within just 2–3 days after a rainstorm, the branches sprout vibrant green clusters of delicate leaves along their entire length, allowing renewed growth. Almost as quickly, the leaves wither and die as groundwater becomes scarce. In this manner ocotillos may leaf out 6–8 times a year.

The PCT continues to climb imperceptibly in and out of innumerable small canyons and gullies, none of which holds running water except during a rainsquall. Still in a very desertlike association of agave, barrel cactus and teddy-bear cholla, you eventually reach the crest of the San Felipe Hills, and cross to their northeastern slopes at a pipe gate (3360-8.5). Now the path descends gently into a small, sandy valley where a sparse cover of scrub oak and juniper would make for adequate but waterless camping. Your trail tread becomes indistinct for a moment as you cross a dry, sandy wash (3210-0.6) which drains the valley, but you can see the trail's switchbacks on the slopes ahead, so navigation is easy.

An ascent of those switchbacks leads gently back to the ridgecrest (3600-1.6). The next leg of your journey stays high on the San Felipe Hills' steep southwestern slopes on an undulating course ranging between 3400 feet and 3600 feet. Just below a ridge saddle you pass a junction (3485-2.1) with an east-branching jeep road, and then your path crosses the next saddle to the north, bisecting another, poorer jeep road (3550-0.8) just beyond a pipe gate.

**Water access:** Here, members of the PCT Section of the Sierra Club's San Diego Chapter established an emergency water cache for PCT thru-hikers. It consists of gallon water jugs secured by a nylon cord. This cache was initially stocked with 55 gallons of water and will be replenished throughout the spring peak-hiking season on a calendar basis, since volunteers have no way of knowing

**See Maps A11, A12**

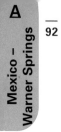
see MAP A14

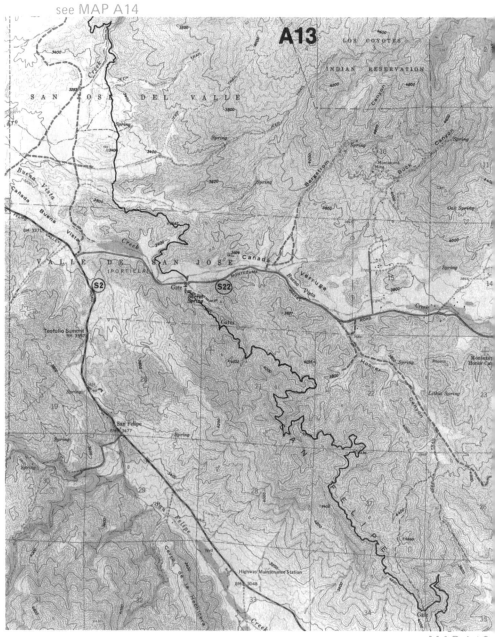

see MAP A12

when all jugs are empty. Please limit individual use to 2 liters of water. Some later hikers may find the jugs empty when they arrive.

Should a desperate hiker find that the water bottles are empty, there is off-trail water in Grapevine Canyon at the W-Bar-W Ranch (Grapevine Spring). To reach it, follow the obvious jeep spur trail leading right (east), down into Grapevine Canyon. Walk about 0.9 mile east to a tall, square fence post by a jeep road. Follow the jeep road to your left until you pass through a wide gate (10 feet or so). Follow the fence line left to reach the caretaker's house. A phalanx of barking dogs will let your presence be known. The caretaker, if in residence, will probably come out to meet you. Both the owner (Richard) and the caretaker (David) are supporters of the PCT and have given their permission for hikers to come on to their private property for water. Hikers should return to the PCT to camp, unless specifically invited by the owner or caretaker to camp in Grapevine Canyon.

Pressing on, you begin a long ascent, again on the eastern slopes of the San Felipe Hills, climbing now past dense chamise. An excruciatingly gentle, time-consuming switchback finally brings you back to the ridgetop and a cattle gate (4155-2.7). A more interesting trail then traverses the headwalls of two treacherously steep canyons, these plummeting 1200 feet to linear San Felipe Valley.

Across that valley the Volcan Mountains rise in pine-green splendor, an enviable cool contrast to your scorched environs. The San Felipe Hills are dry and brown for the same reason that the Volcan Mountains are lush and green: a rain-shadow situation causes moisture-laden Pacific storms to dump their rain on the higher Volcan Moun-

tains, leaving little for the San Felipe Hills. Volcan Mountain is the logical location of the PCT, and in fact was Congress' designated route. Unfortunately, the USFS took the easy way out, and so condemned hikers and horses to a truly dangerous, waterless, desert path on the non-Pacific crest of the San Felipe Hills, rather than wrangle with land owners for right-of-way over the better location. The author urges all PCT users to write their Congress-person and demand a safer relocation of the PCT to Volcan Mountain.

Presently you veer northeast through a gap (4395-1.9), back into dense chaparral on the east side of the San Felipe Hills. Beginning a long, gentle downgrade, the route winds infuriatingly around minor ridges and into nooks, crannies and (it seems) every gully in sight. After a few miles of such mistreatment, most hikers will yearn for a more direct, if steeper, route. But slowly the PCT loses elevation as it circumnavigates a branch of Hoover Canyon, and you gain vistas northeast over sparsely populated Montezuma Valley to San Ysidro Mountain. After only a short eternity you pass through three gates in quick succession, then just a few minutes later, descend under live-oak cover to join a poor road. Now, perhaps marked by a PCT post, your route goes left, west, just a few yards on the road to find Barrel Spring (3475-5.6).

Here, after the first major spring rains, cool water is piped into a concrete trough. Adjacent litter notwithstanding, this good waterhole and a pleasant, shady stand of canyon live oaks make a hospitable campsite, which the Forest Service may improve.

**See Maps A12, A13**

**Water and supply access:** If water is not flowing in the trough, follow the PCT and the feeder pipe back southeast for about 100 yards to an old dirt road that angles uphill to the spring's source. Northbound hikers can be assured of reliable water in 8.7 miles at Warner Springs Fire Station.

Southbound hikers have a longer walk to water—23.8 miles to springtime off-route water at Sentenac Cienaga, 33.0 miles to off-route water on Rodriguez Spur Truck Trail, or 37.9 miles to off-route springs in Chariot Canyon. If no water is available at Barrel Spring, hitch-hike 4.5 miles east on Montezuma Valley Road S22 to Ranchita, which is a small village. One may continue east on S22, 15 miles from the PCT to Borrego Springs, for resupply. On the way, the village of Ranchita, with a single small minimarket, is passed, in about 4 miles.

Resuming your northward trek, you follow the dirt road from Barrel Spring, down through a gate to a dirt-road pullout just south of paved Montezuma Valley Road S22 (3445-0.1). Just across the highway is a poor dirt road, on which you head north just 50 yards to a barbed-wire cattle gate. Just beyond it PCT posts indicate a route leading left (northwest), which quickly crosses the sandy wash of usually dry Buena Vista Creek. The way continues northwest across a sagebrush flat to the southern foot of a ridge. As the trail turns west at the ridge's base, the tread becomes well-defined, soon contouring north into a small canyon. Then the trail begins to climb easily, and you are treated to pleasant views west as you ascend to a 3550-foot ridgetop. The trail next drops easily west along its northern slope and, nearing the southern margin of a narrow, grassy, west-trending valley, the tread abruptly ends. But

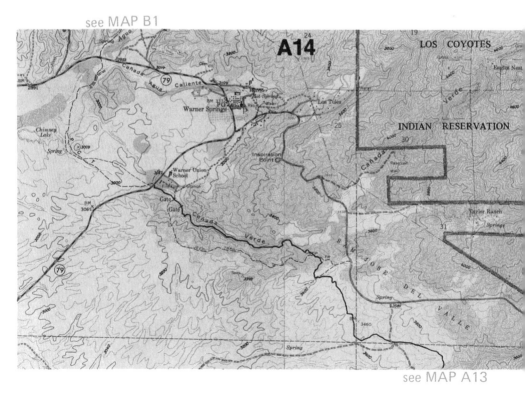

see MAP B1

see MAP A13

**See Maps A13, A14**

ooking north across the pasture, you'll hopefully spot a PCT post marking the crossing of a jeep road (3285-2.1). You'll then note tread immediately to the north, ascending north along the next low ridge. Climb it, then drop northeast to its base on the edge of another, much larger rolling grassland. Thanks to the efforts of PCTA volunteers, trail tread is now well-defined and well-posted from here to San Ysidro Creek. Follow the undulating path almost due north across the meadow, passing some well-trod cattle tracks to angle into the shallow mouth of sandy San Ysidro Creek's chaparral-clad valley. Along the way, you'll pass below a trickling hillside spring seep where cattle often congregate. Later, sweeping levelly through a grove of live oaks near the stream's east bank, you will see just below an 8-foot-diameter concrete cattle trough at a well. The path contours north along the canyon's east slopes, but soon drops to cross San Ysidro Creek (3355-1.7), which usually flows in spring. Like other key points on this trail segment, this crossing is confused by a jeep track just north of the creek but is now marked by a large PCT sign. Anticipate the crossing where San Ysidro Creek first bends northeast, up-canyon, under the first white-barked sycamore tree to shade your path. A fair camp could be made here.

Across San Ysidro Creek, head straight uphill for 20 yards to find the path, which continues up-canyon for only a moment before switchbacking west moderately up out of the shade onto an open hillside. Ineptly built and poorly maintained, the tread ascends from San Ysidro Creek, soon turning north to attain the canyon's rim.

Here you have views west over Warner Valley to Lake Henshaw, a sag pond along the Elsinore Fault, and to famous Mount Palomar Observatory, on the horizon.

After a brief course north the trail turns west and re-enters grassland. It leads gently up, then down, to cross a good dirt road (3495-1.2), then soon it adopts a more northern course as it rolls across a corrugation of ridgelets and dry washes. After crossing a poor jeep trail in one such ravine, the trail climbs through low chaparral and soon crosses a ridgetop jeep road (3510-1.6), which served as part of the temporary PCT route for many years.

From the ridge you descend gently past shady canyon live oaks and cotton-woods which line the pretty valley called Cañada Verde (Spanish for "Green Ravine"). Soon the PCT closely parallels the southern banks of a small stream that flows until late spring of most years. A fine camp can be made almost anywhere along the next mile of creek, in grassy flats adorned with pink wild roses. The Forest Service may develop a formal camping area here. You follow the canyon bottom for almost a mile, and then, near Cañada Verde's mouth, pass through two pipe gates, the second one at a jeep road. Across the jeep road you continue northwest just south of Cañada Verde's banks, and in ¼ mile find the concrete bridge of two-lane Highway 79 (3040-2.0), just west of Warner Springs Fire Station. Although the PCT actually heads under the highway, the bridge clearance is too low for horses, so a pipe gate allows access to the highway. Warner Springs Post Office lies 1.2 miles northeast along the highway.

**Water access:** Water is available at the fire station. The next water for northbound hikers lies in Agua Caliente Creek, in 5.3 miles, while for the southbound, water is next obtained at Barrel Spring, 8.7 miles away.

**See Maps A13, A14**

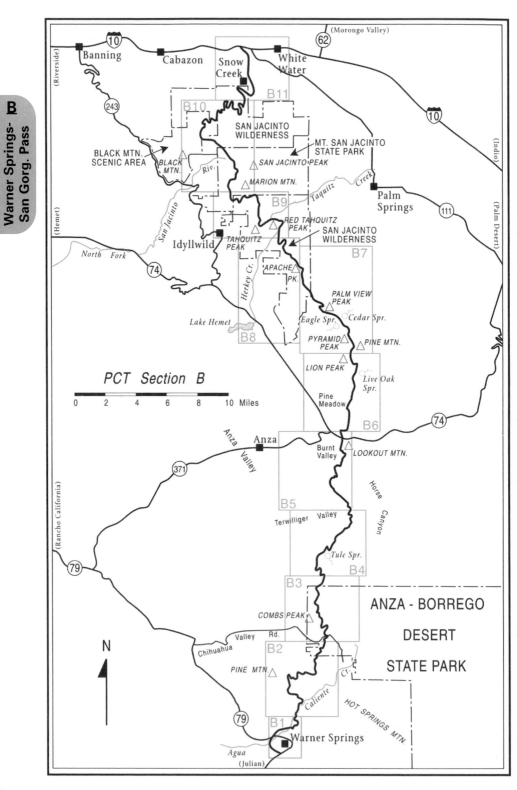

# Section B:

# Warner Springs to San Gorgonio Pass

The San Jacinto Mountains are the high point—and the highlight—of the Pacific Crest Trail's excursion through the northern Peninsular Ranges, and they afford the first true high-mountain air and scenery of your journey. But this section of trail also includes many miles of walking under shady live oaks and through the shadeless chaparral community (see below). On the Desert Divide, where you have your first taste of the San Jacinto Mountains, you find an interesting combination of pine forest, chaparral and desert species. Leaving the San Jacintos, the PCT plunges almost 8000 feet down to arid San Gorgonio Pass, and in so doing passes through every life zone in California save for the alpine zone.

The Peninsular Ranges stretch from the southern tip of Baja California, paralleling the coastline, some 900 miles north to San Gorgonio Pass, which truncates the range along the Banning Fault and lesser faults. The ranges' core, forming the Laguna Mountains, the Anza Upland and the San Jacinto Mountains, where the PCT winds, is made of crystalline rocks—granite and its relatives—which were first intruded in a liquid state several miles beneath the surface and then later solidified. These rocks are similar in age and kind to the granitic rocks of the Sierra Nevada.

Your walk from Warner Springs to San Gorgonio Pass treads mostly upon these rocks, which are usually fine-grained, gray-to-creamy in color, and strongly resistant to weathering, as demonstrated by obdurate monoliths around Indian Flats and Bucksnort Mountain, by outcrops jutting from the alluvium of Terwilliger and Anza valleys, and by the jagged, saurian spine of the San Jacinto Mountains, as on Fuller Ridge. The remainder of the terrain you tread is across either sand and gravel weathered from the granite, found in basins, or metamorphic rocks. These rocks are seen in Agua Caliente Creek's canyon and along much of the Desert Divide.

Section B ends at San Gorgonio Pass, a broad, cactus-dotted trough running east-west, flanked by the San Bernardino and San Jacinto mountains to the north and south respectively. Once a major corridor of

Native American traders, San Gorgonio Pass is bounded by faults on either side. It lies some 9000 feet below the summits of San Jacinto and San Gorgonio, each standing just a few air miles to one side.

Proof that awesome geologic processes are at work today can be seen right at the start of this section, at Warner Springs. Now a tourist spa, but used for centuries past by neighboring Cahuilla and Cupeño Native American tribes, the hot springs here bubble up from deep within the earth's crust and escape along the Aguanga Fault, which cuts just yards behind this small

resort community. Warner's hot spring also served Kit Carson in 1846, and was an overnight stop on the Butterfield Stage Line from 1858 to 1861.

Section B now also traverses the new crown jewel of the Peninsular Ranges—Santa Rosa and San Jacinto Mountains National Monument. Created in October 2000 to protect 272,000 acres of mountains along the vast eastern sweep of those ranges, the monument stretches from the Anza-Borrego Desert State Park boundary on the south to the San Gorgonio Pass on the north. National designation will hopefully give added protection to the natural, historical, and cultural resources found along this rugged mountain crest, and help the diverse agencies that share jurisdiction over the varied landscape coordinate their efforts.

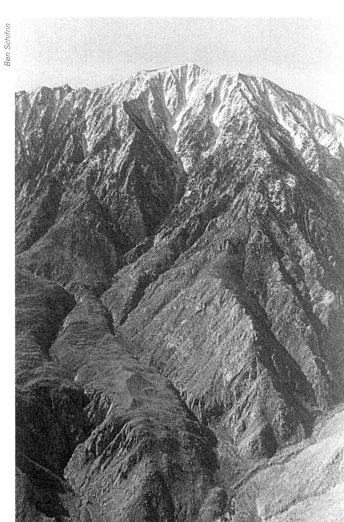

Ben Schifrin

*San Jacinto over
Snow Creek*

# Maps

*Warner Springs*
*Hot Springs Mountain*
*Bucksnort Mountain*
*Beauty Mountain*
*Anza*

*Butterfly Peak*
*Palm View Peak*
*Idyllwild*
*San Jacinto Peak*
*White Water*

# Declination
13°E

| Points on Route | S→N | Mi. Btwn. Pts. | N→S |
|---|---|---|---|
| Highway 79 southwest of Warner Springs | 0.0 | | 101.4 |
| | | 1.8 | |
| Highway 79 west of Warner Springs | 1.8 | | 99.6 |
| | | 3.4 | |
| Agua Caliente Creek ford in Section 13 | 5.2 | | 96.2 |
| | | 3.6 | |
| Lost Valley Rd. to Indian Flats Campground | 8.8 | | 92.6 |
| | | 8.9 | |
| Chihuahua Valley Road to water | 17.7 | | 83.7 |
| | | 10.8 | |
| Tule Canyon Road to Tule Spring | 27.7 | | 73.7 |
| | | 6.5 | |
| jeep road to Terwilliger | 34.2 | | 67.2 |
| | | 8.9 | |
| Pines-to-Palms Hwy. to Anza | 43.1 | | 58.3 |
| | | 6.6 | |
| Live Oak Spring Trail | 49.7 | | 51.7 |
| | | 4.1 | |
| Cedar Spring Trail | 53.8 | | 47.6 |
| | | 6.1 | |
| Apache Spring Trail | 59.9 | | 41.5 |
| | | 7.8 | |
| Tahquitz Valley Trail | 67.7 | | 33.7 |
| | | 1.9 | |
| Saddle Junction and trail to Idyllwild | 69.6 | | 31.8 |
| | | 6.2 | |
| North Fork San Jacinto River | 75.8 | | 25.6 |
| | | 5.8 | |
| Fuller Ridge Trhd. Remote Campsite | 81.6 | | 19.8 |
| | | 16.2 | |
| Snow Canyon Road | 97.8 | | 3.6 |
| | | 3.6 | |
| near Interstate 10 in San Gorgonio Pass | 101.4 | | 0.0 |

## Weather To Go

Traversing the lower, dry chaparral in the southern half of this section is most enjoyable before mid-May. Afterward, it is uncomfortably hot, with springs and creeks rapidly diminishing. The heights of the San Jacinto Mountains, however, can still contain deep snowdrifts and further snowstorms (however brief) can threaten until late May of most years. San Gorgonio Pass, at the end of this section, is uncomfortably warm except in winter.

## Supplies

Warner Springs Ranch is the *town* at the start of Section B. It is a 2500-acre, private, family resort centered around a natural hot spring. Established by John Warner in 1844 on the site of a Cupeño Native American village, the ranch became an important stop for the historic Butterfield Overland Stage. Subsequent visitors have included a large roster of presidents and Hollywood notables. Nowadays, Warner Springs Ranch has a few, simple, inexpensive rooms for hikers as well as plusher accommodations. The Warner Springs Golf Grill is a delightful place to cool off and dine. It is located just south of the gas station, which, in turn, is next to the post office. Pay phones are available. The gas station has limited snack foods. Golf and glider rides are available indulgences. This small ranch is popular, especially in springtime; hikers desiring any services would be wise to make reservations well in advance:

> Warner Springs Ranch
> Box 399
> Warner Springs, CA 92086
>
> Tel: (760) 782-4255
>
> Fax: (760) 782-4284
>
> E-mail: spa@ranchspa.com

Camping food may be mailed to Warner Springs Post Office, located 1.2 miles northeast of the start of this section on Highway 79.

The next possibility for resupply is in the mobile-home community of Terwilliger, a 4.4-mile detour from the PCT, 34.3 miles along this section's stretch. The old Valley Store in Terwilliger was a beacon for a whole generation of PCT hikers. Unfortunately it has closed. Instead, use Kamp Anza Kampground (described on page 109). The owners are very hospitable to PCT hikers and equestrians—they hold packages for thru-hikers. Send them to:

> c/o [Your Name]
> Kamp Anza Kampground
> 41560 Terwilliger Road
> Space 19
> Anza CA 92539
>
> Tel: (909) 763-4819
>
> They have a Web site, *www.jps.net/ thebear1/*, and can be contacted by e-mail at *thebear1@jps.net*.

The larger town of Anza, a 6.0-mile detour from the route 43 miles beyond the section's start, boasts a post office, stores, and restaurants.

At Saddle Junction, high in the San Jacinto Wilderness and 69.6 miles from the start of Section B, most trailers choose to descend the historic Devil's Slide Trail to Idyllwild. This restful mountain resort community has a complete range of facilities, including Nomad Ventures, a mountaineering supply shop, with a very knowledgeable staff and everything for the PCT trekker. PCT travelers are welcome at the San Jacinto Wilderness State Park's "Hike and Bike" campsite near the ranger station in Idyllwild; it's just a minute from downtown. Phone (909) 659-2607.

Ending this section in West Palm Springs Village, a tiny community without any supplies, you have a choice of supply stations. Here, about 102 miles from the start, you can hitchhike east 12.5 miles via Interstate 10 and Highway 111 to revel in the fleshpots of Palm Springs, that famous movie-star and golf-course-studded desert oasis. It offers complete facilities, including a not-to-be-missed tour for PCTers fresh from their conquest of the first major mountain range on the trail: an aerial-tram ride from Palm Springs up 6000 feet to the subalpine shoulder of San Jacinto Peak, for a lavish dinner at the viewful summit tram station!

Alternatively, hikers may elect to hitchhike west on Highway 10 from West Palm Springs Village. From the Verbenia Avenue exit you go 4.5 miles on Highway 10 to the Main Street exit of Cabazon, a small town with a post office and store. It also boasts The Wheel Inn, a good restaurant complete with life-size concrete models of a brontosaurus and a tyrannosaurus. Hadley's, a backpacker's dream market, lies 2 miles farther west on Highway 10 (Apache Trail exit), and it sells an astounding variety of dried fruits and nuts. Near Hadley's is a truly enormous outlet mall, affording the hiker with money to burn a chance to purchase the latest in hikers' couture, sports shoes, and electronic gadgetry, or refuel at some nice chain restaurants. Cabazon Ranch Outfitters, located at 50150 Esperanza Avenue, offers professional pack -animal support and guiding in the San Jacintos and San Bernardinos. Horse feed is available. Also, free of charge, are corrals, water, hot showers, camping and package holds for riders and hikers. Contact: Barbara Gronek, Box 876, Cabazon, CA 92230, or phone (909) 849-2528.

## Water

Water remains scarce in the southern reaches of Section B. Except high in the San Jacinto Wilderness, or at springs where wells have been dug for livestock, do not expect to find water away from civilization. Once you reach the cooler, higher Desert Divide, however, water becomes more plentiful. In fact, many would-be PCT thru-hikes have been ended prematurely by thigh-deep spring snows on the southern flanks of the San Jacinto Mountains. Keep a weather eye out, and be prepared for rough going.

## Permits

The San Jacinto Wilderness consists of two units—the national-forest wilderness and the state-park wilderness. If you are camping in only one of these, you need a permit only for it; if you are camping in both, you need two permits. Obtain the national-forest permit by writing Idyllwild Ranger Station, Box 518, Idyllwild, CA 92549. You can also pick one up at the station, at 25925 Village Center Drive in Idyllwild, which is open between 8 A.M. and 4:30 P.M. Monday through Friday until about June 1, and then 7 days a week through summer. Obtain the state-park permit by writing Mt. San Jacinto Wilderness State Park, Box 308, Idyllwild, CA 92549, or by going to the station at the north edge of Idyllwild on the highway to Banning between 8 and 5 o'clock 7 days a week. No dogs or fires are ever allowed within the state park.

## Special Problems

### The Chaparral

Hikers along the California PCT cannot help but become familiar with the chaparral, that community of typically chest-high, tough, wiry, calf-slashing shrubs and small trees that you meet first by the Mexican border. Draped like a green velvet blanket over most of that part of Southern California reached by ocean air, and extending from close beside the sea up to about 5000 feet, where it mingles with conifers and oaks, chaparral lines most of the PCT south of the Sierra. Chaparral surrounds Warner Springs, at the beginning of this section.

Named by early Spanish Californians, who were reminded of their "chaparro," or live-oak scrub from Mediterranean climes, the California chaparral is a unique assemblage of plants—mostly shrubs—that find this region's long, rainless summers and cooler, wet winters ideal for growth. Chamise, also known as "greasewood" because of its texture and its almost explosive flammability, is the most widespread species, but several species of ceanothus (mountain lilac, buckbrush, tobacco brush and coffee brush), plus ribbonwood, ocean spray, sumac, sagebrush, mountain mahogany, holly-leaf cherry and yerba santa also rank as major members of chaparral, depending on topographic and soil conditions.

All true chaparral plants have small, evergreen, thick, stiff leaves and many have leaves with waxy outer surfaces. The plants' roots are long, to reach deep into rocky subsoil for scarce water. Chaparral plants are suited to survive not only the protracted rainless, hot months, but also a low annual rainfall and a rapid runoff from the thin, poorly developed soils. The plants' main defense against loss of precious water is near-dormancy during the hot, dry summer spells. Almost all photosynthetic activity ceases during this time, but the stiff evergreen leaves are ready to resume photosynthesis within minutes of a rainfall, unlike those plants which lose their leaves or wilt in the face of heat. The small size of the leaves themselves, with the addition of a waxy coat or a hairy insulating cover, plus the presence of relatively few evaporative stomata, greatly reduces water losses.

Not only can chaparral plants vie successfully for, and conserve, scant water resources, but they also win out by thriving in the face of fire. All of the most widespread species are adapted to reproduce well in the aftermath of fast-moving range fires that are a hallmark of Southern California wildlands. In fact, fires actually benefit these species, and most of them contain highly flammable volatile oils, which pro-

mote fires. Before the advent of white people, wildfires burned the Southern California chaparral every 5 to 8 years! Not only does fire exterminate encroaching species, but it returns valuable nitrogen to the soil, thus promoting growth. Some of the species, like scrub oak and ceanothus, need fire to weaken their seeds' coatings to allow germination. Most of the other chaparral plants circumvent the ravages of fire by resprouting—in as little as 10 days—from tough root crowns or by putting out so many seeds that at least some will survive any fire. Chaparral is also unusual in that it succeeds itself right after a fire, unlike other plant communities, such as pine forests, which after a major fire pass through one or more vegetational stages before returning to the final, climax stage.

# THE ROUTE

**Before leaving Warner Springs, northbound hikers must be sure to stock up on water.** The next certain source along the route, barring the seasonal flow of Agua Caliente Creek (reached in 5.2 miles), is Tule Spring, a long, usually hot, 27.7-mile trek away.

Pedestrians can start north on Section B's PCT by simply ducking under Highway 79 via Cañada Verde's streambed, but equestrians must climb through the gate onto the highway shoulder. Then they should follow the highway northeast 200 yards to the entrance to Warner Union School. Across the street from this entrance, a short dirt road along a fence heads left, northwest, 100 yards to a short spur trail that turns south back to Cañada Verde's wash and to the PCT. Your trail departs west away from the wash, quickly crosses a jeep road, and curves gently down into spring-wildflower meadows. Well marked by posts and having a refreshingly well-defined tread, the PCT soon recrosses the jeep road (2960-0.7).

**See Map B1**

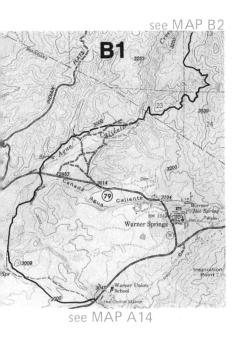

see MAP B2

**B1**

see MAP A14

Next your trail skirts the flanks of low knob 3009, then turns north across sandy flats speckled with mature canyon live oaks to cross the usually dry bed of Agua Caliente Creek (2910-0.6). In just a minute or two, your deep-sand trail recrosses the creek to its east bank and then climbs east a few yards into a cozy oak grove and to a privately operated campground (2925-0.2), which is closed to public use. Here the PCT momentarily joins the dirt road that gives access to the campground's sites, and then it turns northward before branching left to cross another usually dry streambed in Cañada Agua Caliente. Moments later, the PCT passes under Highway 79 (2930-0.3) via a concrete bridge, while simultaneously crossing Agua Caliente Creek, which often flows lazily here.

**Water access:** Warner Springs Post Office and sure water can be found 1.3 miles east along Highway 79.

North of the highway the PCT leaves the western margin of Agua Caliente Creek's sandy bed just beyond a sandbag-reinforced slope. The trail clambers up to pass through a gate, then, ignoring a right-branching path back down to the stream, climbs from a fringe of trees onto a nearly level alluvial terrace covered with sagebrush and dotted with massive live oaks. Follow the terrace northeast, up-canyon, staying some 30 feet above Agua Caliente Creek, which usually flows in this vicinity, if only as a trickle. The PCT dips momentarily in a north-trending wash (ignore a prominent trail down to the creek), then shortly merges with a wider path (an old jeep road) (2960-0.6) that continues eastward, up-canyon, well-marked by PCT posts. A few minutes' walk leads to a junction (2965-0.2) with a dirt road that crosses from the southwest. Beyond this junction the trail, indicated by PCT posts, continues ahead, now paralleling the aforementioned road to its right, and coming slowly closer to the cut banks of Agua Caliente Creek. In a short while, the trail strikes the dirt road at its end, where a large campsite (2975-0.3) is found.

This pleasant, sunny spot has a number of picnic tables and metal fireplaces, a pair of hooks for hanging packs out of the reach of squirrels and raccoons, and an outhouse, all just a few feet from the cool, trickling stream.

The trail resumes at the upstream end of the camp, and descends momentarily to cross via rocks 15-foot-wide Agua Caliente Creek, here burbling among baccharis shrubs, sycamores and cottonwoods. Across the stream, the route climbs north and east away from the creek.

Chia, white forget-me-not and beavertail cacti line the moderate ascent across the Cleveland National Forest border to a terrace, along which the sandy path winds north through ribbonwood chaparral. Then you soon descend to cross Agua Caliente

**See Maps B1, B2**

Creek (3195-2.3), where tall grasses, squaw brush, brodiaea and forget-me-nots grow below screening oaks, sycamores and willows in the narrow, usually watered canyon—a refuge for mourning doves and horned lizards. Particularly in winter and spring, ticks also inhabit the grasses and shrubs, and travelers should check their legs often. You cross Agua Caliente Creek four more times in the next mile, alternating shady, cool creekside walking with hot, yucca-dotted Paleozoic Julian schist hillsides. Unfortunately, heavy rains in Spring 1993 washed out the trail where it made

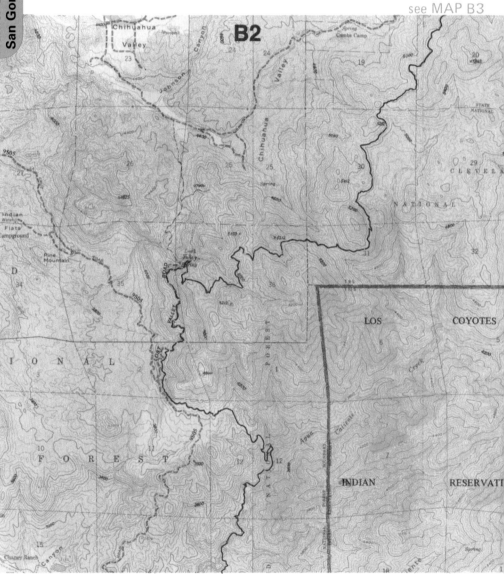

see MAP B3

see MAP B1

**See Map B2**

each crossing of Agua Caliente Creek. This does not confuse the hiker so much as it makes traversing the canyon a chore. The USFS plans to rebuild the trail higher on the slope. Camping possibilities are frequent. A final, shaded traverse north of the seasonal stream leads to a switchback (3520-1.5) in a side canyon, after which the moderately ascending route winds northwest in chaparral laced with deer brush and white sage. Soon the grade eases to contour west, then north, below Peak 4844 and above Indian Flats Road. Here the trail affords good views southwest across Warner Valley to Lake Henshaw, a large sag pond on the Elsinore Fault, and northwest to weathered tonalite outcrops near Indian Flats.

Continuing north, the PCT turns right onto poor Lost Valley Road and ascends it to reach a spur road (4450-1.1).

**Water access:** From here, Lost Valley Road descends north 0.2 mile to reach Lost Valley Spring. The spring has been rehabilitated, and has flow well into all but the driest summers. Small campsites are available, but of poor quality.

From this junction, the PCT climbs northeast above the spring along a 0.3-mile spur—an overgrown jeep track—to reach a continuation of trail tread where the spur ends in a ravine. You ascend briskly to the south to find excellent views back over boulder-dotted Indian Flats and south over Valle de San Jose. Soon the way swings eastward on a gentle, sandy ascent through chaparral and past scattered Coulter pines. After climbing over three low, fire-scarred ridges, you drop moderately east to a saddle (4945-3.2) that lies along the northwest-trending Hot Springs Fault. To the southeast, Hot Springs Mountain's lookout tower rises above tree-lined Agua Caliente Creek.

The PCT ascends east a bit, then turns north to undulate through dry brushland— often sparingly shaded by oaks and Coulter

pines—to the east of a boulder-castellated ridge. After about 2 miles from the saddle you pass into Anza-Borrego Desert State Park, then cross a gap to the sunnier west slopes of the ridgeline. With vistas west over Chihuahua Valley, you contour generally north to yet another gap, then descend quickly east, cross a ravine, and traverse northwest to strike nearby Chihuahua Valley Road (5050-4.6), which drops west into Chihuahua Valley.

**Water access:** Detour here for water: walk east 0.2 mile to a left-branching 0.1-mile dirt spur that descends to a private home. A 20-foot-high, silver water tank with a valve at its base is the source. A sign on the tank in 1999 gave permission from its owners to take some water without first asking at the house, below. Be sure to close the valve!

Directly across the dirt road the PCT starts a sustained, moderate ascent along Bucksnort Mountain's east slopes. The climb ends at the east shoulder of Combs Peak (5595-1.9), where a grove of Coulter pines, now sadly burned, outstanding vistas, and the first level spot for miles combine to make a nice, if waterless, campsite.

The 180° panorama here encompasses a sizable chunk of Southern California real estate. To the north, distant, seasonally snow-capped San Gorgonio Peak peers over the west shoulder of nearer, sometimes snowy San Jacinto Peak. Closer in the north, Thomas Mountain stands behind sprawling Anza and Terwilliger valleys. The rocky spine descending right (southeast) from San Jacinto Peak is the PCT-traversed Desert Divide. To the east-northeast, the dry summits of the Santa Rosa Mountains loom above desert-floored Coyote Canyon, while you spy to the east the vast Salton Sea beyond Anza-Borrego Desert

**See Maps B2, B3**

State Park. The park and the town of Anza to the north both commemorate Captain Juan Bautista de Anza, who in 1774 rejoiced upon entering the valley now bearing his name. He had struggled through the Borrego Desert and Coyote Canyon with a couple dozen men—mostly soldiers—while scouting a route from Sonora, Mexico, to San Francisco. He returned a year later, leading more than 200 settlers and many cattle.

Continuing on, the northbound PCT contours across the steep east face of Bucksnort Mountain, then begins to descend in earnest, on rocky, sandy tread in low chaparral. You eventually cross a usually dry creekbed at the head of Tule Canyon (4710-2.4), just south of where some level spots offer waterless camping. From here your way becomes less steep and rolls northward into a tall brushland dominated by ribbonwood and chamise. The PCT rounds

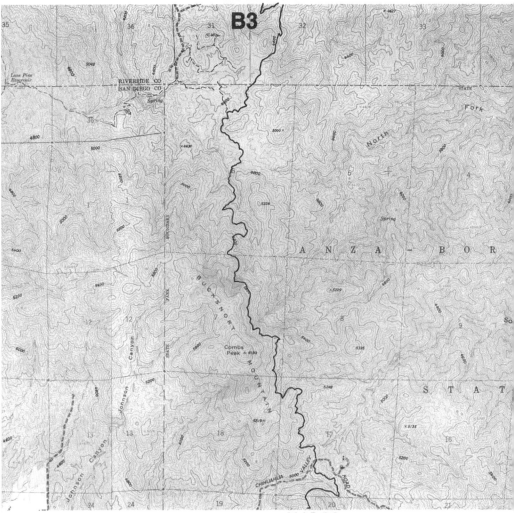

see MAP B4

see MAP B2

**See Maps B3, B4**

the canyon's eastern slopes, drops easily to a broad saddle, then climbs gently north to gain the west end of a low ridge. A few minutes' gentle downhill walk leads to a trail junction (4675-0.9). The north-descending old, temporary-PCT route heads left for 0.3 mile before deadending.

You take the newer, 1987-vintage tread, which first contours east and then drops moderately across the nearby Riverside County line on a northward tack. After traversing east-facing slopes, the PCT descends across to the west side of a small saddle, next descends southwest, and then soon levels to momentarily strike a fair dirt road (4110-2.3) at the Anza-Borrego Desert State Park boundary. Northwest across it the path resumes, making an easy but shadeless descent through Section 30. After an unnecessary switchback the way bends north, still descending.

Some hikers may wonder about the logic of the PCT's route between the county line and the Pines-to-Palms Highway. In order to avoid conflicts with local landowners, the PCT is forced to traverse a checkerboard of public-land parcels. Hence the PCT crosses each section near one of its corners to essentially avoid treading on private property.

Ponder this situation as you continue north, past a white-pipe post marking a section's corner. You then drop for a moment to a shallow, hop-across ford of Tule Canyon Creek (3590-2.1). Water usually flows here, sometimes merely at a trickle, for most of the year. It is more reliable downstream at Tule Spring. Due to land-ownership constraints the PCT is forced to climb very steeply up the sandy hillside north of Tule Canyon Creek. Afterward it side-hills gently northeast, down-canyon, soon to cross good Tule Canyon Road (3640-0.4).

**Water and resupply access:** Just ¼ mile southeast down this dirt road is year-round Tule Spring, the only reliable waterhole on the PCT for miles. Thanks to the work of the PCTA and CDF, water is now easily available from a metal-handled spigot found 50 feet below the 10,000-gallon water tank, on the edge of Tule Canyon creek's high cut bank. Should the water tank or spigot not be operational for some reason, check in the high grass to the left of the tank—a seep is always present, even during the late 1980s' drought years. Floods in Spring 1993 caused destruction of most of the lovely cottonwoods and flat areas hereabouts, but camping is still possible. In the morning quiet, one may see desert bighorn sheep watering here, having escaped the scorching heat of the Borrego Sink. Everyone should fill water bottles here. Northbound hikers have 22.0 usually hot miles until the short detour to Tunnel Spring, on the Desert Divide, while southbound hikers have an even hotter 22.5 miles to Agua Caliente Creek in Section 13.

One may also choose to resupply at Terwilliger or Anza from Tule Springs. Ascend Tule Canyon Road past the PCT, reaching a locked gate 0.3 mile west of the trail, at the boundary of Anza-Borrego Desert State Park. Continue up the sandy, rutted road, which steadily improves, past a home or two to a junction with larger dirt Terwilliger Road (4045-2.5), where the road is signed, "Tule Canyon Truck Trail". Turn right, north, and follow this busier way past numerous smaller junctions and a handful of homes to a T-junction with larger dirt Ramsay Road (3921-1.3). Now swing right, east, to the paved continuation of Terwilliger Road (3920-0.2). Swing left, again due north, on the shoulder of Terwilliger Road to paved Bailey Road (3859-0.2). Kamp Anza Kampground (3990-1.6) is farther north on Terwilliger Road. Find the town of Anza (3920-5.1) beyond Kamp Anza as described in more detail in the next "water & supply access" paragraph.

Return to the PCT's northward continuation on a sandy, hillside traverse, undulating through rocky ravines. It overlooks the environs of Tule Spring, then bends northeast. After dipping to a broad valley, the trail climbs to a small pass with a

self-replenishing wildfowl "guzzler" water tank, then drops on sandy, indistinct tread to nearby Coyote Canyon Road (3500-2.9). Across it you continue down a ravine to a single switchback leading to the pleasant grassy floor of Nance Canyon. Step across its seasonal creeklet (3350-0.5) to find some small flat spots that offer potential dry camping. Ignore a spur trail going right, downstream, after crossing the creek. Instead, go left, upstream. Beyond, a mod-

see MAP B5            see MAP B5

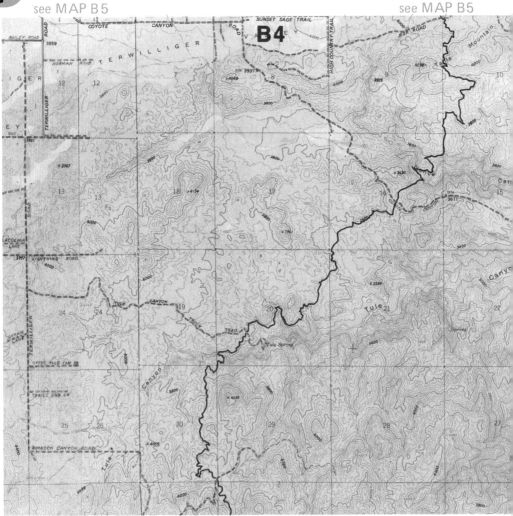

see MAP B3

erate grind leads up around a low knob, then across a rugged bluff. The trail was unnecessarily routed here, at the expense of much dynamite and at least one badly injured worker. This route offers panoramas south and east over Anza-Borrego Desert State Park's wild, northern canyons, which are visible through a haze of heat waves and salt particles from the Salton Sea. Continue the ascent, making two small switchbacks and passing a faint use-trail through a chain link fence to reach a chamise-covered gap (4185-2.4) on the south end of Table Mountain. Now you wind north and descend gently to a narrow, very sandy jeep road (4075-0.7). Table Mountain Truck Trail is now obscured by a wider dirt road, cut in 2001 to access new homes. The PCT passes the large Anza Hiker Oasis' water cache (reliable through the normal spring season) just before striking a swing-gate in a barbed-wire fence. A few feet later, the trail reaches old Table Mountain Truck Trail, followed left or west a few feet to the new, wider Table Mountain Truck Trail. On it, turn back right, north, 15 yards to the obscure resumption of PCT tread, branching left, northwest, downhill of a 10-foot plastic post.

**Water & resupply access:** This jeep road is so important that it leads out to Terwilliger and its Hikers' Oasis, and on to Anza—both logical resupply sites. To reach Terwilliger, turn left on the new, wider Table Mountain Truck Trail, following it due south, up to a junction with signed dirt Eagle Nest Court (4165-0.4). There is a water trough at this junction, but it is usually dry, except after rain. Head right, west, undulating down across a hillside on Table Mountain Truck Trail, passing south-branching dirt Old Cattle Trail in 0.4 mile, and then a more-obscure merger with the old Table Mountain Truck Trail in another 0.5 mile. A brief westward ascent, 0.1 mile, leads to a good dirt road, signed HIGH COUNTRY TRAILS.

Turn right on it, and walk north ¼ mile easily up to a broad road, Sunset Sage Trail, branching left, west. Take this dirt road ¾ mile down past numerous north-branching dirt roads and several homes to its end at Yucca Valley Road (3925-2.1). Turn left and follow this dirt road briefly south to a four-way junction. Here Coyote Canyon Road heads south and west. Follow this road right, west, across the arid, level grassland, finally making a small dogleg before ending at paved Terwilliger Road (3870-1.8).

On Terwilliger Road, you can walk north to Kamp Anza Kampground (3990-1.3), (phones, groceries, laundry, hot showers and campsites available at reasonable cost). On 41790A Gassner Road, just behind Kamp Anza to its east, is The Bear's PCT Hikers' Oasis, hosted by two delightful trail angels, The Bear and Ziggy. The Oasis has a complete range of services for hikers in the spring season (telephone, computer and internet access). The Bear offers shuttling throughout the Anza Valley and San Jacintos to trailheads, post offices or shopping and has on-site water, toilets, camping and minor first aid. Hikers intent on an Anza resupply can continue north past the trailer park to Wellman Road (4245-1.5). Take it west to Kirby Road (3935-1.0), then Kirby north to Cahuilla Road (Highway 371) (3970-1.0-8.7). Turn left, west, and head to the small town of Anza (3920-1.6-10.3), with a post office, grocery stores, restaurants and a laundromat.

If you don't want to backtrack from Anza to the PCT at the far eastern part of Terwilliger Valley, walk east back along Cahuilla Road, passing Kirby Road and later crossing a 4855-foot summit just before reaching a junction with Pines-to-Palms Highway 74 (4790-6.0). Then go southeast on this highway, which starts southeast and then climbs gently through a grassy valley to reach the PCT just short of a dirt parking turnout (4919-1.0-17.3).

**See Maps B4, B5**

From the obscure jeep-road junction at the far eastern part of Terwilliger Valley, the PCT ascends indistinctly northwest for a moment before good tread resumes. It leads moderately and persistently uphill, in an ascending traverse along the granitic, boulder-strewn southwestern flanks of Table Mountain. You gain excellent views over Terwilliger Valley and south to your PCT's route along Bucksnort Mountain. On a breezy day this stretch is quite enjoyable, particularly in spring when it's likely to be flanked by clusters of California poppy, purple chia, baby-blue-eyes, and feathery

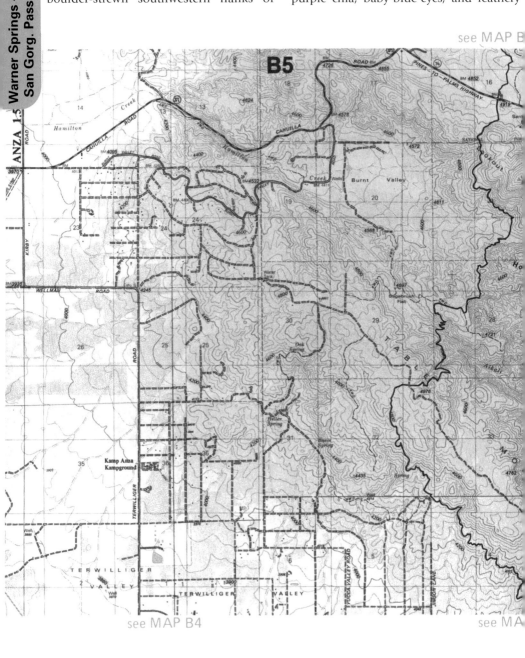

**See Map B5**

green ribbonwood shrubs among white boulders. At one point, you pass a side trail that leads south to a dirt road serving some hillside homes. Beyond, your climb continues, eventually rising to top Table Mountain's shoulder. You cross a dirt road (4910-3.9) at a point just northwest of the long mountain's highest point.

The route drops and leads into a narrow ravine, switchbacks once to cross it, then descends to the bottom of the dry head of Alkali Wash (4540-1.2). A steep, rocky and sometimes hot quintet of switchbacks accomplish the ensuing ascent of the far slope. They lead to a chaparral ridge, where your trail swings east over a low saddle into a grassy flat. Now the path winds north, right along the raw, precipitous lip of Horse Canyon.

Uplifting of the area with each passing earthquake is making the course of Horse Canyon's stream steeper. It is aggressively eroding into the red and white strata of the surrounding uplands,. resulting in a badland of tortuous ravines and ridgelets, stretching east to Vandeventer Flat, at the foot of Toro Peak. This erosive process will result in a drainage rearrangement in Burnt Valley, to your northwest, as Horse Canyon's stream advances into that valley.

Walk along a narrow divide, enjoy views, then push on across the flanks of Lookout Mountain. Eventually the trail finds a low pass (5070-3.3) on the peak's northwestern shoulder, and you have a delightful panorama north over the San Jacinto Mountains. In the left-most distance the rounded form of lofty San Jacinto Peak reigns, usually with a regal coat of snow in spring. Leaving the gap you descend into San Bernardino National Forest. The trail levels and then turns north across a sandy, sagebrush-matted valley to quickly strike 2-lane Pines-to-Palms Highway 74

(4919-0.5) at a point just west of Santa Rosa Summit.

**Water access:** Water may be obtained by detouring left, northwest, for 1.0 mile to a restaurant at the junction of Highway 74 and Cahuilla Road (Highway 371). For supplies, one could walk 6.0 miles farther west on Highway 371 to Anza.

Across Pines-to-Palms Highway 74, you skirt a dirt trailhead parking area and ascend through a recently burned brushland. A mileage sign and a 6-foot stone monument diagram the PCT's route through the San Jacintos and commemorate the death of a trail worker. Beyond, you walk north to a ridgetop, then switchback once down its north side, soon engaged in a sandy, fitful ascent into and out of numerous small ravines and around picturesque blocky cliffs of crumbling granite. You pass close along the western face of a low ridge, then descend short switchbacks to hop across the usually dry creek (5040-3.7) that drains Penrod Canyon.

Here, a comfortable waterless camp could be made under Coulter pines and live oaks.

The track winds up-canyon, crossing the streambed twice more then climbs to sunnier chaparral for a contour of the canyon's eastern slopes. The PCT eventually strikes Road 6S01A (5700-2.0), ascending from the west to reach an open-pit limestone quarry just above your trail. Your way proceeds directly across the road; resume the ascent, now steeper, along Penrod Canyon's east wall. Thomas Mountain and Bucksnort Mountain are visible on this stretch, just before you swing east around a nose to abruptly encounter marble bedrock. The first leg of the PCT's climb into the San Jacinto Mountains ends soon, as

**See Maps B5, B6**

you first go through a stock gate, then pass southeast-traversing Trail 3E15 to Bull Canyon, and in 50 yards top out at a saddle on the Desert Divide (5950-0.9). Here are junctions with Live Oak Trail 4E03, right,

and the Tunnel Spring Trail, left. Here, too, you reach the boundary with the brand-new Santa Rosa and San Jacinto Mountains National Monument, whose western edge is defined by the crest of the Desert Divide.

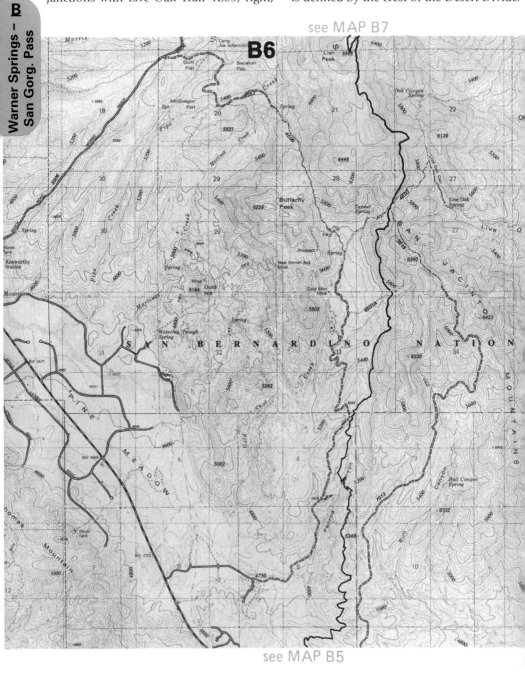

see MAP B7

see MAP B5

**See Map B6**

You will pop into and out of this new reserve, until you finally descend into San Gorgonio Pass, at the end of Section B.

**Water access:** Travelers low on water are advised to go to Live Oak Spring, if they also plan camping or lunch, but to Tunnel Spring—half the distance—for emergency water only. Live Oak Spring is reached by a sunny 1-mile, well-graded path that descends east from the saddle, eventually finding two nice campsites under an enormous gold-cup oak and box elders. It has much better camping than Tunnel Spring, and delightful clean water in a circular concrete trough.

The Tunnel Spring Trail descends southwest from the PCT atop the gap. Steep, rocky tread leads down 0.3 mile to where the trail moderates in a grove of oaks and four tall Coulter pines, which have scattered their huge, clawed cones on the ground. Now look right, north, to a shallow streambed and a faint trail along a black PVC pipe. This goes up a few yards to the metal cattle trough at Tunnel Spring, shaded by box elders. Poor camping is the best that can be found nearby.

Resuming your northbound trek, you turn north along the east face of the Desert Divide. Shady interior live oaks and Coulter pines alternate with xeric chaparral areas (look for shaggy Mojave yuccas) as the trail ascends gently across Julian schist to the east slopes of Lion Peak. Expect to cross a few bulldozed jeep roads on this traverse—the area south of Lion Peak is private property, used for cattle range. You get sporadic vistas down Oak Canyon to subdivided upper Palm Canyon, then a rough switchback leads to the ridgetop north of Lion Peak. For the next 2 miles the route remains on or near the divide, traversing gneiss, schist, quartzite and marble bedrock and skirting past low chaparral laced with rabbitbrush and cacti. Little Desert Peak

(6883') offers panoramas east and north to the Coachella Valley and Palm Springs, and west to coniferous Thomas Mountain and pastoral Garner Valley. Moments later, a short descent ends at a saddle where you cross the Cedar Spring Trail 4E17 (6780-4.1).

**Water access:** Most hikers ignore the southern branch of this good trail, which switchbacks southwest to Morris Ranch Road. Instead, head north a short mile down to delightfully shaded flats and clear water at Cedar Spring Camp (6330')—the only permanent water along the southern Desert Divide. This is your best choice for a first night's camp in the San Jacintos. The next morning, simply retrace your steps to the PCT. Old trails that could reconnect hikers with the PCT via Lion Spring or Garnet Ridge have fallen into disrepair after brushfires in the 1980s, and are not recommended. Be sure to carry a full load of water away from Cedar Spring—the day's ridgetop walk is hot, sunny, and entirely waterless.

**Alternate route:** In the face of high snowpack or early-spring snowstorms on the Desert Divide, northbound hikers should consider leaving the PCT via the Cedar Spring Trail, exiting south to the Pines-to-Palms Highway, then going north to Idyllwild and Cabazon. The Tunnel Spring Trail down to Penrod Canyon may also be used for the same purpose. In the face of severe storms, another option would be to go east on the Pines-to-Palms Highway to Palm Springs, and thence northwest to White Water.

The route, however, steeply ascends the ridgecrest, then it briefly descends to another saddle (6945-0.6). Continuing northwest, you soon pass Trail 4E04 (7080-

**See Maps B6, B7**

see MAP B9

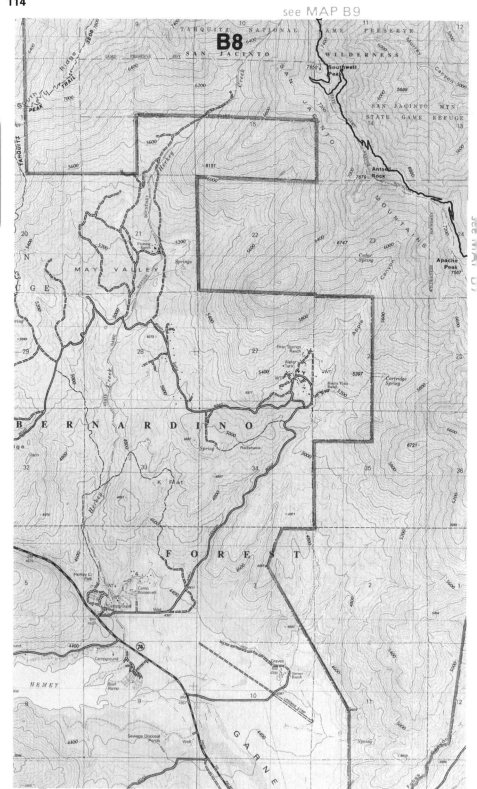

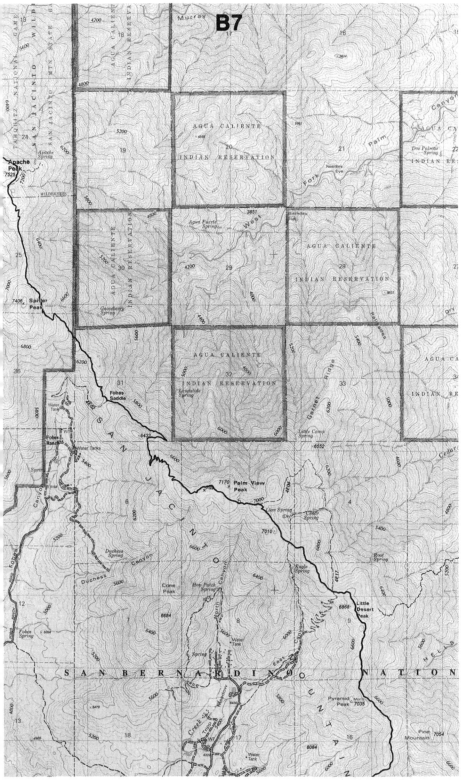

**B7**

see MAP B6

0.5), which starts east from near Palm View Peak, then drops north toward Garnet Ridge. Then, past a 7123-foot summit, you descend, often steeply, on a rocky, nebulous tread back into a cooler environment of white firs growing at the head of the spectacular West Fork Palm Canyon. Presently the route emerges on brushy Fobes Saddle and meets Fobes Ranch Trail 4E02 (5990-2.4), which descends west.

The PCT north from this saddle ascends steeply to the upper slopes of Spitler Peak, where one encounters a charred forest of black oak, white fir, incense-cedar and Jeffrey pine, gloomy mementos of a massive 1980 blaze that blackened almost the entire upper West Fork Palm Canyon and Murray and Andreas canyons. One will find evidence of it all the way to Red Tahquitz. Along your climb you enter San Jacinto Wilderness and then beyond some very steep pitches the PCT levels to wind around to the north of Spitler Peak. It then descends just east of the rocky spine that forms the ridge between Spitler and Apache peaks. Gaining this knife-edge col, where the PCT was widened by fire fighters to form a fuelbreak, the trail wastes no time in attacking the next objective: Apache Peak. Steep rocky-sandy tread leads up its southern slopes to emerge on a black, burned summit plateau.

**Water access:** Here you find a sign marking the Apache Spring Trail (7430-2.6), which descends steeply east ½ mile to poor camps at burned-over but viewful, flowing Apache Spring. From your junction too, a short use trail ascends northwest to the viewful, if ugly, summit of Apache Peak.

The PCT now begins to descend gently along the eastern flanks of Apache Peak, passing through a ghost forest of immense, burned manzanitas. After a useless 0.2-mile-long switchback you reach a fine overlook of the northern Coachella Valley and of Joshua Tree National Park, which lies well beyond the valley in the Little San Bernardino Mountains. A well-constructed stretch next leads west along a cliff face to a gap, where one can dry-camp, at the head of Apple Canyon. To circumvent the granitic ramparts of Antsell Rock, the PCT's next leg follows a dynamited path under its sweeping northeast slopes, which are thankfully shaded by conifers spared from the 1980 fire. This same shade, however, often creates dangerously icy conditions for springtime PCT thru-hikers—use caution and an ice axe! Once north of Antsell Rock's major buttresses, you take switchbacks for a 400-foot elevation gain to reach the San Jacinto's crest at a pleasantly montane gap (7200-2.9). Big-cone spruce, close relative of Douglas-fir, plus white fir and mountain mahogany provide pleasant cover as the often-dynamited path ascends another 400 feet, first on the east and then on the southwest slopes of South Peak. Notice Lake Hemet, lying just east of the active Thomas Mountain Fault, at the head of Garner Valley, to your southwest.

North of South Peak the rocky PCT is dynamited to traverse under precipitous granitic gendarmes, and the ascending hiker can gaze northwest to Tahquitz Peak and north to Red Tahquitz, or east down rugged Murray Canyon. The ascent ends (8380-3.4) above Andreas Canyon's deep gorge, where your route turns west to descend gently on duff and sand and eventually to cross South Fork Tahquitz Creek in a forest, and then join, moments later, the Little Tahquitz Trail (8075-1.5).

**Water access:** This trail descends north ⅓ mile to good camps and water in Little Tahquitz Valley, and then traverses to Tahquitz and Skunk Cabbage meadows.

From your junction the PCT climbs southwest through dense groves of lodgepole pines to manzanitas and western

**See Maps B7, B8, B9**

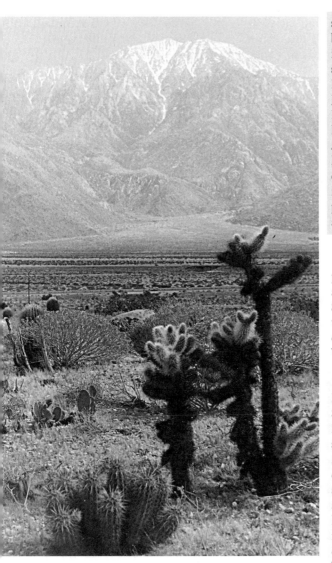

B
Warner Springs –
San Gorg. Pass

San Jacinto Peak from San Gorgonio Pass

such as Strawberry Valley below, are eroding back into the high, rolling landscape that lies between Red Tahquitz and San Jacinto Peak. Tahquitz Peak commemorates a legendary Cahuilla Native American demon who lived hereabouts, dining on unsuspecting Indian maidens and, when displeased, giving the weather a turn for the worse.

Those who need to press on will turn north and ease down the PCT to Saddle Junction (8100-1.3), the crossroads for an array of trails into the San Jacinto Wilderness.

**Resupply access:** From the saddle Devils Slide Trail 3E05 descends 2.5 miles west past three springs to Fern Valley Road 5S22. The mountain-resort community of Idyllwild— a good place to resupply and take a layover day— lies 2 miles down this road. Also leaving the saddle are two more trails, the Willow Creek Trail branching northeast to Long Valley, and the Caramba Trail heading southeast, back to Tahquitz Valley.

of decomposed granite. Presently you come to a junction with the Tahquitz Peak Trail 3E08 (8570-0.6), which offers a side trip ½ mile up to the peak's airy summit lookout.

**Side route:** This trip is well worthwhile, for from the 8846-foot summit you can get an idea of how steep canyons,

The PCT continues north, soon switchbacking out of the forest to slopes that offer excellent over-the-shoulder vistas toward Tahquitz (Lily) Rock, a magnet for Southern California rock climbers. Almost 1000 feet higher than Saddle Junction, the PCT levels

**See Map B9**

to turn left from a junction with the Wellmans Cienaga Trail (9030-1.8), just within the confines of Mount San Jacinto State Park.

    Please note that all camping within the state park must be in designated sites only. Along the PCT there is only one approved campsite: Strawberry Junction Trail Camp. USFS Wilderness Permits are *not* valid for camping in the state park; get a separate camping permit for a specific date, to use these campsites. No dogs or fires are ever allowed within the state park.

**Side route:** This trail arcs about 2 miles northeast to Round Valley Trail Camp and beyond to 10,804-foot San Jacinto Peak, a recommended side trip.

    From the junction the PCT immediately leaves the state park and descends on a generally westward bearing above Strawberry Valley's steep headwall to Strawberry Cienaga (8560-0.9), a trickling sphagnum-softened freshet and a lunch stop with a great view. "Cienaga" is a Spanish word, often seen in Southern California, meaning "swamp" or "marsh." Further descent leads to a forested junction with Deer Springs Trail 3E17 (8070-1.4), formerly known as the San Jacinto Peak Trail and described that way on Map B9. Just before this junction, Strawberry Junction Trail Camp is found on a small ridge south of the trail, a pleasant and viewful, but waterless camp. There may be some trickles of water until midsummer in heads of canyons nearby.

**Side route:** As an alternative to the Devils Slide Trail, one can use the Deer Springs Trail to descend 4.3 miles to Highway 243, just ½ mile west of downtown Idyllwild. Multiple dry flats in open pines and firs 2–3 minutes below the

PCT's junction with the Deer Springs Trail could also offer dry camping.

    Now out of the Federal wilderness and back in Mount San Jacinto State Park, the PCT turns north to ascend Marion Mountain's pleasant mixed-conifer slopes, and eventually passes two closely spaced trail junctions.

**Side route:** The first, the Marion Mountain Trail, descends west-southwest to the environs of Marion Mountain and Fern Basin campgrounds. The second, the Seven Pines Trail, descends generally northwest, then west to a saddle, from which Road 4S02 switchbacks almost 2 miles down to Dark Canyon Campground.

    Soon after the second lateral your trail heads heads up along a marshy dank creek: the reliable North Fork San Jacinto River, which you cross (8830-2.1), below Deer Springs. This used to be a campsite, but is now closed to allow revegetation. Before leaving, hikers should restock their water bottles, since the next water along the route is from Snow Creek, at the northern base of the San Jacinto Mountains, a punishing 25-mile descent away.

    A minute beyond the infant San Jacinto River, you climb to a nearby junction with the San Jacinto Peak Trail (aka the Deer Springs Trail), which is the return route of the recommended side trip to the peak's summit. From the junction you switchback down to Fuller Ridge (8725-1.9), a rocky, white-fir-covered spine separating the San Jacinto and San Gorgonio river drainages.

    Here the northbound trekker gets his first good view of the San Bernardino Mountains' 11,499-foot San Gorgonio Peak, to the north, which is Southern

**See Maps B9, B10**

California's highest point. Separating that range from ours is San Gorgonio Pass, 7000 feet below you, lying between the Banning Fault and other branches of the great San Andreas Fault (also known as the San Andreas Rift Zone).

The PCT's route along Fuller Ridge is a tortuous one, composed for the most part of miniature switchbacks, alternately descending and climbing, which wind under small gendarmes and around wind-beaten conifers. It can also be as treacherous as it is tortuous, when shaded, early spring snow patches are icy hard. Poles or an ice axe are often required for safe footing. In a little over 2 miles, though, the route takes to north-facing slopes, and, exchanging state wilderness for a brief stint in the Federal wilderness, it gently descends to a small dirt-road parking circle at Fuller

Ridge Trailhead Remote Campsite (7750-3.9). Pleasant but waterless, the sites lie in open stands of ponderosa pine and white fir. The PCT, marked by a post, resumes on the west side of the road loop, heading due north past a site. It rounds northwest above, then drops to cross, well-used Black Mountain Road 4S01 (7670-0.2).

**Water access:** Those low on water may opt to follow this road left, descending 1.3 miles to Black Mountain Group Campground.

The trail leaves the road on a gentle-to-moderate descent north along a ridge clothed in an open stand of mixed conifers. You switchback down three times across the nose of the ridge separating Snow Creek from chaparral-decked Brown Creek.

see MAP B10

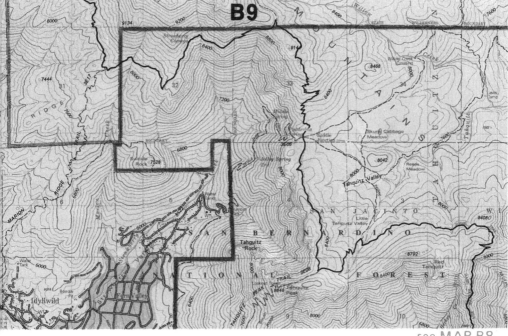

see MAP B8

**See Maps B9, B10**

**B** Warner Springs – San Gorg. Pass

**B10**

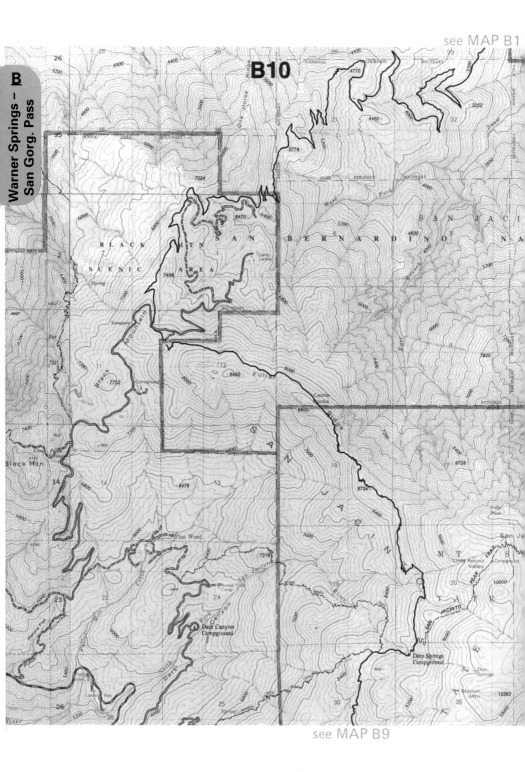

More-open conditions on the west side of the ridge allow for sweeping vistas: hulking San Gorgonio Peak looms to the north, above the desert pass that bears its name, while, stretching to the northwest, the San Bernardino and San Gabriel valleys, flanked by the lofty summits of the San Gabriel Mountains, extend toward the Los Angeles basin. On a clear day in winter or spring, snow-flecked Mount San Antonio (Mount Baldy) and Mount Wilson are both visible in that range.

You re-enter San Jacinto Wilderness and presently your sandy, lupine- and penstemon-lined path meets a switchback in a dirt road (6860-1.9), which winds eastward into a shallow basin. Marked by large ducks the trail leaves the northwest side of the open gap containing the road, but soon your route turns south to descend alongside and just below that road. After a bit your course veers from the road and winds east down dry washes and under the shade of low scrub oaks to a narrow gap (6390-1.3) in a sawblade ridge of granodiorite needles. Four long switchbacks descend the east face of this prominent ridge, depositing us in noticeably more xeric environs.

Initially, Coulter pines replace other montane conifers, and then, as the way arcs north in continual descent, you enter a true chaparral: yerba santa, buckwheat, holly-leaf cherry, scrub oak, manzanita and yucca supply the sparse ground cover, while scarlet gilia and yellow blazing star add spring color. Unlike chaparral communities moistened by maritime air, the desert-facing slopes here force these species to contend with much more extreme drought conditions. As a result, many more of the plants growing here are annuals, which avoid drought by lying dormant as seed, while others, such as yerba santa, wilt and drop their soft leaves to prevent water loss during sustained dry periods.

A continued moderate downgrade and another set of long switchbacks soon allow you to inspect the awesome, avalanche-raw, 9600-foot north escarpment of San Jacinto Peak, which rises above the cascades of Snow Creek.

To your northeast the confused alluvial terrain beyond San Gorgonio Pass attests to recent activity along the San Andreas Fault. Beyond, suburban Desert Hot Springs shimmers in the Coachella Valley heat, backdropped by the Little San Bernardino Mountains.

Inexorably, your descent continues at a moderate grade, presently switchbacking in broad sweeps across a dry ravine on slopes north of West Fork Snow Creek. After striking a small saddle (3200-8.6) just west of knob 3252, the trail, now taking an overly gentle grade, swings north, then northwest down a boulder-studded hillside. You note the small village of Snow Creek lying below you at the mountain's base before your way makes three small switchbacks and then heads back southeast toward Snow Canyon. After winding your way through a veritable forest of 20-30-foot high orange, granitic boulders, you negotiate a final set of switchbacks before dropping to cross a dry creekbed on the western edge of Snow Canyon. Soon after, you strike narrow, paved Snow Canyon Road (1725-4.2).

**Water access:** A 3-foot-tall concrete water fountain stands at the trail junction. This permanent water source is a welcome respite after the usually baking-hot descent.

**See Maps B10, B11**

Snow Canyon is both a game refuge and a water supply for Palm Springs, so camping here is not allowed.

Make a moderate descent along narrow Snow Canyon Road, which winds north down Snow Canyon's rubbly alluvial fan, often near a small, usually flowing western branch of Snow Creek. This stream may be dry by April of drought years. If so, the closest water is available from homes in Snow Creek village, but there is no camping currently allowed thereabouts. Eventually the road simultaneously leaves San Bernardino National Forest and its San Jacinto Wilderness at a Desert Water Agency gate, and then it veers northwest to hop across the western branch. Just beyond, your route joins paved Falls Creek Road (1225-1.0) at the outskirts of the small village of Snow Creek.

**Water access:** Southbound hikers should note that this community is their last certain water source until North Fork San Jacinto River, a grueling 24 miles and a 7600-foot climb away high in the San

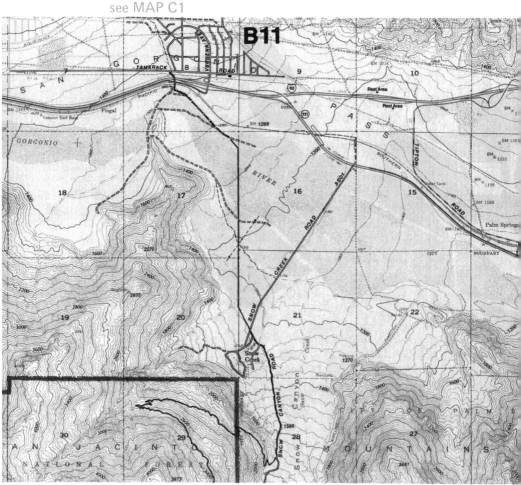

see MAP C1

see MAP B10

**See Map B11**

Jacintos. For the northbound, the next water is at Mesa Wind Station, 6.5 miles (an emergency source only), or better, at the Whitewater River, a long, hot 13.3 miles away.

Now you briefly follow Falls Creek Road northwest to a junction with Snow Creek Road 3S01 (1230-0.2). From here the permanent PCT route starts a contour northwest. Constructed by Sierra Club volunteers and the Bureau of Land Management, the next 2 miles of PCT are not really trail at all. Because of shifting sands and the possibility that off-road-vehicle enthusiasts might abuse an actual trail, they decided not to build an actual trail across broad San Gorgonio Pass. Instead, the PCT route is indicated by a row of 5-foot-tall 4x4 posts, some metal, some redwood, each emblazoned with the triangular PCT shield and with white directional arrows. Standing beside one post, you can usually see the next one without much difficulty. The first metal post stands a few yards northwest of Snow Creek Road, in a field of foxtails. It indicates the way (330° bearing) to the first of a long line of redwood posts that march due north along a section boundary.

The actual route is somewhat more tortuous, winding through well-spaced head-high yellow-flowered creosote bushes on a very gentle descent. A few minutes' walk leads across a sandy wash, which at about 1188 feet elevation is the PCT's lowest point south of the Columbia Gorge on the Oregon–Washington border. Another few minutes finds your not-a-trail intersecting a pair of crossing jeep roads (1195-0.7) under a high-tension powerline. Beyond, the wooden posts continue north, now across a more cobbly desert floor with mixed shrubbery. You cross a good gravel road (1210-0.2), then proceed across numerous sandy washes that constitute the ephemeral San Gorgonio River. Usually no water at all is to be found, but often there is a strong westerly wind, which throws stinging sand in your face. Also it sets hundreds of power-generating wind turbines flapping like alarmed sea gulls, these standing to the north, across Interstate 10. In the rainy season, look for purple-flower clusters of sand verbena hereabouts.

Eventually metal posts indicate a bend northwest in the route to soon cross a sandy dirt road (1265-0.7). Now you hike left, northwest, slowly diverging from the road and climb to hike atop a narrow, sinuous 20-foot high alluvial bank. It was built to protect the busy Southern Pacific Railroad, which parallels our route, just to our north. Shortly, you drop off the north side of the alluvial bank, heading sandily over a level treadles route marked by 4x4 posts, west towards a tangle of roads at the mouth of Stubbe Canyon Creek (1320-0.7), which you were able to see from atop the rise. Here the route emerges from three concrete bridges, one of Southern Pacific Railroad and two of Interstate 10. Now you follow a dirt road that goes north under the bridges, then clamber up a road bank to paved Tamarack Road (1360-0.1). By passing under these bridges you finally leave Santa Rosa and San Jacinto Mountains National Monument behind.

**Resupply access:** A slowly dying suburb, West Palm Springs Village, is centered ⅓ mile east along Tamarack Road, at Interstate 10's Verbena Avenue offramp. Although water might be obtained in an emergency from a few homes there, the village has no other resources for PCT travelers. To resupply, hitchhike, as recommended under "Supplies," 12.5 miles east to Palm Springs or 4.5 miles west to Cabazon.

**See Maps B11**

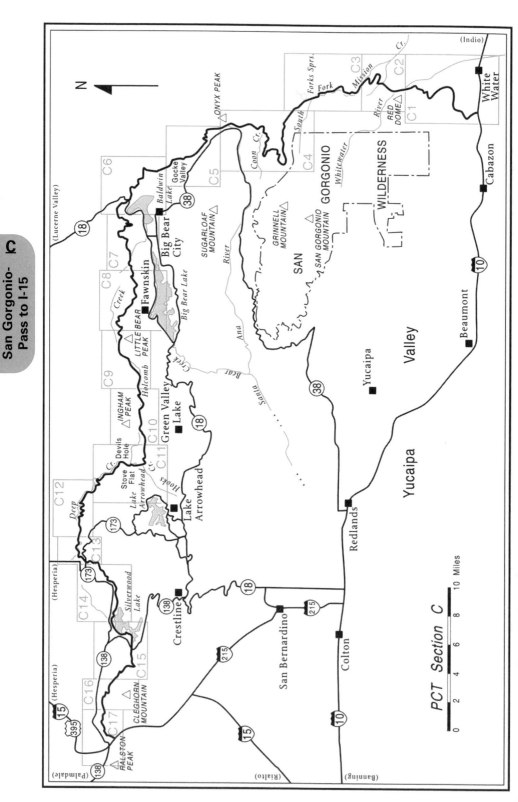

*Section C:*

# San Gorgonio Pass to Interstate 15 near Cajon Pass

Running the entire length of the San Bernardino Mountains, this long trail section samples most of the diverse ecosystems found there. Beginning in San Gorgonio Pass in the sweltering heat of a typical Colorado Desert (Lower Sonoran Zone) ecosystem, the Pacific Crest Trail crosses the San Andreas Fault and then climbs through a sparse, drab chaparral of bayonet-sharp cacti and thorny scrub along the Whitewater River and Mission Creek. Though sprung from subalpine snowbanks high in the San Gorgonio Wilderness, these streams almost all evaporate or sink beneath desert gravels before reaching the foothills.

As you climb higher, small drought-tolerant pinyon pines, favored food source of Native Americans and various animals, soon border the trail, heralding your passage through the Upper Sonoran Zone. These trees gradually mingle with Jeffrey pines and incense-cedars until, at about 7000 feet, you find ourselves in the crisp air and enveloping forests of the Transition Zone. Just north of Coon Creek, at the 8750-foot apex of the PCT in the San Bernardino Mountains, the route touches the Canadian Zone, where isolated snow patches might linger into early summer. Hikers traversing the high San Bernardinos in April or May should expect possible hail or snow and nightly subfreezing temperatures. Bring warm clothing and carry a tent. From the high point, one can turn southwest to scan the San Gorgonio Wilderness' high summits, where hardy subalpine conifers huddle below gale-screening ridges. The PCT was routed around the highest elevations of the wilderness because its backpacker population was already excessive.

Nearing dammed Big Bear Lake, a popular resort area, the PCT alternates between Jeffrey-pine and pinyon forest. In this northern rainshadow of the San Bernardinos, plant and animal life is much more influenced by proximity to the high Mojave Desert, stretching northward, than by the terrain's elevation, which would normally foster a uniform montane Jeffrey-pine-and-fir forest. Instead, Joshua trees, cacti, mountain mahogany and sagebrush share the rolling hillsides with dry pinyon-pine groves, and drive Jeffrey pines, incense-cedars and white firs away to higher summits or to the cold-air microclimates of streambeds.

North of Big Bear Lake the PCT begins to trend west, following the main axis of the San Bernardino Mountains. A part of the Transverse Range Province, which includes the San Gabriel Mountains and other mountain chains stretching west to the Channel Islands, the San Bernardinos cut conspicuously across the lay of other California physiographic features, which trend northwest-southeast. Long before being intruded by molten rock that solidified to form granitic plutons, the region now straddled by the San Bernardinos had been alternately low land and shallow sea floor. Evidence of this lies in two rock types you will encounter often: the Furnace marble—derived from marine carbonates that

became limestone—and the Saragossa quartzite—derived from sand that became sandstone. The limestone and sandstone were then altered under heat and pressure, perhaps several times, to reach their present metamorphic states.

Near Lake Arrowhead, another reservoir originally constructed to store water to irrigate foothill orange groves, the PCT again veers north, now down Deep Creek, a permanent stream feeding the ephemeral Mojave River. The floral composition of the Mojave Desert, seen here and also later as the PCT skirts Summit Valley, differs strikingly from the lower Colorado Desert flora seen farther south. Bitter-cold, windy winters here account for many of the differences.

Section C ends unremarkably under 6-lane Interstate 15 in Cajon Canyon, overshadowed by massive workings of humanity—the freeway, the powerlines from the Colorado River, and the multiple railroad tracks. These in turn are dwarfed by an awesome artifact of nature—the cleft of the San Andreas Fault, which slashes through Cajon Canyon and bends east to demarcate the southern base of the San Bernardino Mountains.

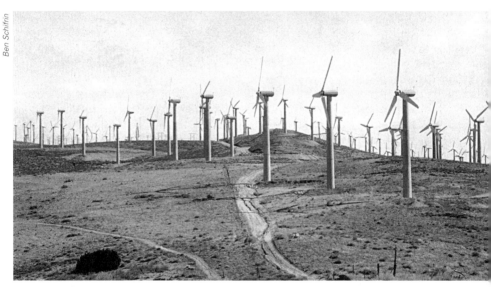

*Ben Schifrin*

*Mesa wind farm*

# Maps

| | |
|---|---|
| *White Water* | *Fawnskin* |
| *Catclaw Flat* | *Butler Peak* |
| *Onyx Peak* | *Lake Arrowhead* |
| *Moonridge* | *Silverwood Lake* |
| *San Gorgonio Peak* | *Cajon* |
| *Big Bear City* | |

# Declination
13°E

| Points on Route | S→N | Mi. Btwn. Pts. | N→S |
|---|---|---|---|
| near Interstate 10 in San Gorgonio Pass | 0.0 | | 132.9 |
| | | 3.9 | |
| Mesa Wind Station | 3.9 | | 129.0 |
| | | 6.8 | |
| camps by Whitewater River ford | 10.7 | | 122.2 |
| | | 5.2 | |
| East Fork Mission Creek Road | 15.9 | | 117.0 |
| | | 6.4 | |
| Forks Springs | 22.3 | | 110.6 |
| | | 7.2 | |
| Road 1N93 and Mission Creek Trail Camp | 29.5 | | 103.4 |
| | | 6.6 | |
| Coon Creek Jumpoff Group Camp | 36.1 | | 96.8 |
| | | 5.7 | |
| dirt road just east of Onyx Summit | 41.8 | | 91.1 |
| | | 4.1 | |
| Arrastre Trail Camp at Deer Spring | 45.9 | | 87.0 |
| | | 9.5 | |
| Highway 18 near dry Baldwin Lake | 55.4 | | 77.5 |
| | | 2.5 | |
| Doble Trail Camp | 57.9 | | 75.0 |
| | | 6.4 | |
| Van Dusen Canyon Road to Big Bear City | 64.3 | | 68.6 |
| | | 3.5 | |
| Holcomb Valley Road to Fawnskin | 67.8 | | 65.1 |
| | | 7.2 | |
| Little Bear Springs Trail Camp | 75.0 | | 57.9 |
| | | 6.8 | |
| Crab Flats Road | 81.8 | | 51.1 |
| | | 1.9 | |
| Holcomb Crossing Trail Camp | 83.7 | | 49.2 |
| | | 4.1 | |
| Deep Creek Bridge to Lake Arrowhead | 87.8 | | 45.1 |
| | | 9.4 | |
| Deep Creek Hot Spring | 97.2 | | 35.7 |
| | | 5.0 | |
| Mojave River Forks Reservoir Dam | 102.2 | | 30.7 |
| | | 1.7 | |
| Hwy. 173 above Mojave River Forks Reservoir | 103.9 | | 29.0 |
| | | 9.4 | |
| Road 2N33 near Cedar Springs Dam | 113.3 | | 19.6 |
| | | 6.0 | |
| Silverwood Lake Area's entrance road | 119.3 | | 13.6 |
| | | 7.1 | |
| Little Horsethief Canyon's dry creek bed | 126.4 | | 6.5 |
| | | 6.5 | |
| Interstate 15 near Cajon Pass | 132.9 | | 0.0 |

## Weather To Go

The San Bernardino Mountains customarily offer clear warm weather and snow-free trails throughout May and June. By then, however, the lowlands at either end of this section—especially in Mission Creek at the start—typically have daytime temperatures in excess of 100 degrees. March and April are the best times to explore those areas, if you aren't thru-hiking.

## Supplies

West Palm Springs Village, at the beginning of Section C, has nothing for hikers. Supplies may be purchased 4.5 miles west on Interstate 10, in Cabazon, which has a post office, market, and a smattering of motels. It also boasts a few nice restaurants, including the quirky Wheel Inn, complete with life-sized concrete dinosaur statues, and Hadley's, famous for their date milk shakes and mind-boggling array of dried fruits. Cabazon is now home to an enormous designer outlet mall, where almost any conceivable need for clothing, shoes, electronics, or sporting goods can be fulfilled. Cabazon Ranch Outfitters, located at 50150 Esperanza Avenue in Cabazon, offers professional pack animal support and guiding in the San Jacintos and San Bernardinos. Contact Barbara Gronek, Box 876, Cabazon, CA 92230, or phone (909) 849-2528. Horse feed is available at their facility, and they host, free of charge: corrals, water, hot showers, camping, and package holds for riders and hikers.

Fully 10 miles west of West Palm Springs Village on Interstate 10 is Banning, which has even more complete services than Cabazon. Palm Springs lies 12.5 miles east via Interstate 10 and Highway 111. It has a dazzling array of markets, hotels, and fine eateries.

Big Bear City, 3 miles south down Van Dusen Canyon Road from the 64.3-mile point on the PCT, is the next convenient provisioning stop. It boasts a post office, stores, restaurants, motels and laundromats beside shallow, picturesque Big Bear Lake. In recent years, the fire station has offered showers to PCT hikers.

Fawnskin, another resort community, is located on the northwest shore of Big Bear Lake, and it is 3.7 miles off-route along Holcomb Valley Road, 67.8 miles from the start. It has a post office, stores, restaurants and motels. It is also accessible via the Cougar Crest Trail, at the 67.0-mile point of this PCT section, by way of a 2-mile detour.

The next chance for supplies lies in Lake Arrowhead, 3½ miles from the PCT's crossing of Deep Creek, 87.8 miles from the start. Access to Cedar Glen, on the east shore of Lake Arrowhead, is facilitated by a very popular hikers' access at Hook Creek roadend—getting a ride is usually very easy. That road leads up to the convenient Cedar Glen Post Office and nearby supermarket, restaurants, shops, and motels.

Upon descending Deep Creek to Mojave River Forks Reservoir, about 103 miles into this section, walkers may opt to head for the desert community of Hesperia. Arrowhead Lake Road leads north 2.8 miles to Hesperia Lake Park, a delightful enclave with lawn-cushioned camping under deep shade, fishing in a small lake, and a small mini-mart. Downtown Hesperia lies about 3 miles farther, with all modern amenities.

Crestline, a mountain village similar to Cedar Glen, also offers similar accommodations for hikers who hitchhike south 10 miles on Highway 138 from the 119.1-mile point of the PCT, at Silverwood Lake State Recreation Area. Travelers with less extensive needs may avail themselves of a small store and cafe a short distance off the trail in the recreation area, or Summit Valley Store, reached via a short detour from the Mojave-scorched PCT in Summit Valley, at the 109.5-mile point.

Section C terminates at a roadend just shy of Interstate 15 in Cajon Canyon. This paved spur road leads 0.6 mile northwest to meet Highway 138 about 200 yards east of its overpass of Interstate 15 at Cajon Junction. Hikers will find three gas stations, three well-stocked mini-marts, and a pleasant motel. Also sited there are two of the objects of many hikers' fantasies: a Del Taco restaurant and the inexplicably ever-popular McDonald's. Tiffany's Restaurant, the old landmark of the Route 138 cloverleaf, is now closed.

The owners of the motel, the ECONOmy Inn, located west of the overpass, hold supply boxes for hikers who rent a room for at least one night. This is an excellent option, because camping nearby is generally terrible, and, besides, they have a swimming pool and a hot tub! Resupplying here lets you avoid the lengthy descent to Wrightwood. For details, contact:

ECONOmy Inn
8317 US Hwy. 138
Phelan, CA 92371

Tel: (760) 249-6777
Manager: Mr. Vinod Somani

From the Cajon Junction overpass, Highway 138 continues northwest 8½ miles to Highway 2, which goes 5½ miles to Wrightwood. This pleasant mountain community has a post office, stores, restaurants, motels and a laundromat. Those who don't mind a return to true civilization—smog, congestion, street lights and concrete—may go south 17 miles on Interstate 15 to San Bernardino, which has all the dubious advantages of a hectic metropolis.

## Water

Carry ample water north from West Palm Springs since the Whitewater River and the lower reaches of Mission Creek that the PCT traverses are often dry by June of drought years. The most certain water source is Fork Springs, a mind-broiling 22.3 miles into the journey. For most of the remainder of this San Bernardino Mountains section, however, water sources are encountered regularly, even if they are not numerous. This situation changes for the last leg, along the rim of the Mojave Desert. Be sure to leave Deep Creek and Silverwood Lake with a few liters of water per person—the stretches of dusty chaparral along Summit Valley, and over to Cajon Pass, are usually bone-dry.

## Permits

Day-hikers and section-hikers, but not thru-hikers, will be affected by the National Forest Adventure Pass system now in effect for all parked cars within Southern California's national forests. This pass is required for all vehicles, while parked along any road or even at a designated trailhead, in Angeles, Cleveland, Los Padres and San Bernardino National Forests. It is not required for PCT travelers, per se. Cost is $5 per visit to one forest, or $30 per year (good for all four forests). Plans are to return 85% of collected monies to the individual forest for human-use enhancing projects. Passes can be purchased from the USFS, from Southern California outdoor shops and vendors near or in the forests.

No wilderness permits are required for overnight PCT campers in the BLM portion of the San Gorgonio Wilderness.

## Special Problems

### Ticks

Ticks are ubiquitous in the grassy fields and brushy slopes of the PCT as it traverses Southern California. Bites by these blood-sucking arachnids cause two general problems for hikers and equestrians: 1) How to get them off and what to do to the wound; and 2) rare infections. The recognition of Lyme disease has raised concern about infections from tick bites; thankfully, tick bites in California's inland mountains are more nuisance than risk.

Ticks burrow their headparts into the skin of the groin, armpits, hairline or other body areas, especially where there is a constriction created by snug clothing, such as the waistband. The trick is to get them out of you, whole, without doing further injury. Countless lore has been retold in Scouting and woodcraft manuals about the task of removing embedded ticks from the body. Home methods abound, such as applying the tip of a hot match to the tick's derriere, or smothering it with vaseline, margarine or nail polish, or to irritate it with a dollop of gasoline or alcohol. Equal argument has arisen as to whether they should be tugged on with fingers or tweezers, or unscrewed clockwise, or the reverse. Scientific investigation has shown that *all of the above methods work*, but the most effective one is also the simplest—simply grasping the tick, with tweezers or fingers, as close to its attachment to you as possible, and pulling gently, but firmly, until the tick lets go.

Once removed, examine the tick to make sure that you haven't ripped its head off, and examine the skin wound for a black or brown dot that might represent a tick head left behind. If seen, remove it with tweezers. In any event, try to prevent infection: wash the wound with soap and water, apply a small amount of antibiotic ointment, and try to keep it clean. No further preventive treatment is necessary.

Tick-borne infections are the feared hazard of tick bites. All are sometimes difficult to diagnose, even by doctors, so prompt hospital attention is recommended for anyone who has symptoms that suggest such an infection. **Lyme disease** is exceedingly rare in any mountains of California, and particularly unlikely in the southern Sierra and Southern California ranges. This is because most nymphal ticks feed on Western fence

lizards, the most common "blue-belly" lizard of the Southern California chaparral and mid-elevations of the Sierra range. The fence lizards' immune systems clear the Lyme disease parasites from the ticks. In any event, it is almost impossible for ticks to transmit the Lyme parasite to humans unless one is embedded for more than 24 hours—a rare occasion, indeed. Hence, prevention is possible by checking carefully for ticks once or twice daily. Lyme disease is characterized by a migrating rash, fevers, flu-like symptoms, and worsening joint pains. It is easily treated by antibiotics.

**Spotted Fever** is marked by high fever, headache, and a red spotty rash that becomes purple over time. This very serious illness is promptly treated by antibiotics. It is quite rare throughout the Pacific West. "Spotless" forms of the fever are also occasionally contracted. Though difficult to diagnose, the victim's history of a prolonged tick bite will help steer the doctor toward the correct diagnosis.

**Tick Paralysis** is a rarer condition of progressive severe weakness. It is usually completely reversed by removal of the tick. It rarely affects adults, and is almost never seen outside of the Pacific Northwest.

Prevention of tick bites is the best medicine. In tick country, wear long-sleeved clothing, with cuffs tucked under sox or into boots. Insect repellent is also of some use for ticks—apply it liberally, and often, to skin and clothing.

# The Route

Reach the southern terminus of Section C via Interstate 10's Verbenia Avenue exit. Head briefly north to Tamarack Road, which parallels the freeway, and follow it ⅓ mile west to the posted PCT, just west of Fremontia Road.

Easy-to-follow PCT trail tread climbs gently north from Tamarack Road, first just west of dry Stubbe Canyon Creek, then on a low levee to its east. You wind past many roads of a failed subdivision, then pass under a powerline and its attendant road. Across a second such road (1475-0.5) the tread may be vague, but it is marked by 4x4 PCT posts and it runs just west of a green-wire fence. Beyond it, you wind up to a dirt road over the buried Colorado River Aqueduct (1580-0.4). A minute later, you cross a better road. Here a crude sign and PCT Association trail register indicate an important dirt road that branches left, northwest, to an important seasonal water supply. Walk through a junkyard of a dozen cars and trailers and other metal debris, then about 200 yards north up a sunny hillside to Don & Helen Middleton's "Pink Motel." It consists of a pink stucco structure cobbled to an assortment of travel trailers, which afford welcome shade, cooking and sleeping areas, and an outhouse. Even more importantly, the Middletons graciously truck a large supply of bottled water up to the site for northbound hikers each spring, and will store resupply packages sent to them, there, as well. For more information about the Pink Motel, contact Don & Helen Middleton: 13010 Cottonwood, HCR-1, Box 2001, Whitewater, CA 92282, or phone (909) 849-8440.

Keeping to a low bench with knee-high scrub, you traverse a succession of jeep roads, then cross better Cottonwood Road (1690-0.6). The PCT turns left, north, uphill alongside Cottonwood Road, keeping within 10 yards of it, in a delightful, thigh-high garden of silver-flannel-leaved, yellow-flowered brittlebush, a drought-tolerant shrub of the sunflower family. Nearing the mouth of Cottonwood Canyon, the trail passes around a metal-signed Cotton-wood Trailhead, a dirt parking area, then crosses two side-by-side roads (1850-0.6) then makes a slightly indistinct ford of the almost always dry stream that drains Cottonwood Canyon. Across it, the way merges with a jeep track to strike east to the mouth of Gold Canyon. Its unusual east-west orientation is due to erosion along the Bonnie Bell fault, a splinter of the great San Andreas rift.

Entering Gold Canyon, your jeep track strikes Gold Canyon Road (1845-0.2). You wind south of it on trail constructed by the Sierra Club. In the next long mile, you recross the road, pass through a stock fence at a corral, then cross the road, now blocked, twice more, all in desert vegetation of Mojave yucca, rabbit-brush, creosote bush and multiple species of cacti. Presently, you see windmills of the Mesa Wind Farm, and the canyon bends north. Here, a large trailside map and a list of mileages through the San Bernardinos stand beside a now-blocked spur trail (2310-1.6) to a dirt road junction near the metal headquarters shed.

**Water access:** The water fountain that once existed at this road junction was dismantled in November 1994, due to traces of uranium contamination found in the 400-foot-deep well. Workers at the wind farm now bring in their own bottled water. If you are dangerously low on water at this point, walk 100 yds east and 80 yds north, to the large metal building, and ask for water. It comes from a well that you walk past: just south of the road, at an electric control panel for the transformer station, a blue-domed cylinder sits atop the wellhead, with numerous valves and taps. Camping—in the company of range cattle—could be done anywhere nearby.

Sometimes vague, your path now leads more moderately up a small parallel ravine west of the road. Later, you come back alongside the main ravine and momentarily join a rough jeep road (2470-0.5). The way leads easily up-canyon, keeping just west of its dry wash and braiding with a network of cattle paths. After passing through a stock drift fence, the path steepens to climb the head of Gold Canyon.

**See Map C1**

Mostly, the way is unrelentingly shadeless, but occasional, small laurel sumac trees do offer respite. During the wet season, a profusion of wildflowers may sprinkle the route, including many members of the sunflower family, and also white, blue and lavender phacelias, chia and popcorn flower. Lizards too numerous to count also scurry from underfoot. Finally, four small switchbacks help you gain a narrow pass (3225-1.3) between Gold and Teutang canyons. This pass is now the approximate southern boundary of the expanded San Gorgonio Wilderness Area, which the PCT will climb through, until the head of North Fork Mission Creek. The most impressive vistas are southeast, contrasting the granite and seasonal snow of the San Jacinto massif with the Colorado desert sands of Coachella Valley.

Starting north, you descend moderately to a ridge nose, down which small, tight switchbacks descend. These bring the PCT to a dry crossing of the streambed in Teutang Canyon (2815-0.7), just upstream of a chasm of gray granite. Next you round an intervening promontory to step across another canyon tributary, which has a seasonal spring ¼ mile up-canyon, then proceed fairly level down-canyon. When you gain a narrow ridgetop, your path doubles back on itself to climb northwest, perhaps indistinctly, up an open grassy slope, before resuming a traversing line high above the canyon's floor. This stretch does afford interesting panoramas east over the cleft of Whitewater Canyon to the sun-browned Little San Bernardino Mountains.

Eventually you descend, first directly along a ridgelet, then in a sweeping arc that leads to the lip of Hatchery Canyon. Now on switchbacks that are susceptible to erosion, you drop quickly to the floor of Hatchery Canyon, where you step across its dry streambed. The trail now heads sandily downstream, soon passing through a stock gate, and then striking an old jeep road (2285-2.7) at the canyon's mouth in

Whitewater Canyon, just beneath an impressive conglomerate scarp. Here you turn left, north, on sandy alluvium of the west bank of the Whitewater River, which is a raging torrent true to its name in early season, but more often is a noisesome brook. Southbound trekkers must fill their canteens here—the next safe, certain on-route water lies across desertlike San Gorgonio Pass at the west branch of Snow Creek, 14.3 long miles way. The Whitewater River usually has water throughout summer, but may be dry by early May of severe drought years. The route—essentially a jeep road—winds across sandy washes where the flanking scrub is alive with phainopeplas, which are crested silky flycatchers closely related to waxwings.

Hikers should ignore a beckoning oasis of trees and lush mowed grass, just across the Whitewater River, to the east. This is the private Whitewater Trout Farm, where hikers have been consistently unwelcome for many years. Please avoid this private property and camp west of the river.

Just past red basalt outcrops of Miocene age that mark two good camps (2605-1.6), large ducks and a sign lead you northeast across the Whitewater River's bouldery granite and marble bed to a narrow canyon peppered with boulders of basalt and gneiss, among junipers, catclaws and bladderpods patrolled by collared lizards. Here the best jeep track jogs northwest, paralleling the river bed for a moment, to find a resumption of trail at an old California Riding and Hiking Trail (CRHT) signpost. From the post your path ascends moderately northeast in a terrain not unlike Death Valley, soon switchbacking to gain a ridgetop (3075-1.3) in deeply incised gneiss and fanglomerate. Ignore a short deadend trail climbing south along the ridge from here. Fiddleneck and foxtail brush against

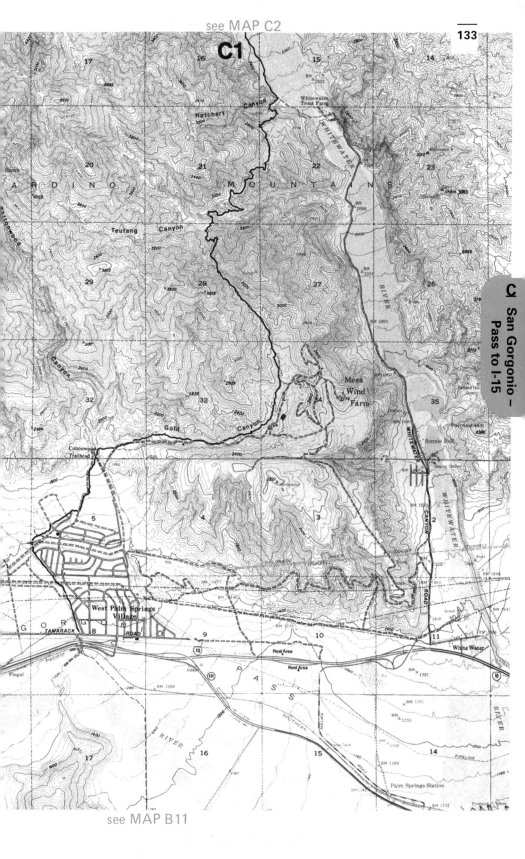

**C** San Gorgonio –
Pass to I-15

Ben Schifrin

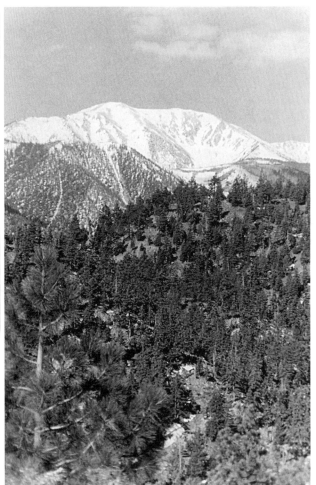

*San Gorgonio Peak, from east fork Mission Creek*

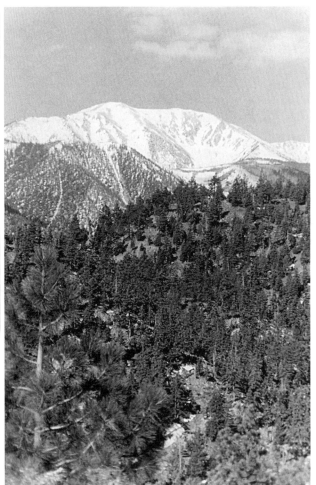
Atop this ridge, views are panoramic and startling. The southern horizon is dominated by 10,804-foot San Jacinto Peak, often frosted in winter and spring with snow and contrasting markedly with the red, yellow and gray hues of the desert's alluvial landscape, in the foreground. To the west, gneissic rocks support Kitching Peak, while the Whitewater River Canyon ascends as a rocky scar northwest to the Jumpoffs below barren San Gorgonio Peak. The gully just north of the ridge that you ascended, plus West Fork Mission Creek, Catclaw Flat, and Middle Fork Whitewater River are all aligned with the north branch of the San Andreas Fault, which is partly responsible for this region's varied geology.

The PCT continues to wind northwest up the ridgetop dividing the East and West forks of Mission Creek, then the ascent gives way to a moderate descent east down a chaparralled nose to East Fork Mission Creek Road (3060-3.1). Here you turn northwest up-canyon to cross usually flowing East Fork Mission Creek in about ½ mile. Continue along its shadeless north bank to the end of the dirt road (3360-1.4). From this point your hike up Mission Creek is often difficult, despite reconstruction efforts by C.C.C. trail crews, who in 1993 installed boulder bridges across each of the stream fords.

one's legs on the descent northeast from this saddle, and one soon reaches and turns north beside West Fork Mission Creek Road (2918-0.6). Just minutes later the PCT veers north away from this dirt road (3010-0.2) in a dry, sandy wash. Look for CRHT posts and follow them east into a side canyon, then up, arcing across the north side of the small valley, across its head, and then ascending its south wall to an east-ascending nose, eroded from Quaternary and Tertiary sediments.

**See Maps C1, C2**

see MAP C3

C2

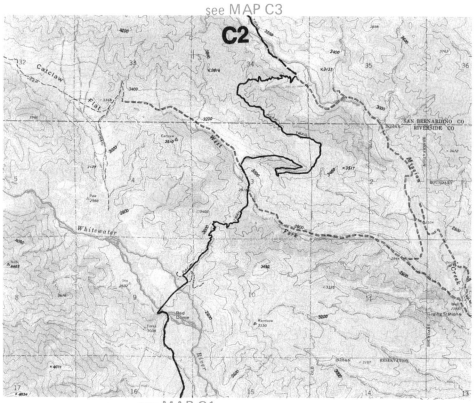

see MAP C1

Mission Creek's narrow gorge, incised in tortured granite gneisses, leaves little room for a trail, so washouts are frequent and the path is often vague through alluvial boulder fields and jungles of baccharis (false willow), alder, willow and cottonwood. Rattlesnakes inhabit the grassy stream margins, as do garter snakes, racers, horned lizards, antelope ground squirrels, summer tanagers and bobcats—so keep an eye open while making any of the 20+ fords of Mission Creek lying south of Forks Springs. Note too where prominent faults cross the canyon—at 3400 feet, at 3900 feet and at 4080 feet, where the Pinto Mountain Fault further tortures the banded gneisses.

Chia, yerba santa, catclaw, baccharis, and bladderpod are the most frequent plants, but you also see notable specimens of Joshua tree, yucca, and cactus.

One species that hikers thankfully won't have to see anymore are cattle. Mission Creek Ranch, which owned land traversed by the PCT, alternating in a checkerboard fashion with BLM, has now been purchased by the Wildlands Conservancy. All cattle grazing has been eliminated from the area, which should make campsites and water much cleaner. The bad news, for some, is that, since the area is now being managed with a more-aggressive pure-wilderness ethic, the once-popular "Hiker Haven," a private wilderness hostel in

See Maps C2, C3

upper South Fork Mission Creek canyon, has been dismantled. There are numerous other, more primitive options for camping, anywhere along the lower reaches of Mission Creek, however.

Just below the confluence of the South and North forks of Mission Creek you pass nice campsites, then cross this major creek (4830-5.0), which is fed just up-canyon by Forks Springs. Water is generally available here year-round, but may not be elsewhere in Mission Creek due to the porous sediments of its bed. North of Forks Springs, the now discernible PCT keeps usually to northeastern banks in an ocean-spray chaparral. Near 5200 feet the path crosses granitic bedrock emplaced at the same time as Sierran granites, and later, at 5600 feet, the tread turns to sugar-white and yellowish Saragossa quartzite. Near 5900 feet the PCT veers away from Mission Creek into a side canyon and quickly reaches a pleasant creekside camp (6110-3.1) shaded by alders, incense-cedars, Jeffrey pines and interior live oaks. Eight switchbacks lead west from this spot, elevating you to atop a phyllite-and-quartzite promontory. The friability and instability of the quartzite bedrock are demonstrated both by vegetational scarcity and by a massive landslide cutting across your path as you contour a steep slope shortly after gaining this ridge. Just past this slide, you leave BLM jurisdiction for San Bernardino National Forest.

White firs and Jeffrey pines soon shade the PCT as it resumes its ascent close beside Mission Creek, which usually has flowing water near its headwaters. Tank up here, for there might not be water at Mission Creek Trail Camp. A rough jeep road, built to log the forested flats south of Mission Creek, is met at a junction (7490-3.0) which may still be marked by yellow paint-daubs on nearby trees. Follow its overgrown tracks west up along willowy creekside meadows to meet gravel Road 1N93 (7965-1.1) at a PCT marker. A sign

here pretentiously announces MISSION CREEK TRAIL CAMP, which is merely a pleasant flat spot with fire rings, located south of North Fork Mission Creek.

**Water access:** Fill your water bottles here, since the next water on route is at Arrastre (Deer Springs) Trail Camp, in 16.4 miles.

PCT trail tread resumes here, starting north up from Road 1N93 on a well-graded trail in an open stand of pines. The route rounds northeast, with some fine backward glimpses of subalpine Ten Thousand Foot Ridge in San Gorgonio Wilderness. Soon you reach a sandy gap and cross Road 1N05 (8240-0.6). Now you have some fine views northwest to rounded Sugarloaf Mountain and its smaller western sibling, Sugarlump. Next on your agenda is a pleasant, level traverse, first northward, then southeastward, in cool forest on the north side of the divide, which here separates the Santa Ana River and the Whitewater River drainages. Eventually the trail dips easily to a post-marked crossing of Road 1N05 (8115-0.8) at a saddle. Now, the easy route leads east under a forested summit, and you have panoramas northwest to Sugarloaf Mountain. Later, dropping rockily, the PCT finds a junction (7980-0.8) with a CRHT-marked trail that descends northwest from just below a forested saddle.

**Water access:** Travelers low on water may trace this trail about ½ mile down to usually flowing Heart Bar Creek.

The PCT proceeds north from this junction, contouring at first, then making a sustained moderate ascent through a woodland of mountain mahogany, manzanita, pinyon and Jeffrey pines and scraggly white fir. Vistas gradually unfold southwest over to San Gorgonio Peak and Ten Thousand Foot Ridge and west down Heart Bar Creek

**See Maps C3, C4**

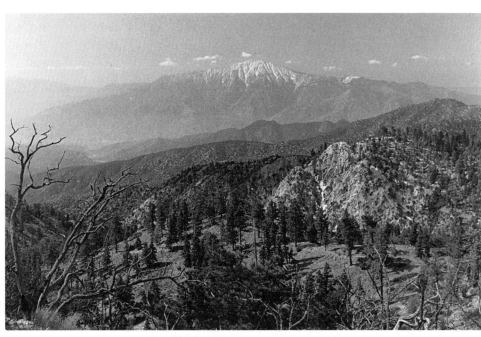

*Ben Schifrin*

*San Jacinto Peak, from divide north of Coon Creek Jumpoff*

to lush Big Meadows and the popular Barton Flats camp area. Bending northwest, the path soon levels out atop the long west ridge of Peak 8828, and then it swings east into shady mixed-conifer forest lying north of that summit.

For a few minutes the PCT skirts across white, granular Furnace marble, and the surrounding vegetation also changes markedly: edaphic effects (see Chapter 3's "Biology") allow only hardy whitebark pines and junipers, the former normally found in higher, colder climes, to muster a scattered occupation of the crumbly slopes.

Rounding to the east of Peak 8828, you descend gently to a ridgetop and join Road 1N96 (8510-2.5), where good views southeast over North Fork Mission Creek to the San Jacinto Mountains and the Coachella Valley help to make a pleasant, but waterless, camp surrounded by lupine and purple sage.

You continue east down the poor dirt road to a road junction (8340-0.6) located on the ridge east of Peak 8588. From here the PCT continues east along the ridgeline as Road 1N96, while a better dirt road, 1N95, branches northwest, downhill. The route soon crosses onto north slopes, becomes a trail, and drops gently around Peak 8751 to Coon Creek Jumpoff—a spectacular, steep, granitic defile at the head of a tributary of North Fork Mission Creek.

The raw scarp here points to rapid erosion east of the Jumpoff and illustrates the process of stream capture. The small stream draining the Tayles Hidden Acres basin and part of adjacent Section 20, to your northeast, used to connect with Coon Creek, to the west, but accelerated headward erosion of Mission Creek at the Jumpoff has intercepted that stream. Its

**See Map C5**

see MAP C5

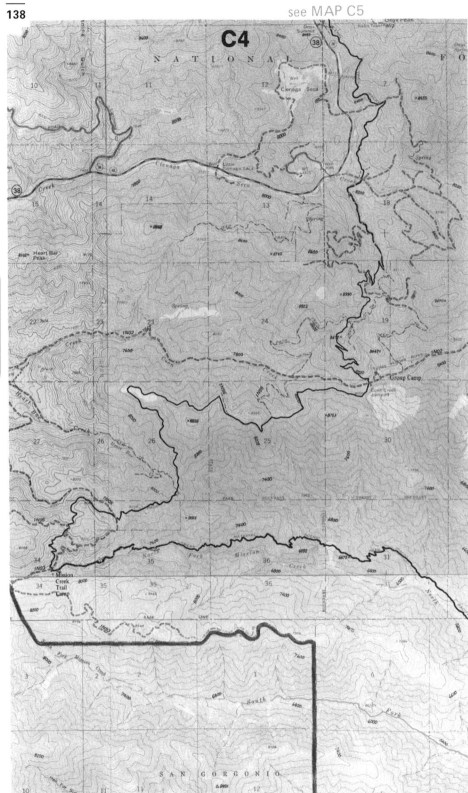

C4

see MAP C3

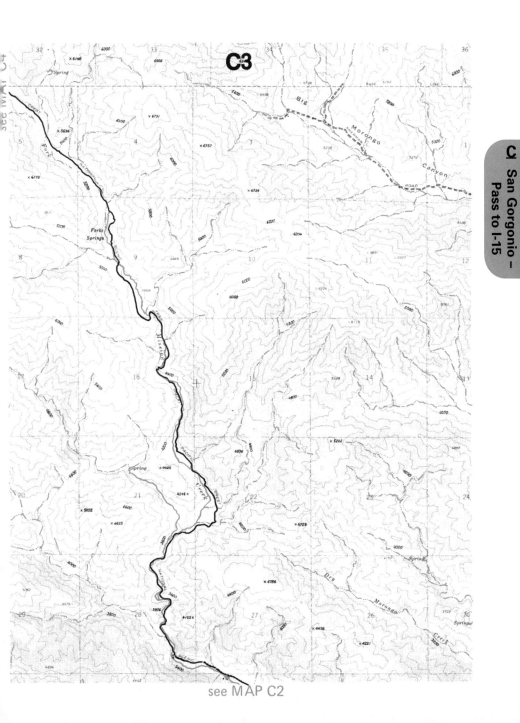

**C3**

see MAP C2

**San Gorgonio – Pass to I-15**

waters now flow southeast, eventually to the Salton Sea, rather than west to the Santa Ana River and the Pacific Ocean.

From this thought-provoking overlook, the trail climbs gently for a moment to Coon Creek Road 1N02 (8090-1.3). Coon Creek Jumpoff Group Camp, with toilets but no water, is just to the east.

**Water access:** Until midsummer, water may be obtained by walking as much as 1.5 miles west down the dirt road.

The way now attacks, via moderate switchbacks through scattered pines, firs and montane chaparral, the south slopes of the ridge dividing Coon and Cienaga Seca creeks.

Extensive views compensate for the climb. Seasonally snowy Grinnell and San Gorgonio mountains loom in the southwest, Mounts Baldy and Baden–Powell mark your upcoming travels west, and glimpses of the Santa Rosa Mountains and Palm Springs shimmer in the southeast.

Rounding north of a conifered hillock alive with mountain bluebirds, Clark's nutcrackers, white-headed woodpeckers and dark-eyed juncos, you strike a trail (8610-1.3) which cuts perpendicularly across your route and meets a jeep road immediately east of your trail. The PCT continues ascending for ⅓ mile, passing under small, granitic cliffs before reaching a viewless, forested ridgetop. This 8750-foot point is the highest spot your trail reaches in the San Bernardino Mountains.

Now the way drops sandily on a gentle gradient to cross a dirt road (8635-0.7), then it switchbacks down into a canyon, the path flanked by tall mountain-mahogany shrubs. At the mouth of a gully in the canyon bottom, you cross a jeep road (8390-0.6), and then the PCT momentarily parallels its northward course before routing itself onto this road. Private land in Section 18 prevents the Forest Service from constructing PCT trail tread at this time, so you continue north on the jeep road/CRHT right-of-way. Soon the jeep road yields to a better dirt road (8260-0.4), which you trace north down-canyon to a five-way junction—four roads and a trail—(8100-0.6) located beside often dry Cienaga Seca Creek. The PCT rises north from this junction out of lodgepole pine into stands of juniper and mountain mahogany, then descends west along a dirt road for 130 yards to a junction (8440-1.0). Here the trail picks up again to contour the west slope of Onyx Peak over to a dirt road (8510-1.1) that is just east of Highway 38 and Onyx Summit.

The PCT crosses the road and climbs gently-to-moderately above Road 1N01, gaining increasingly good views of Baldwin Lake and Gold Mountain, in the northwest. Presently the path levels and crosses Road 1N01 (8635-1.0), then descends, first north, then west below a ridge. Lower, the well-marked route crosses a jeep road twice in quick succession before a switchback drops the trail to Broom Flat Road 2N01 (7885-2.2), a good dirt road running alongside shaded Arrastre Creek. Now you enter fragrant white-fir groves to descend easily northwest along the seasonal creek, and soon find Arrastre Trail Camp at Deer Spring (7605-0.9). This has a fire pit, toilet, hitching posts, benches, and the last water until Doble Trail Camp, 12 miles away.

Two minutes onward, you turn north at a junction with a jeep road that leads to Balky Horse Canyon. The route continues down Arrastre Canyon to Balky Horse Canyon and crosses Road 2N04 (7155-1.5).

One can appreciate the subtle changes in vegetation that have occurred

**See Maps C4, C5**

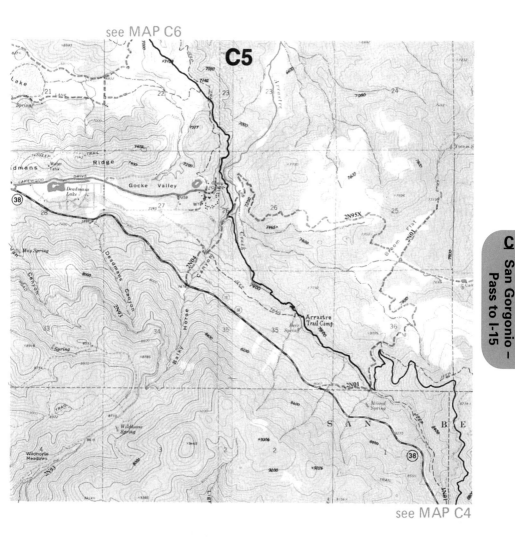

see MAP C6

C5

see MAP C4

on the descent into this region, which are influenced more by the Mojave Desert's parching winds than by moisture-laden ocean breezes.

Minutes later, you reach wooden berms that lead under Camp Oakes' rifle range, and then you climb gently across Saragossa quartzite in a true high-desert plant community: pinyon pines, buckwheat, and ephedra, a shiny yellow-green shrub with wiry stems called Mormon Tea—after its use by Mormon pioneers. Atop a 7240-

foot shoulder, you gaze eastward and see gold mines near Tip Top Mountain's summit and also see a high-desert woodland of Joshua trees and pinyon pines.

Now paralleling an expansive, desert-like ridge, the PCT crosses two jeep roads and first gives you views west over seasonal Erwin Lake and east to the Mojave, then later views west to large, shallow, some-times completely dry Baldwin Lake. Even-tually the sandy path descends to cross Arrastre Creek Road 2N02 (6775-3.8) amid pinyon pines, Joshua trees and sagebrush.

**See Maps C5, C6**

From that road the PCT climbs north, then contours northwest for alternating vistas of desert and mountain as it wanders among pinyon pines and crosses the Doble Fault just northeast of Peak 7057.

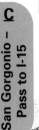 Here the rock underfoot abruptly changes from banded Precambrian gneiss to whitish Paleozoic quartzite. The Helendale Fault, stretching from north of Victorville southeast to Tip Top Mountain, runs parallel to Nelson Ridge, lying below you to the northeast.

Presently, with fleeting glimpses of Baldwin Lake you descend to meet High-way 18 (6829-4.2) just yards west of some interesting mining prospects.

North of the highway, find the trail angling left of a metal gate across a jeep road at the edge of a small pinyon forest, just west of a bulldozed-bare slope. The PCT next switchbacks to cross the jeep road, then contours north of Nelson Ridge before angling west down through a dense stand of pinyon pines to meet Doble Road 3N16 (6855-2.0) just south of the county dump. West across Doble Road the trail curves and contours south across three jeep tracks in sagebrush and rabbitbrush, affording good views of Baldwin Lake's playa surface beyond the ruins of Doble.

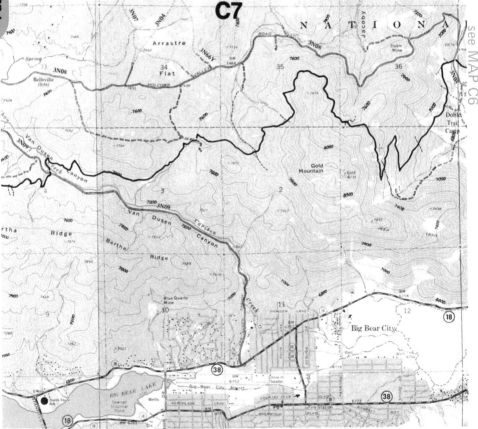

**See Map C6**

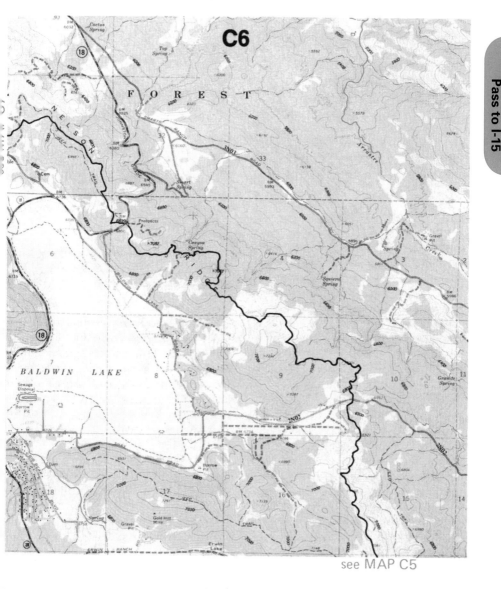

Baldwin Lake is named for Elias J. "Lucky" Baldwin, owner of the prosperous Doble Gold Mine, located high on the slopes above you.

The PCT contours low on Gold Mountain, and soon reaches a short, inobvious and unsigned spur trail (6880-0.5) down to signed Doble Trail Camp. Look for the first lush patch of rushes and iris under scattered pinyons and junipers to mark the junction. The camp has a pit toilet, corral, campfire ring and good piped water.

Continuing on, you make a gentle ascent in scrubby vegetation, crossing two jeep roads and making three switchbacks to gain a saddle on the northeast ridge of

see MAP C5

**See Maps C6, C7**

Gold Mountain. Here you leave pinyon pines behind for incense-cedars, Jeffrey pines and junipers. A gentle traverse around Gold Mountain's northern flanks bisects a jeep road and offers vistas over Arrastre and Union flats, scenes of the fevered Holcomb Valley mining excitement in the 1860s.

This gold rush began when William F. Holcomb discovered flecks of placer gold at the head of Van Dusen Canyon, one mile west of Arrastre Flat. Hired by other prospectors for his ability with a rifle, Holcomb and a companion trailed a wounded grizzly bear north from Poligue Canyon. His experience prospecting in the mines of the Sierra Nevada's Mother Lode paid off when his bear-tracking led to the alluvial flats on Caribou Creek. Soon the sagebrush-and-pine-dotted basin swarmed with prospectors, and a camp, named Belleville, was erected.

History records that this settlement was one of the least law-abiding of the California gold camps—over 40 men died by hanging or gun battles. Causes for argument included not only the usual charges of claim-jumping and theft, but also political affiliations in the Civil War. Southern sympathizers were particularly numerous, as they had been forcibly ejected from many pro-Northern mining camps in the Mother Lode. Although the site of fevered and hectic activity for almost a decade, Holcomb Valley was relieved of most of its readily accessible placer gold by 1870, and its inhabitants moved on to greener pastures. Belleville was soon a ghost town. Interest in the region revived, however, when hard-rock mines opened to seek the local Mother Lode—the source of the Holcomb Valley placer gold. Soon shafts and their adjunct tailings dotted the land. Lucky Baldwin's Doble Mine was one of these, but, like the other hard-rock mines, it failed to locate the Mother Lode, and it is doubtful that Baldwin recouped his $6 million purchase price for the mine.

The PCT veers south along Gold Mountain's flanks to strike one jeep road, then a second (7630-3.9), which leads north ⅔ mile down to Saragossa Spring. About ¼ mile beyond the next small rise you cross a better road (7560-0.7), then turn southwest down to a tributary of Caribou Creek, dotted with mining ruins.

**Water access:** A mile-long contour then leads to Caribou Creek itself, which rarely flows later than early June, but offers good camping before then. The next water for northbound PCT hikers is not until Little Bear Springs Trail Camp, 10.8 miles; for the southbound, at Doble Trail Camp, 6.3 miles.

Just 0.1 mile beyond Caribou Creek the trail bisects Van Dusen Canyon Road 3N09 (7260-1.8), which leads southeast 3 miles to Big Bear City.

**Resupply access:** Big Bear City, the best resupply town in this section, is closest from this point.

More mountain mahogany, Jeffrey pines and junipers shade the PCT as you leave Van Dusen Canyon, crossing numerous jeep tracks as you make a gentle ascent west under Bertha Ridge. Finally, a switchback leads to a saddle north of Bertha Peak, where you cross a jeep road (7720-1.6), then another (7735-0.7), leading to the summit, in excellent exposures of marble. West of the second road, sweeping vistas open up to the south across dammed Big Bear Lake to Moonridge and to the high summits of the San Gorgonio Wilderness. Just beyond these vistas, the PCT junctions with the Cougar Crest Trail 1E22 (7680-0.4).

**See Maps C6, C7, C8**

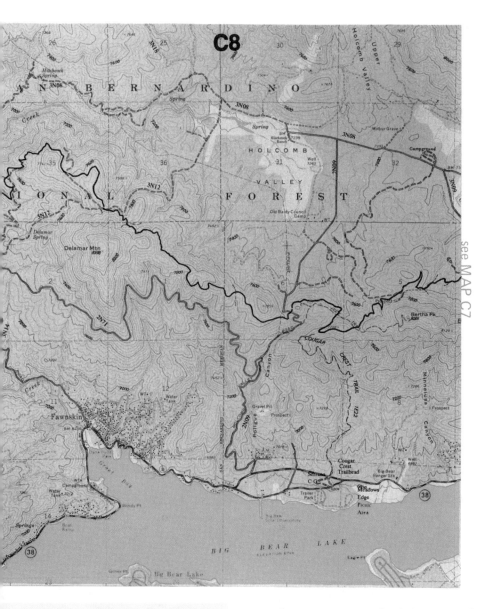

**Resupply access:** This enjoyable path starts west, then heads south 2.0 miles to Highway 38, near Serrano Campground on the north shore of Big Bear Lake—a convenient place from which to hitch-hike either west to Fawnskin, with its limited supplies, or east to Big Bear, with more complete provisions.

The PCT recrosses the last jeep road midway down to wide Holcomb Valley Road 2N09 (7550-0.8).

**Resupply access:** From here travelers can head 3.7 miles to Fawnskin for supplies by first walking south along the dirt road, which descends Poligue Canyon to reach Highway 38 beside Big Bear Lake, then walking west along the highway.

From Holcomb Valley Road the PCT continues its traverse of the San Bernardino Mountains' spine by continuing west, easily up along the south side of Delamar Mountain's east ridge. This pleasant and viewful walk under open conifers and oaks ends after a long mile when the route crosses to the shadier north side of the ridge to traverse past an east-ascending jeep track, then descends to Road 3N12 (7755-2.8), atop a saddle.

**Water access:** Delamar Spring, with poor camping nearby, lies 0.9 mile west down this dirt road.

The PCT contours north from Road 3N12, then arcs west around a nose covered with mountain mahogany before crossing another good dirt road (7610-0.8). Dropping gently, the trail rounds north on a steep hillside with vistas east over Holcomb Valley, but soon turns southwest and eventually strikes a jeep road (7305-1.1), which you follow downhill for 35 yards before resuming trail tread. Next, continued descent for 0.3 mile leads into a small canyon, then northwest along its south wall, then into another similar canyon, now just below a dirt road. Later, near the bottom of Holcomb Creek's wide canyon, the route switchbacks, crosses one poor dirt road, then another, and immediately reaches Little Bear Springs Trail Camp (6600-2.5).

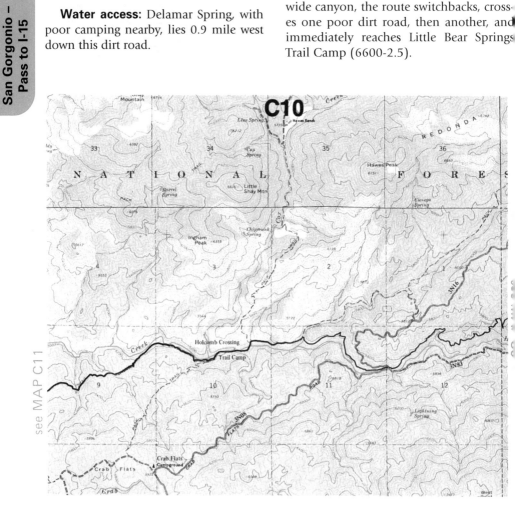

**Water access:** Little Bear Springs Trail Camp has a corral, toilets, benches and piped water. Southbound PCTers should tank up here, since the next seasonal water is 10.8 miles away, at Caribou Creek in Van Dusen Canyon.

Most wilderness lovers will likely not pend the night at this poorly sited camp-ground, which is a haven for buzzing motocross enthusiasts, but rather will sack out farther down Holcomb Creek.

From the trail camp the PCT turns northwest down a creek's mouth to quickly reach the willow-lined, sagebrush-dotted banks of year-round Holcomb Creek. The trail follows its south bank, crossing a jeep road leading to the trail camp, then parallels the lower shoulder of Coxey Road 3N14

as it descends west a few yards to a culvert bridge over Holcomb Creek (6510-0.3).

The PCT resumes above Holcomb Creek's north bank, 35 yards up Coxey Road, and proceeds gently down-canyon in an open ponderosa-pine forest, staying just above canyon-bottom dirt Road 3N93, which is repeatedly drowned under beaver-dammed pools. The trail passes two dirt roads and a jeep track, and then about ½ mile later it turns west up a side canyon, climbing moderately to a saddle (6485-2.1). From it a gentle descent southwest in warm groves of conifers and black oaks leads across a dirt road (6350-0.9), beyond which the route follows a sunny, rock-dotted divide north of Holcomb Creek. Drier conditions prevail as the easy descent continues, eventually leading to a rock-hop

**C** San Gorgonio – Pass to I-15

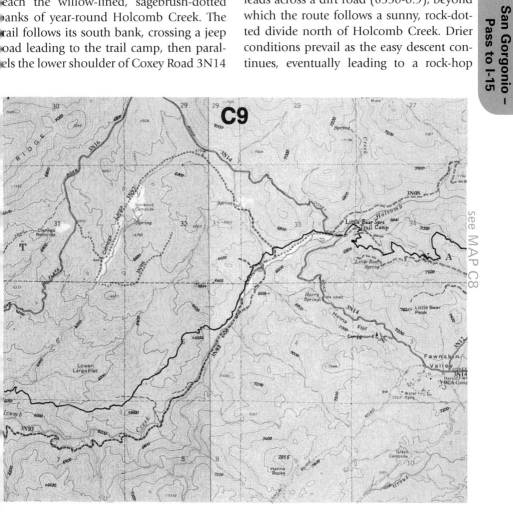

see MAP C8

**See Maps C9, C10**

crossing of the Cienaga Larga fork of Holcomb Creek. From it the trail parallels some 50 feet above shaded, bouldery Holcomb Creek, soon passing some nice campsites and dropping to cross it via boulders. Moments later the streamside canopy of willows and cottonwoods opens where wide Crab Flats Road 3N16 (5465-3.5) has a junction with rough Road 3N93.

The PCT now continues on Holcomb Creek's south bank, via very rocky tread under white alders.

> Most of the alders hereabouts were spared, but the surrounding hillsides are charred by the massive and devastating Willow Fire, which began August 28, 1999. The PCT from this point, all of the way down Holcomb Creek and Deep Creek, to Mojave River Forks Reservoir dam, was blackened by that blaze, started by a thoughtless camper. Much of the streamside vegetation is living, but beware of blow-downs and falling limbs.

Pushing on, you soon enter a sandy flat with adequate camps and again cross Holcomb Creek (5430-0.2). The trail now winds northwest above it in a dry chaparral of mountain mahogany, buckwheat, and yellow, fleshy-petalled flannelbush. Turning more westward, the way drops once again alongside Holcomb Creek, traverses the perimeter of a bouldery sand flat with a good camp, and then crosses the permanent Cienaga Redonda fork of Holcomb Creek to find the north-branching Cienaga Redonda Trail (5325-1.0). Many horned lizards might be seen as the trail continues its gentle descent west on rotting granitic rock along Holcomb Creek and soon enters a grassy flat to reach a junction with the Hawes Ranch Trail (5230-0.4), just shy of the PCT's bouldery fourth ford of Holcomb Creek. Minutes later, one finds Holcomb Crossing Trail Camp (5190-0.3), with fire-

pits and a toilet under large Jeffrey pines thankfully unburned.

A few minutes later, on a side-hill traverse we pass the now-enormously-rutted Crab Flats Trail, which has been heavily abused by motocross riders. Nearing the alder-and-cedar-shaded banks of Holcomb Creek once again, we pass less-appealing signed Bench Camp, and then a few nice ersatz campsites. Soon afterward, the trail ascends onto burned-almost-bare hillsides. In a mile the trail begins to descend, and eventually heads northwest, dropping via four oak-shaded switchbacks to a beautiful 90-foot steel and wood bridge (4580-4.1) spanning Deep Creek. Here the beautiful stream drops between large granitic boulders, and harbors a good population of rainbow trout. Note that all of Deep Creek is a Wild Trout Area (with a two-fish-daily limit, minimum 8″ each, no bait allowed and barbless hooks required).

**Resupply access:** Just beyond the bridge, a good, signed trail strikes left, back upstream, briefly to cross diminutive Bear Creek and hit the end of dirt Hook Creek Road 3N34C. The very busy trailhead, called, "Splinters Cabin," has toilets, tables, and a shady ramada—a perfect lunch spot while waiting for a ride up to Lake Arrowhead. Hook Creek Road leads west, up-canyon 0.5 mile to cross Road 3N34, then later becomes paved and designated 2N26Y, climbing 3½ miles in all past numerous homes and cabins to Lake Arrowhead. Here you find the Cedar Glen Post Office and supermarkets just before meeting Highway 173 near the lakeshore.

After crossing Deep Creek the PCT briefly climbs northeast, then contours under live oaks and near crumbling granitic parapets. Unfortunately, the Willow Fire thoroughly scorched Deep Creek in 1999, and you can expect the entire gorge to be shadeless. After ½ mile the path

San Gorgonio – Pass to I-15

see MAP C12

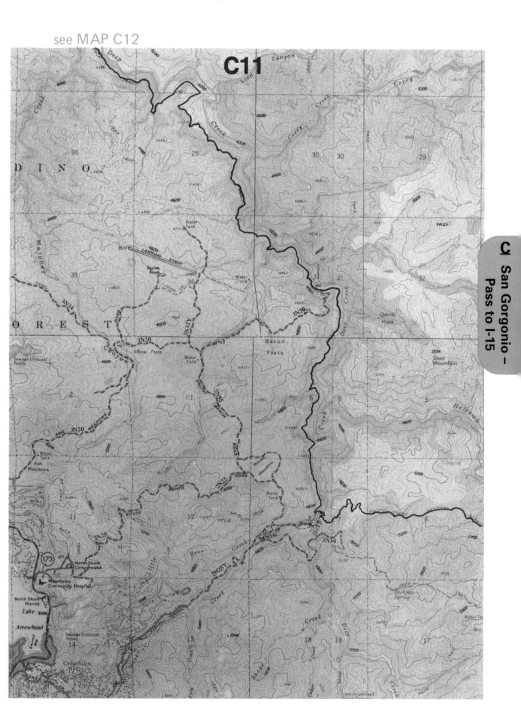

descends gently, matching the gradient of Deep Creek, which is flanked by spruces and pines 140 feet below. The way presently becomes hot and exposed near ocean spray and holly-leaf cherry, and many will wonder why the trail wasn't routed lower, along the cool streamside. Soon you get your answer, in the form of steep, friable bluffs, above which the PCT must skirt. Later, the route bends west and strikes Bacon Flats Road 3N34D (4255-2.6), just above the popular Devil's Hole fishing area. It offers the last chance to head out to Lake Arrowhead to resupply.

Across Bacon Flats Road the PCT winds along the canyon walls, well above quietly flowing Deep Creek and its streamside willows, cottonwoods and alders. Though sometimes shaded by steep, granitic bluffs, your route soon becomes more exposed to sun and seasonally stifling heat.

Your proximity to the Mojave Desert is reflected in both the shimmering heat and in the flora and fauna. Coarse chamise chaparral, harboring flitting phainopeplas and somnolent horned lizards (see picture page 158), lines your way, while scurrying insects and pursuant roadrunners share your sandy path. Rattlesnakes are also seen, although not in the heat of day—their cold-blooded metabolism cannot stand extreme ground temperatures, but they love to bask when shadows are long.

Soon after passing a streamside terrace where the Forest Service plans an equestrian camp, your undulating descent alters its northwest-ward course to a more westward one. Shortly thereafter, it passes a jeep road that rolls ½ mile east to Warm Spring, and then it drops ¼ south to Deep Creek Hot Spring (3535-6.8), which is situated on a prominent northeast-southwest fault. The hot spring, with its bubbling water, high-diving rocks, warm sunbathing,

and green grass, is a surprisingly popular and crowded spot at almost any time of the year.

Trail-dusty would-be swimmers should heed this caution, however: a very rare, microscopic amoeba living in the hot water has caused deadly amoebic meningoencephalitis by invading a few swimmers' bodies through their noses. Swimming may cut your hike short! Be advised that camping is not allowed in this area, and rangers patrol the trail frequently.

Taking leave of the skinny-dippers, you eventually cross Deep Creek via an arched bridge (3315-2.0), and then start a traverse west along the almost barren north wall of Deep Creek canyon, tracing the route of an old aqueduct. This walk ends at the spillway of the Mojave River Forks

see MAP C14

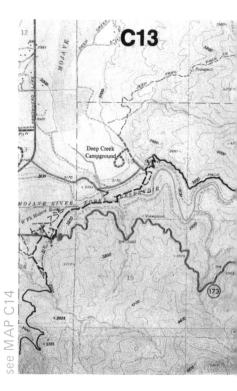

eservoir dam (3131-3.0). This mammoth ood-control dam, over a mile long, is an xample of overkill, since West Fork Mojave tiver and Deep Creek don't have that much low.

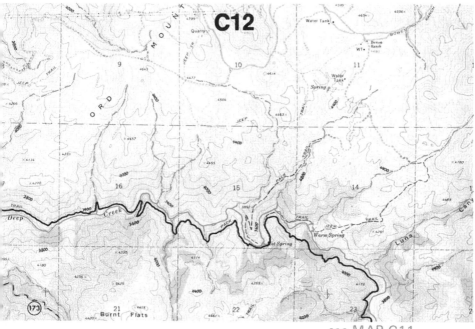

Standing in the maw of the spill-way, we find a small exhibit that describes efforts to save the endangered arroyo southwestern toad. Fair camping exists below the dam's spillway, in groves of willow and cottonwood beside a pooling oxbow in Deep Creek. Pick your campsite with care, since 2-, 3-, and 4-wheeled off-road vehicles can be anywhere. This is the vicinity of an old Mojave Native American village called Atongai. It was visited by Padre Garces, a member of de Anza's expeditions, in 1776. A mission was built hereabouts in 1819. Rallying, the indige-nous tribes massacred the missionaries a

few years later. Their efforts against the Army Corps of Engineers were apparently less successful.

The next morning, rejoin the PCT atop the dam. The designated PCT route from this point actually drops southwest back to the foot of the dam, on flats beside Deep Creek, but an overgrowth of brush, fields of nettle and foxtails, and a welter of dirt-bike paths have essentially obliterated the way. Instead, cross the spillway, then turn up to the crest of the dam at a paved spur. Now proceed left, in a westward arc across the top of the boulder-faced dam, treading a one-lane paved road. The dam ends on the eastern shoulder of Hill 3353 at a road junction (3170-0.6), close beside a small concrete building with a tall radio mast.

**Resupply access:** Hesperia can be reached from this point. Continue walk-

**C** San Gorgonio – Pass to I-15

**C12**

see MAP C11

**See Maps C13, C14**

ing westerly on the paved road, swinging north around Hill 3353, then across the top of another dam segment, eventually reaching busy, two-lane paved Arrowhead Lake Road (0.7). Now walk right (north), gently down past increasing numbers of homes, about 6 miles to downtown Hesperia.

Hesperia Lake Park is found on the right in just 2.8 miles, offering cool, shady camping beside a small lake, with showers, phones, and a small convenience store. For more information contact Hesperia Recreation and Parks District, 7500 Arrowhead Lake Road, Hesperia CA 92340, or call (619) 244-5951.

From the western end of Mojave River Forks Dam, the PCT turns left, southeast from atop the dam's paved road, dropping moderately down a gravel road that traces the edge of the dam's face. This road services a paralleling row of 4-5-foot-high white and black posts that mark theoretical depths of the reservoir, after some future biblical rainfall. At the base of the dam, a 10-foot-tall, white-metal depth marker (3000-0.2) indicates the point where the now-more-visible original PCT route joins levelly from the left (east). Turn right (southwest), on the sandy trail, and in just a moment plunge through a phalanx of willows to a usually shallow but wide and rocky ford (2295-0.1) to the south side of Deep Creek. Now scramble up a sandy bank to a low alluvial terrace, just west of the mouth of a small, rocky canyon. Here the trail—an old jeep track—becomes more distinct. Trace it west above a fringe of baccharis and willows before dropping again to the creekside. Here, Deep Creek is sucked north through the dam, down a massive, iron-gated outlet tunnel.

From here, you're back on a trail, which winds west in a thicket of willows

and cottonwoods that show evidence of beaver cuttings. These trees are just south of another sandy arroyo, this one draining ephemeral West Fork Mojave River. Presently you cross the base of a narrow ravine where your trail begins to trace the grade of an abandoned, torn-up paved road (3010-0.4). This is followed moderately uphill, southwest, giving you a fair overlook of the "reservoir." Soon you level out on a terrace to strike a wide turnout on a curve of Highway 173 (3190-0.4).

Across Highway 173, pick up a new segment of signed PCT and follow it almost levelly south along a fence line in open chaparral. After a bit, the path begins an easy, sandy ascent, soon striking the end of a little-used jeep road (3205-0.4). Now the path climbs briefly south into a small canyon, then ascends around several ridges on a southward, winding course, soon leveling in the process to undulate at about 3500 feet. Just after heading around a north-dropping ridge, you reach a small canyon that spawns a trailside spring (3470-1.7). This flows through late spring of most years, but has no nearby camping. Turning more westward, the route traverses hillsides clothed in an open, desert-dry low chaparral of chamise, buckwheat and flannelbush, with panoramas northwest over the broad expanse of Summit Valley to the aberrant alluvial scarp forming its northern limit.

This long, steep-faced ridge is actually the upslope edge of an early Pleistocene alluvial fan, whose sediments originally came from canyons of the San Gabriel Mountains, seen far to the west. However, subsequent right-lateral movement along the San Andreas Fault displaced the range northwest, thereby cutting off the fan's source of sediments. Continuing lateral and vertical movement along the San Andreas Fault and associated parallel faults not only altered the

**See Map C14**

San Gorgonio – I-15 Pass to I-15    C

landscape but also brought about drastic changes in the stream-drainage pattern.

The PCT drops slightly as it winds south into a broad valley, then climbs to a ridgetop saddle where it joins a jeep road (3430-1.5) serving a powerline. You follow this road south down to an easy ford of Grass Valley Creek (3330-0.3), which flows most summers. Unfortunately, private lands prohibit camping here. The trail resumes just across the stream, on the jeep road's east (left) side, and momentarily it crosses a second, poor jeep track before climbing northwest. Around a nose, the trail hairpins south across another steep jeep road (3480-0.7), then undulates interminably west in and out of gullies and ravines in shadeless chaparral. About halfway to Silverwood Lake, you come to a flat area where an ascending jeep road from Highway 173 seems to terminate upon reaching the PCT (3480-2.6).

**Resupply access:** This road can be followed 0.2 mile north down to two-lane, paved Highway 173, clearly visible along the south margin of arid Summit Valley. Follow Hwy. 173 left (west), 0.1 mile to Summit Valley Country Store, with a good selection of snacks, well-deserved cold drinks, and camping foods, and a telephone. The store sits 1.7 miles east of where the PCT later strikes Highway 173 at the spillway of Cedar Springs Dam.

Back on the PCT and refreshed by a cool drink, you continue winding almost levelly west. Eventually the way strikes Road 2N33 (3400-2.2), a paved road ascending west to the nearby east end of Cedar Springs Dam. Walking a few minutes up to that end will give you vistas over giant Silverwood Lake, which is part of the California Aqueduct system. From Road 2N33 the PCT descends steeply, then turns south around a sharp ridge and joins a west-branching dirt road close under the base of 249-foot high, rockfill Cedar Springs Dam.

PCT travelers lacking a fast mode of transportation might be less than enthused to learn that the active Cleghorn Mountain Fault lies not far south of the damsite: the reservoir's northern east-west arms lie along the fault.

Now, possibly with a brisker stride, you turn west down the dirt road for a few yards to the end of a poorly paved road (3170-0.4) that bridges the canyon bottom and continues northwest to some dam-maintenance facilities. Follow the poor road left, gently up onto a sandy flat, to a paved road just east of the large maintenance sheds. Turn right, north, along that short road's west shoulder, through a hurricane fence and out to two-lane paved Highway 173 (3175-0.3) at a line of junipers. Now walk left, west, on the highway shoulder, crossing a bridge that straddles the concrete spillway flume of Cedar Springs Dam. Pass dirt Las Flores Ranch Road and an access road to new Mojave Siphon Power Plant, to the next road on the south (3200-0.5), a very poor dirt road angling southwest, up the brushy hillside. Here the PCT's overgrown trail tread resumes, climbing parallel to the dirt road, which is immediately above it.

Many hikers have complained that the start of this trail segment is indistinct, and it is, though it is marked by a PCT post at the roadside. The segment is also quite overgrown with brush farther on, as is much of the route around Silverwood Lake.

Entering Silverwood Lake State Recreation Area, the PCT continues below the road for a bit, then crosses it and switchbacks southeast to a nearby saddle (3460-

**See Maps C14, C15**

C San Gorgonio – Pass to I-15

0.6), on which it crosses a similar road. Here northbound hikers gain their first vistas over windy Silverwood Lake. The warm water will likely prove irresistible to most, as the PCT route traverses near the reservoir's western shoreline. Twice you follow jeep roads for 60 yards as the route winds through sparse chaparral, crossing many gullies. North of the westernmost arm of northern Silverwood Lake, a meager spring wets the trail, then the path meanders south before climbing moderately east above the Chamise Boat-in Picnic Area, which lacks running water. Now 200 feet above the reservoir, you pass onto a hillside scorched by a fire that started at the picnic area, then the trail bends south to an

unsigned spur trail (3580-2.5) that drops south to another trail and to Garces Overlook—an octagonal hilltop gazebo—which makes a fine, albeit waterless, picnic spot.

Back on the PCT, you descend easily west across a jeep road (3455-0.8) and eventually come to a paved, two-lane bike path (3390-0.7) next to a paved road leading east to Cleghorn Picnic Area, which has water, tables, bathrooms and telephones. This junction is not signed, but is easy to spot, coming southbound on the PCT, if you look carefully: It is 80 yards east of where the infant, usually dry West Fork Mojave River passes under the bike path via a cattle grate. The trail leaves from

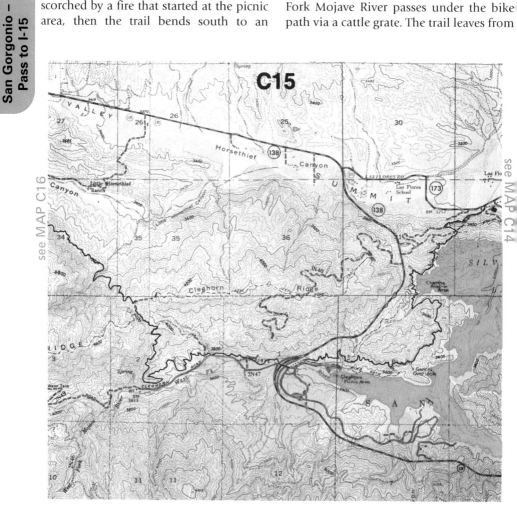

a curve in the path that is farthest from the paved road to the picnic area. Heading toward Oregon on the PCT, walk southwest across the Mojave River's wash and slightly up to a signed junction (3380-0.1) with another paved bike path that leads west, towards the group-camp complex. Follow the path up to the paved Silverwood Lake State Recreation Area's entrance road (3390-0.1).

**Resupply access:** This road may be traced south to the entrance station and then 1.7 miles east beyond it for camping, water, showers, telephones and a small store and cafe at the reservoir's marina. Northbound hikers must note

that the next certain water lies in lower Crowder Canyon, 13.2 miles west of the SRA, while, except for the reservoir, the next water for those southbound flows in Grass Valley Creek, 11.5 miles east.

Continuing on the PCT route from the SRA entrance, you first walk west under the Highway 138 overpass to its offramp (3395-0.1). From here one may hitchhike southeast to Crestline for supplies at its post office and stores. Here too, the trail resumes at the offramp's junction with the SRA's entrance road. PCT posts and ducks lead northwest from a concrete culvert across a small grassy field to five sycamores,

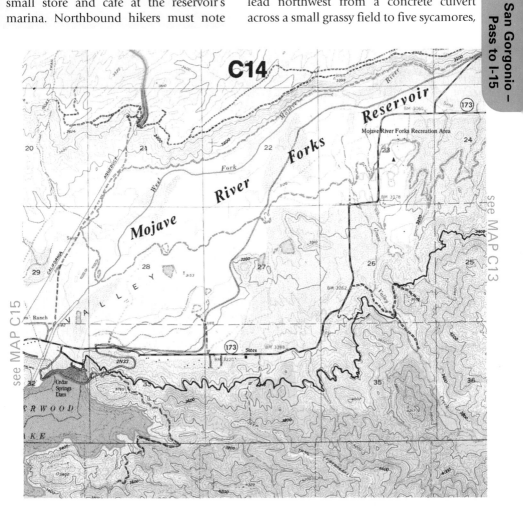

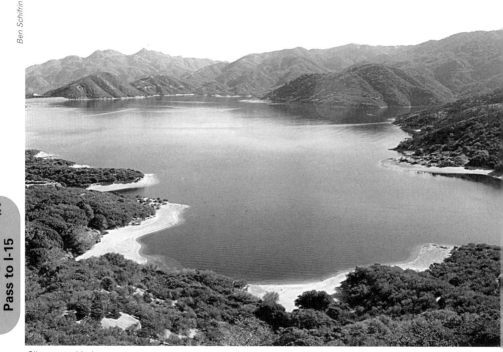

*Silverwood Lake*

clustered against the northern hillside. Here tread becomes more distinct. The PCT leads gently up-canyon, then dips into West Fork Mojave River's sandy wash for a moment before crossing a dirt road that serves a small picnic area (3440-0.4). From it the route continues up along the base of a canyon wall cloaked in chamise, buckwheat and pungent yerba santa. The trail's tread is interrupted as you follow the paved group-camp access road for 25 yards, then it resumes to strike a narrow paved road (3530-0.4) that climbs steeply to a water tank. Three lavish group camps lie just down this road, in Silverwood Lake State Recreation Area.

Now you leave the SRA and begin climbing in earnest, winding southwest up numerous dry gulches, then around an east-jutting nose, and finally turning north up to join a jeep road (4040-2.2) at a small promontory. Here the PCT turns west, fol-

lowing the track which climbs moderately to its junction with a road (4160-0.3) atop viewful Cleghorn Ridge.

Eastward gazes take in the Lake Arrowhead region, Miller Canyon, Silverwood Lake and West Fork Mojave River, the last three aligned along the east-west Cleghorn Fault, which separates Mesozoic granitic rocks, found here, north of the fault, from older Precambrian metamorphic rocks south of the fault.

Resuming your trek, you follow the ridge road north 100 yards down to where the trail's tread resumes. The way descends moderately northwest across hillside gullies, presently reaching a deeper canyon with a small stream (3830-0.9), which usually flows through late spring. No camping is possible, however. The next leg winds

**See Map C15**

northwest across numerous similar ravines while it contours above ranches in Little Horsethief Canyon.

This canyon and Horsethief Canyon to its north commemorate Captain Gabriel Moraga's pursuit of a Native American band whom he suspected of horsethievery in 1819. The first known crossing of nearby Cajon Pass occurred in 1772, and this key pass was heavily used by the Mormon Battalion and Death Valley borax teams.

Eventually the route drops into the canyon's head, where PCT posts show the way through a grassy flat. The Forest Service plans to build a trail camp with well water here.

Your trail turns north across Little Horsethief Canyon's dry creek bed (3570-2.8), ignoring a use-trail that continues up-canyon, then climbs again, up to a narrow ridgecrest, which you traverse in low, bedraggled chamise chaparral—an impoverished indicator of your proximity to the Mojave Desert. Another fire has charred this area. It did not affect navigation but certainly adds to the feeling of desolation. The PCT then proceeds west up into another draw, and near its head strikes a road (3840-2.5) under a huge power-transmission line. You walk across the road, then west along a spur beneath a mammoth power pylon. Trail tread continues west from here, vaguely at first along a gravelly wash, then more obviously as it climbs to an overlook of spectacularly eroded badlands above Cajon Canyon.

**C San Gorgonio – Pass to I-15**

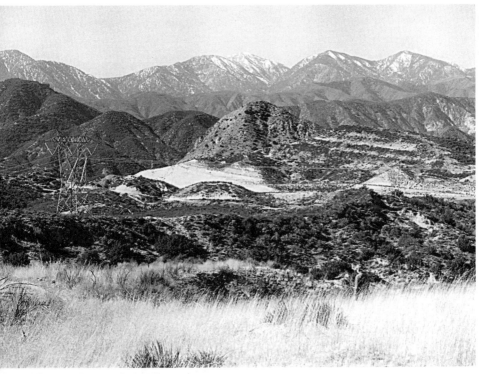

Ben Schifrin

*Mount San Antonio from Road 3N44*

**See Maps C15, C16**

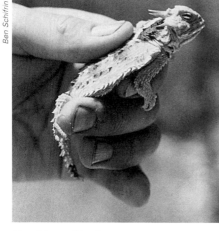

*Coast horned toad*

Because these sediments have been removed from their source of rejuvenating alluvium, stream flow has easily incised their once gently sloping surfaces into a dramatic series of razorback ridges.

The path climbs to top the most spectacular of these ridges, then winds tortuously down, west, along it, giving you superb vistas of the San Gabriel Mountains' crown, Mount San Antonio, and of Lytle Creek Ridge, which you will climb on the PCT one day hence. Presently you cross Road 3N44 (3355-2.4) and minutes later you pass through a burnt gate on a saddle, and then descend easily southwest. You quickly cross another road (3300-0.4), from which well-marked trail tread resumes to lead west, momentarily passing under power-transmission pylon #63 to strike the previous descending dirt road (3265-0.2). Here the PCT turns left, south, down the road as it drops steeply into quiet Crowder Canyon, dotted with baccaris and willows.

The Pliocene sediments here were eroded from the infant San Gabriel Mountains, then shifted east, relatively speaking, along the San Andreas Fault, which now cuts through Cajon Canyon, below.

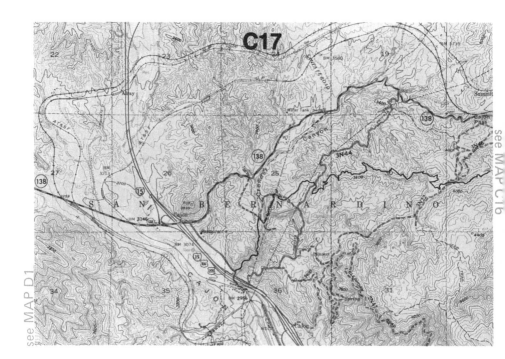

**See Maps C16, C17**

There, just shy of a hop-across ford of sandy, always-flowing-a-little Crowder Canyon Creek, you end the descent at a post-marked merger with a better dirt road (3140-0.3), which goes briefly down-canyon to another power pylon.

A cluster of cottonwoods and baccharis, teeming with birds, at this three-way junction would make the best camp since Silverwood Lake. You follow the PCT, which proceeds right, northwest, directly across the cress-decked creekbed, then leads 90 yards uphill across a buried gas pipeline to a wood PCT post, which marks the resumption of trail heading left, south, onto an alluvial bench.

**Water access:** This pleasant path winds along the narrow, shady gorge of lower Crowder Canyon, where pools and trickles of water (3045-0.3) afford the last on-route water until Guffy Campground, a long 23 miles away.

The trail ends abruptly at six-lane Interstate 15 (3000-0.4) in Cajon Canyon, just south of a roadend memorial to Santa Fe Trail pioneers.

**Resupply access:** No facilities are available here (save for a weighing station on the freeway if your backpack loads are "over gross"), but they are found in Wrightwood and San Bernardino, as described in the introduction to this section. Just 0.5 mile northwest up the access road to the trail's terminus, just 0.1 before the Route 138 cloverleaf, is a Chevron gas station with a large convenience market, and a McDonald's restaurant. If no palatable water is available in lower Crowder Canyon, this restaurant is a recommended detour. Just west of the cloverleaf are two more gas stations, another mini-mart, a Del Taco restaurant, and the ECONOmy Inn motel (described on page 129).

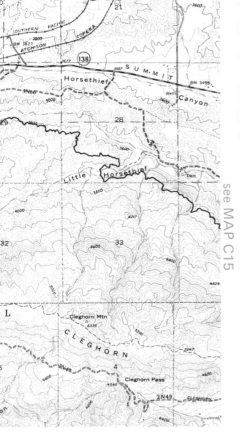

**See Map C17**

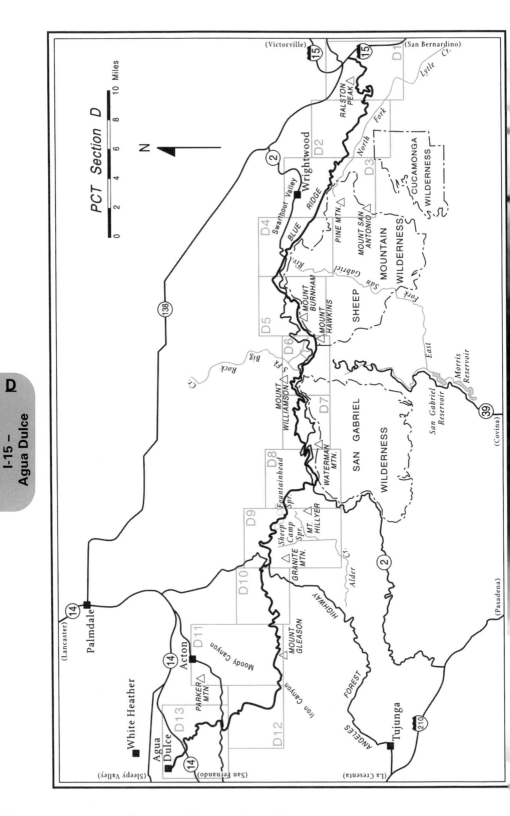

# Section D:

# Interstate 15 near Cajon Pass to Agua Dulce

True to its name, the Pacific Crest Trail through the San Gabriel Mountains remains on or close to the watershed dividing streams that flow into the Pacific Ocean from those that run north, losing themselves in the sand or evaporating from muddy playas in the Mojave Desert. The PCT climbs quickly from smoggy, arid Cajon Canyon to the subalpine reaches of the San Gabriel Mountains, and soon ascends its Southern California apex—wind-torn, 9399-foot Mount Baden–Powell. Most of the PCT's winding route lies between these two extremes, treaded in pine-needle duff under groves of shading, hospitable Transition Zone forest trees: Jeffrey pine, incense-cedar, black oak, sugar pine, white fir and water-loving white alder.

Except for frequent roads and resorts that the PCT skirts, much of the trail route traverses country unchanged, at first glance, by the encroachment of modern man. But on closer inspection, the San Gabriels are seen to be no longer the wild and remote range that moved legendary mountaineer John Muir to call them "more rigidly inaccessible than any other I ever attempted to penetrate." Man has tamed the San Gabriels' clawing chaparral and steep-walled gorges with miles of highway, and has prevented once-devastating floods with dams and catchment basins. Bears and bighorn sheep, which once roamed the range, have been driven by thousands of hikers, skiers, picnickers, hunters and loggers into the most remote and forbidding canyons. The forests, however, show the most insidious and far-reaching effects of California's burgeoning population. Smog, that yellow pall that has made Los Angeles infamous, now rises well into the surrounding mountains, and the pollutants are severely damaging trees—yellowed needles on thousands of acres of dying pines and firs are mute testimony.

A part of the Transverse Ranges geologic province, the San Gabriels are thought to be rather young, at least in their present stature. Despite their relative youth, geologists state that some of California's oldest rocks lie in the San Gabriels. Precambrian anorthosite (a light-colored, plutonic rock composed almost entirely of plagioclase feldspar and high in aluminum content) and gabbro estimated to be 1.22 billion years old both line the PCT route in the vicinity of Mt. Gleason. These rocks are much older than most of the rocks along the San Gabriel Mountains segment of the PCT. Most of the trail tread lies in familiar granitic rocks of Mesozoic age; these were intruded at the same time as similar rocks in the Sierra, San Bernardino and San Jacinto mountains, and in Baja California. Other rocks, like the Pelona schist, which you first encounter on Upper Lytle Creek Ridge as you enter the San Gabriels, are metamorphic rocks, once volcanic and ocean-bottom sediments, which may have been altered by the intruding granites.

The present-day San Gabriels are a complex range, cut by and rising along numerous faults that occur along their every side. The major San Andreas Fault is the most famous, and it bounds the San Gabriels on their northern and eastern margins. This great fault stretches from near Cape Mendocino southeast about 1000 miles into the Gulf of California. Geologists now know that hundreds of miles of horizontal shift along the fault (with the western side moving north) have occurred in the last 30 million years, since about the time the fault first formed. Where the San Andreas Fault slashes through Cajon Canyon, at the start of this section, one can see an example of long-term motion along the fault: the bizarre Mormon Rocks and Rock Candy Mountains, all sedimentary rocks, lie northeast of the fault about 25 miles east of related rocks at the Devils Punchbowl, on the fault's southwest side. The Punchbowl and the trace of the San Andreas Fault can be seen easily atop Mount Williamson, a short side hike from the PCT.

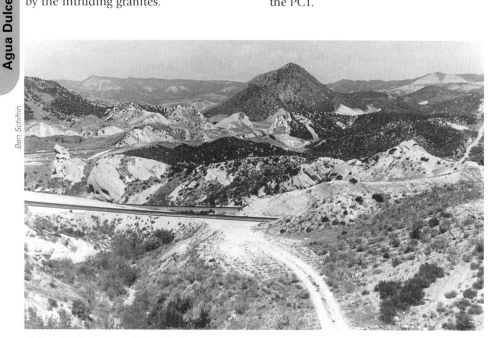

Railroad at Cajon Pass–Sullivan's Curve

# Maps

| | |
|---|---|
| *Cajon* | *Waterman Mountain* |
| *Telegraph Peak* | *Chilao Flat* |
| *Mount San Antonio* | *Pacifico Mountain* |
| *Mescal Creek* | *Acton* |
| *Valyermo* | *Agua Dulce* |
| *Crystal Lake* | |

# Declination
13½°E

| Points on Route | S→N | Mi. Btwn. Pts. | N→S |
|---|---|---|---|
| Interstate 15 near Cajon Pass | 0.0 | | 112.5 |
| | | 5.5 | |
| Swarthout Canyon Road | 5.5 | | 107.0 |
| | | 4.4 | |
| Sharpless Ranch Road 3N29 | 9.9 | | 102.6 |
| | | 11.3 | |
| Acorn Canyon Trail to Wrightwood | 21.2 | | 91.5 |
| | | 0.9 | |
| Guffy Campground | 22.1 | | 90.4 |
| | | 6.1 | |
| Grassy Hollow Family Campground | 28.2 | | 84.3 |
| | | 1.3 | |
| Jackson Flat Group Campground | 29.5 | | 83.0 |
| | | 4.0 | |
| Lamel Spring Trail | 33.5 | | 79.0 |
| | | 5.7 | |
| Lily Spring Trail | 39.2 | | 72.4 |
| | | 2.0 | |
| Little Jimmy Campground | 41.2 | | 71.3 |
| | | 7.2 | |
| Rattlesnake Trail | 48.4 | | 64.1 |
| | | 4.1 | |
| Cooper Canyon Trail Campground | 52.5 | | 60.0 |
| | | 7.5 | |
| Three Points | 60.0 | | 52.5 |
| | | 3.3 | |
| Sulphur Springs Campground | 63.3 | | 49.2 |
| | | 12.3 | |
| Mill Creek Summit Picnic Area | 75.6 | | 36.9 |
| | | 11.8 | |
| Messenger Flats Campground | 87.4 | | 25.1 |
| | | 5.5 | |
| North Fork Saddle Ranger Station | 92.9 | | 19.6 |
| | | 8.7 | |
| Soledad Canyon Road | 101.6 | | 10.9 |
| | | 7.0 | |
| Antelope Valley Freeway at Escondido Canyon | 108.6 | | 3.9 |
| | | 3.1 | |
| Vasquez Rocks County Park entrance | 111.7 | | 0.8 |
| | | 0.8 | |
| Agua Dulce | 112.5 | | 0.0 |

**D**

**I-15 –
Agua Dulce**

## Weather To Go

Mount Baden–Powell and the other San Gabriel crest peaks usually maintain a heavy snowpack until mid-May. But May is otherwise the nicest time to traverse this section. Before then, expect most of the trail to be snowbound. By June, the trail's lower reaches, at either end of the section, can be oppressively warm.

## Supplies

At the Start of Section D, minimal supplies can be purchased at either of two convenience stores at the freeway overpass 0.6 mile north of the trail's beginning. A complete selection of needed items may be purchased in San Bernardino, 17 miles south on Interstate 15. Be sure to restock on water before leaving Cajon Canyon, since the next water won't be found until Guffy Campground, high in the San Gabriels, about 22 miles away. Wrightwood, a ski-resort community with a post office, stores, restaurants, and motels, is the next possible supply point. In the past, a PCT register has been kept at the pharmacy. Check with the Methodist Church camp— they sometimes offer bunks, showers and laundry facilities. Wrightwood is a 4.4-mile round-trip detour down from the PCT via the Acorn Canyon Trail, 21 miles from Interstate 15. Alternately, reach it by hitch-hiking east on busy Angeles Crest Highway 2, 27.2 miles from the start of this section. From Wrightwood, inexpensive public buses leave four times daily to Victorville. This large, sprawling Mojave Desert community has neither Wrightwood's charm nor cool temperatures, but it does afford many more conveniences.

Acton, a small town with a post office, grocery stores and motel, lies 5.8 miles east off the PCT route in Soledad Canyon, about 100 miles from Interstate 15. Saugus, a larger town with complete amenities, lies west of the PCT some 12½ miles from the

same point in Soledad Canyon. Agua Dulce, at the end of Section D, is the most logical resupply point, and a long carry from Wrightwood. Now a rapidly growing ranching center, the village of Agua Dulce has a small convenience store but, as of 2001, neither a full grocery store nor a post office (the closest is in Acton). It does have three great restaurants, a hardware store, a feed store, a veterinarian, and a hair salon. This area may also have the largest concentration of dedicated "trail angels" anywhere along the PCT. Ask at the store or any of the restaurants for a referral to one of these families, or subscribe to the Internet's PCT-List at *PCT-L@mailman.backcountry.net*, for up-to-date seasonal contact information.

## Water

While generally well-watered, the San Gabriel Mountains nonetheless pose a challenge to the PCT walker in search of regular water sources. This is especially true at either end of the mountain chain, where lower elevations and the proximity to the fiery Mojave Desert create an arid chaparral, with few permanent springs or streams. Carry plenty of water for the long, hard uphill day at the start of this section, to reach water at Guffy Campground. From there, you should encounter water a few times a day, from natural sources or campgrounds. By summertime, however, don't count on stream-flowing water in most creeks. West of North Fork Saddle Ranger Station, the pickings again become slim—don't count on water, except at human-made facilities.

## Permits

Day-hikers and section-hikers, but not thru-hikers, will be affected by the National Forest Adventure Pass system now in effect for all parked cars within Southern California's national forests. This pass is required for all vehicles, while parked along any road or even at a designated trailhead, in Angeles, Cleveland, Los Padres and San Bernardino National Forests. It is not required for PCT travelers, per se. Cost Is $5 per visit to one forest, or $30 per year (good for all four forests). Plans are to return 85% of collected monies to the individual forest for human-use enhancing projects. Passes can be purchased from the USFS, from Southern California outdoor shops and multiple vendors near or in the forests.

No wilderness permits are required for overnight PCT campers, since the route just barely touches the borders of the Sheep Mountain and San Gabriel wilderness areas.

## Special Problems

### Fires

Note that, even with a campfire permit, open fires are NOT ALLOWED at any site outside of a designated campground in the Angeles National Forest, due to the extreme fire danger. This is a compelling reason for all hikers to carry a gas stove throughout their trip.

### Poison Oak

See this section of Chapter 2.

# The Route

The beginning of Section D is reached by taking Interstate 15 north 17 miles from San Bernardino to the "Palmdale Highway 138/Silverwood Lake" exit. Atop the offramp, turn right and head 12 yards east along Highway 138 to paved Wagon Train Road, the frontage road that branches south. Paralleling Interstate 15, take this road down past a gas station, mini-market, and a McDonald's restaurant,

0.6 mile to its end beside a stone monument to Santa Fe Trail pioneers. This spot is just short of narrow Crowder Canyon, the PCT's route. Just south of the memorial plaque, the Pacific Crest Trail curves south under the freeway via a boxed culvert, emerging on the other side in a verdant thicket. The author has found water running here even in midsummer of severe drought years. The route becomes a sandy-muddy jeep track paralleling the freeway. Moments later, you pass under the wooden Atchison-Topeka and Santa Fe Railroad trestle, then turn right, to follow a jeep road west, just below the tracks, well-marked by PCT posts. Just north of a fenced private home, PCT trail tread resumes (2930-0.4) branching obliquely left, west-southwest, from the jeep trail, and marked by a yellow PCT post. The path winds levelly through a desert chaparral, soon to encounter a welter of faint side paths. This is San Bernardino County's Elsie Arey May Nature Center. Hikers should spend a few minutes here, walking the trails, to learn to identify the common chaparral plant species that are here described on trailside plaques. Beyond this instructive herbarium, the PCT swings south, up and over a sandy ridge on a well-signed route, then dips to a rough dirt road that heads west to Sullivan's Curve, an historic railroad grade. Cross this road, then walk down a short trailless wash to a culvert under another AT&SF railroad track. Now walk right, southwest, up a faint path that parallels the rails, to find the PCT climbing south once again, via two small, overgrown switchbacks.

Soon the trail crosses the newer Southern Pacific Railroad tracks (3020-0.8) and swings to the right along a dirt access road for 30 yards, before bending southwest to wind among the hills and sandstone-conglomerate outcrops of the Mormon Rocks, a badland of Miocene alluvium. At one point you amble south along a jeep road (keeping to the right where the

**See Map D1**

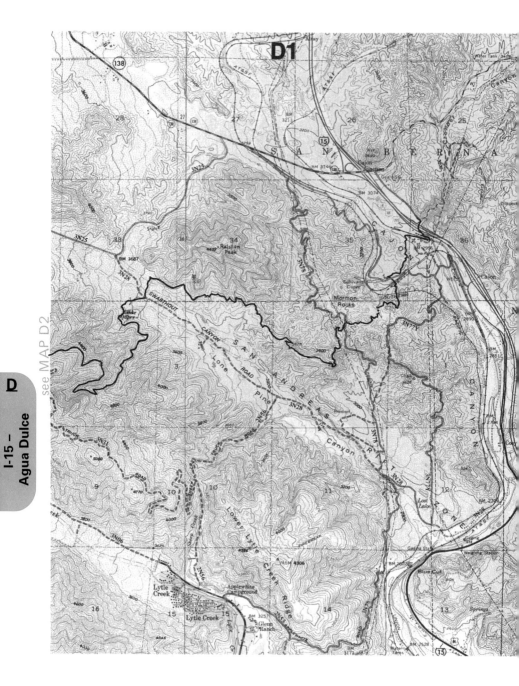

see MAP D2

road forks) for 100 yards, before trail tread resumes on the right side of the road.

The Mormon Rocks commemorate Mormon pioneers who were among the first Caucasians to utilize Cajon Pass, and who settled San Bernardino Valley. Pedro Fages, who on one trip discovered the Colorado Desert and the San Jacinto Mountains, crossed the mountains in this vicinity when he tired of leading a contingent to capture Army deserters, and an urge to explore captured him. The De Anza-Garces forces passed near here 4 years after Fages, in 1776, on their way north from Sonora, Mexico. By 1813 the Cajon Pass route, part of the Santa Fe Trail, was seeing frequent use by American trapper-trader Ewing Young and others. The Mormon Battalion used this route both coming from and going to the Great Salt Lake, and borax teams from Death Valley and the Santa Fe Railroad also crossed here.

Pushing on, you cross first one powerline road, Road 3N78, and then in ¼ mile cross another (3360-1.2) amid bush sunflower, chamise and scattered cacti. Upon reaching the second powerline road, ascend south up the road for 150 yards before resuming trail tread on the right side of the road. Next the PCT ascends to a sandy ridge dominating lower Lone Pine Canyon, eroded along the San Andreas Fault. The path traverses this ridge, which presents some striking blue clays, then cuts across sandy washes under the south face of Ralston Peak to dirt Swarthout Canyon Road 3N28 (3560-3.1). The PCT route strikes invisibly west from the road, marked by 4x4 posts in the cobbly alluvium, then turns south across a bouldery wash to a jeep road (3700-0.5). Two vandalized concrete tubs at Bike Springs are found just yards north, but they have been dry more often than not in recent years. Even when water is running, its heavily polluted nature relegates it to emergency use only. Four white PVC pipes have been driven here in the dry wash, and will eventually be developed as a well, hopefully with a horse camp. No reliable water is available yet, as of Spring 2002.

Attacking the chaparral-clothed eastern flanks of Upper Lytle Creek Ridge, the trail swings into a canyon, then switchbacks north, up across three canyons to finally strike dirt Sharpless Ranch Road 3N29 (5150-3.9) near the ridge's crest. Now, on a segment of trail built in 1994 by PCTA volunteers to avoid a shooting-range on the south side of Upper Lytle Creek Ridge, you round a nose and amble more-or-less levelly west on the cooler northern slopes, just yards below ridgetop Sheep Creek Truck Road. At the next gap in the ridge (5260-1.0), you find remains of the old south-side PCT tread, and might choose to walk up to the ridgetop, where cooling vistas are had of the snow-dappled Mt. San Antonio massif and the rugged Cucamonga Wilderness, to the west and southwest, above North Fork Lytle Creek.

In the 1890s Lytle Creek was the setting for a spirited but short-lived gold rush.

Continuing on, your path ascends gently, keeping to the ridge's steep north side, where you parallel arid Lone Pine Canyon from a slightly cooler vantage. Eventually, you cross dirt Sheep Creek Truck Road 3N31 (6300-3.2), at an intersection where it turns northwest to drop into Lone Pine Canyon. **Now your chia-lined path crosses to the south side of the ridge, and in a few minutes finds a small, viewful ridge-top flat (6350-0.2), where, under a cluster of shady big-cone spruce, one could make the first nice camp west of Cajon Pass.** Unfortunately, the site is waterless. Beyond it, you wind south around a

**D**

**I-15 – Agua Dulce**

**See Maps D1, D2, D3**

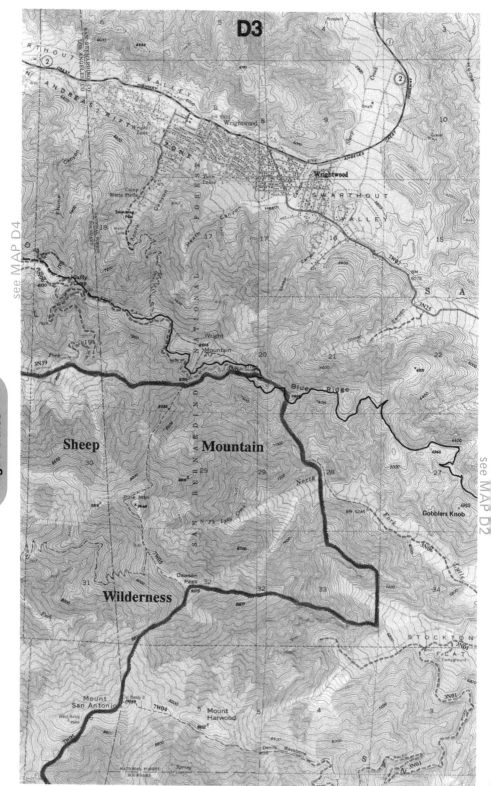

see MAP D4

see MAP D2

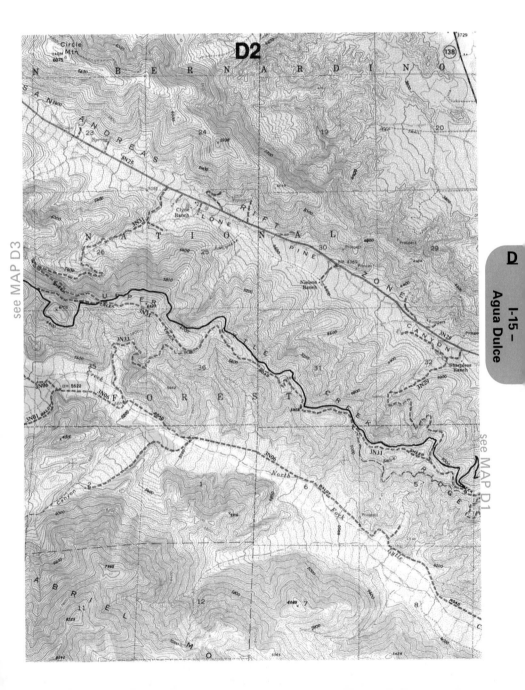

see MAP D3

see MAP D1

D

I-15 –
Agua Dulce

prominence to a roadend (6480-0.9) just east of Gobber's Knob.

Above this point the way used to be more shaded, by frequent groves of big-cone spruce, mountain mahogany and some juniper. Sadly, a man-caused fire here in the early 1990s burned many of the trees.

As the route swings under Blue Ridge, both the Devils Backbone and Dawson Peak dominate the southern horizon, thrusting ridges of platy brown Pelona schist above tree line. These points mark the eastern boundary of Angeles National Forest's new Sheep Mountain Wilderness, a 43,600-acre preserve which protects the rugged San Gabriel River drainage, just west of Mt. San Antonio.

Look for black-granular phyllite and outcrops of white quartz and fibrous green, shiny actinolite, a close relative of asbestos, in the schist before the PCT switchbacks east up to a jeep road (8115-4.3) atop Blue Ridge. This road climbs northwest up to a posted trailhead (8176-0.1) just north of the jeep road's intersection with Road 3N06. Here you can gaze north down to Wrightwood, across the north face of Wright Mountain, where cycles of mudflows, triggered by the melting of winter snows, have cut a spectacular, barren swath. The PCT contours south around Jeffrey-pine-forested Wright Mountain, staying just above dirt Road 3N06.

Soon Prairie Fork San Gabriel River comes into view, incised along the San Jacinto Fault. Mount Baden–Powell dominates the western horizon, while San Gabriel Valley smog is partly screened by the Pine Mountain Ridge to the south.

West of Wright Mountain you meet the Acorn Canyon Trail (8250-1.6).

**Resupply access:** This path descends 2 miles north to a road that drops 1½ miles to the western edge of Wrightwood. The next possibility for reprovisioning on the route lies in Agua Dulce, about 89 miles ahead.

The PCT continues west up Blue Ridge, sometimes on Road 3N06, but often to its north on short trail segments. It enters Angeles National Forest and arrives at Guffy Campground (8225-0.9).

**Water access:** Guffy Campground has water at a good spring reached by a side trail 270 yards down Flume Canyon to the north. Trekkers have frequently complained that water here, the first logical campsite west of Interstate 15, was hard to find. It can be, especially during the summer of drought years. A better strategem for thru-hikers in those years would be to detour to Wrightwood, the best resupply point in this section, and avoid the uncertainty.

Continuing, the trail, often sited on old, narrow dirt roads, continues mostly north of Blue Ridge's crest, offering vistas to the north over Swarthout Valley and the San Andreas Fault Zone to pinyon-cloaked ridges abutting the Mojave Desert. You descend easily in fine mixed-conifer forest around Blue Ridge's high point, eventually reaching a dirt road (8115-2.3) beside an artificial lake, enclosed by a high fence. This is one of two reservoirs serving the snowmaking operations of the Mountain High Ski Area, which has ski-lift terminals that you will pass in the next mile. Here, turn left, south, briefly up over the ridgecrest, through a large white pipe gate to Road 3N06, which you follow right, west, for a minute to access a resumption of PCT pathway (8120-0.1) on the west side of the reservoir. This leads back up to the ridgetop, from which you wind down in nice fir forest, beside a ski run, to again strike Road 3N06 (7955-0.4). As indicated by white metal PCT posts, you cross the road and descend a few feet to traverse the western perimeter of pleasant but waterless Blue Ridge Campground (7910-0.1). Beyond the campground, you parallel the boundary of Sheep Mountain Wilderness, the rugged chaos of mostly trailless ridges and gorges to your southwest.

The Narrows Fire, a 9,437-acre wildfire, burned a large portion of the headwaters of East Fork San Gabriel River canyon hereabouts during August 1997. It was started by a hiker who was conscientiously but unwisely burning toilet paper. Suppression of the blaze required an estimated $8 million. You'll encounter burned terrain off and on along upper Blue Ridge, to Grassy Hollow Visitor Center.

Atop the second hill along your way, you find the second artificial lakelet and some more ski lifts, and the path is forced directly onto the brink of Bear Gulch's steep headwall. Beyond, you cross or swing next to now-paved Road 3N06 several more times. Black oaks and white firs join the ecosystem as you near Angeles Crest Highway 2 (7386-2.2), just east of Inspiration Point, a sweeping overlook of the East Fork San Gabriel River basin.

Carefully cross the highway to a paved parking area, which has bathrooms but no water. Here a white metal PCT post marks your route, branching left, west, from short Lightning Ridge Nature Trail. Ascend easily past a returning loop of the nature trail, then drop west through flats of whitethorn and bitter cherry to reach forested Grassy Hollow Visitor Center (7300-1.0), with water, toilets, and a large, new interpretive center and part-time ranger station.

About ½ mile northwest of the campground the PCT route goes along Jackson Flat Road 3N26 for 100 yards before returning to trail tread on the north side of Blue Ridge. Next on the itinerary is a short spur (7480-1.3) to walk-in Jackson Flat Group Campground, in shading pines and firs. It has piped water and toilets throughout summer, even in drought years. After passing north of Jackson Flat and turning Blue Ridge, the PCT drops south across Road 3N26 (7220-1.5), then switchbacks moderately down past interior live oaks and ocean spray to Angeles Crest Highway 2 at Vincent Gulch Divide (6585-0.8).

South of the highway, beside a parking area and a trail east to the interesting Bighorn Mine, is Mount Baden–Powell Trail 8W05—a popular pilgrimage for Southern California Boy Scouts. You take this trail, which starts southwest before switchbacking gently-to-moderately up in Jeffrey-pine/white-fir groves on crunchy Pelona schist tread. After a number of switchbacks you reach a side trail (7765-1.7) that contours 100 yards south to Lamel Spring. This marks a good rest stop, and one might choose to camp at either of two level spots a minute farther along the main trail. With care, adequate camping for a dozen hikers can be found hereabouts.

Above, the switchbacks become tighter, the air grows crisper, and firs give way to lodgepole pines, which yield in turn, above 8800 feet, to sweeping-branched, wind-loving limber pines. These hunched, gnarled conifers, believed by some botanists to be 2000 years old, are the only obvious living things at the Mount Baden–Powell Spur Trail (9245-2.1).

**Side route:** Take this side hike to the 9399-foot summit for superlative views north across desert to the southern Sierra, west to Mt. Gleason, south down Iron Fork San Gabriel River (in Sheep Mountain Wilderness) to the Santa Ana Mountains, and east to Mts. San Antonio, San Gorgonio and San Jacinto. On the clearest days, Mt. Whitney, still 3–4 weeks to

**D**

**I-15 – Agua Dulce**

**See Maps D4, D5**

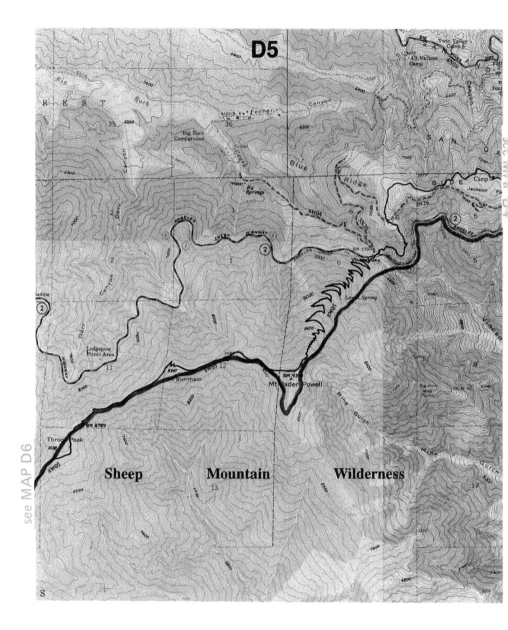

your north, and Telescope Peak, overlooking Death Valley, can be seen. A concrete monument here is a tribute to Lord Baden–Powell, founder of the Boy Scout movement. This summit marks the terminus of the Silver Moccasin Trail, Scouting's 53-mile challenge through the San Gabriel Mountains, which is congruent with the PCT until Three Points, about 23 miles away.

Back on the PCT, your route bears west, descending the steep ridge under Mt. Burnham. **A number of small, exceptionally scenic but waterless camps can be made along the ridgeline between Mount**

**See Map D5**

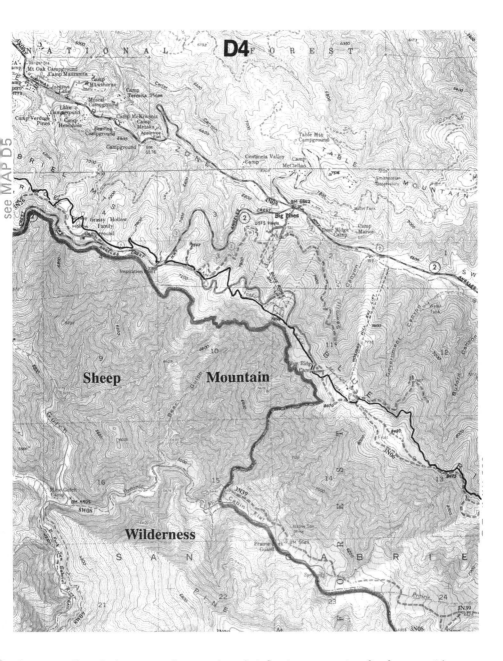

**Baden–Powell and Throop Peak.** In early season, melting snowdrifts might be a source of water. Later, ascend two small switchbacks and pass a signed spur trail that heads north down the shoulder of Throop Peak to Dawson Saddle. You climb briefly in open pine-fir forest, with an understory of manzanita, whitethorn and sagebrush, to navigate Throop Peak's east and south slopes, where you briefly enter Sheep Mountain Wilderness. More descent follows, past a signed lateral to the summit

**See Map D5**

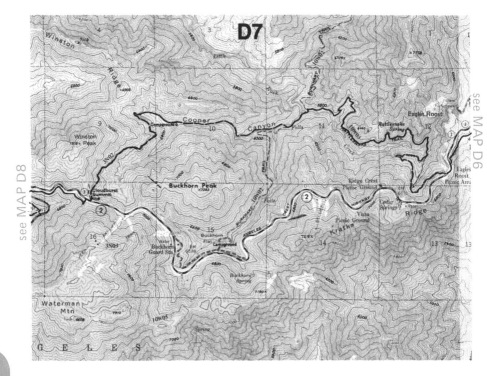

of Mt. Hawkins. Then, on the sparsely conifered ridge west of that peak, you pass a lateral (8540-3.6) that drops ⅓ mile north to Lily Spring. Just a bit later, you pass another signed lateral trail, this one south to South Mt. Hawkins, before an aggressive descent ensues, bringing you to aptly named Windy Gap (7588-1.6), from where a trail drops south to campgrounds in the Crystal Lake Recreation Area. From here the PCT descends north off the ridge to Little Jimmy Spring (7460-0.2), lying just below the trail. This is the last water until Little Rock Creek, in 7.7 miles. Little Jimmy Campground (7450-0.2) is just a couple of minutes farther, with toilets, tables and firepits.

Beyond the campground you curve west on a trail that soon passes above Windy Spring. Now your route parallels dirt Road 9W03, keeping some distance below it. Presently, the road hairpins across

the trail (7360-1.2), and here you should find a sign identifying the PCT route. The trail heads west moderately down to Angeles Crest Highway 2 (6670-1.0), reaching it just east of its Islip Saddle intersection with now-closed Highway 39. Just west of the parking area and restrooms on Islip Saddle, turn right on Mount Williamson Trail 9W02 and ascend moderately northwest past white firs and whitethorn ceanothus to the Mount Williamson Summit Trail (7900-1.6), which climbs 0.4 mile north to good views of fault-churned Devils Punchbowl. While you switchback west down from your ridgetop, you can look south down deep ravines in the friable tonalite to the San Gabriel Wilderness, which is a Southern California refuge of mountain bighorn sheep. Ending the descent, the route merges with a jeep road for 200 yards, and then crosses Angeles Crest Highway 2 (6700-1.3).

**See Maps D6, D7**

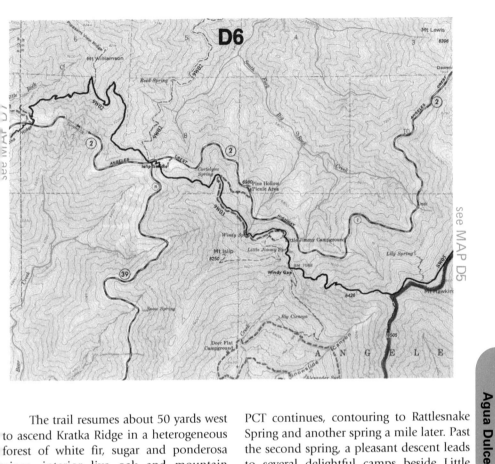

The trail resumes about 50 yards west to ascend Kratka Ridge in a heterogeneous forest of white fir, sugar and ponderosa pines, interior live oak and mountain mahogany. Soon, you descend back to Angeles Crest Highway, where you walk along the southern road shoulder, past a large tan metal highway-maintenance shed for 180 yards to waterless Eagles Roost Picnic Area (6650-0.9). At its entrance just west of the highway, turn west down a rocky, unsigned and unused dirt road and descend to its end at Rattlesnake Trail 10W03 (6165-1.2), in a shady gully. This little-used path drops north under the stone gaze of the cliff now known to rock climbers as Williamson Rock (leaving behind an older, poor path that climbs south), and crosses melodious Little Rock Creek (6080-0.3) in cedar-lined Rattlesnake Canyon. A cozy camp can be made here by the stream, but no more campsites are available as the

PCT continues, contouring to Rattlesnake Spring and another spring a mile later. Past the second spring, a pleasant descent leads to several delightful camps beside Little Rock Creek, where the PCT merges with Burkhart Trail 10W02 (5640-2.3) and turns south across the stream to ascend southwest into Cooper Canyon. Past a pristine waterfall and the south-branching Burkhart Trail (5730-0.3), which climbs to Buckhorn Flat Campground, the PCT route becomes an often steep jeep road, Road 3N02. You ascend it to pleasantly shaded Cooper Canyon Trail Campground (6240-1.2), with reliable water. Here PCT trail tread branches right, northwest from the still-climbing road, briefly paralleling it before turning north up a ravine. In a sunny open forest of Jeffrey pine amid tufts of silvery-leaved, multi-hued lupine, the way winds up and across a hillside, merges subtly with a disused jeep road, and winds to a ridgetop

**See Map D7**

gap (6700-1.0) at the head of Winston Ridge. Here you can look west down brushy Squaw Canyon to the Sulfur Spring vicinity. Now the jeep-road-cum-trail ambles gently up over the eastern shoulder of Winston Peak, then drops momentarily to cross the better dirt road (6640-0.6) that returns to Cooper Canyon Trail Campground. Below that road, your way traverses southwest back into Cooper Canyon, where a tier of sandy flats, shaded by pines, fir and cedar next to the permanent, trickling headwaters of Cooper Canyon Creek (6530-0.4) affords the last nice camps before Sulfur Springs Campground. Now, via small, steep switchbacks, the PCT tackles the finals slopes to gain the better dirt road just below its end at Cloudburst Summit (7018-0.8). Here, you cross the Angeles Crest Highway again.

On the west side of this forested gap, the path drops to contour just south of the highway in open forest, then crosses the highway (6735-0.9) again below a hairpin turn. Now you follow another gated jeep road, Road 10W15, which makes a switchback down into the head of Cloudburst Canyon, where you find a road junction (6545-0.6) with a dirt spur leading west down to Camp Pajarito. Here brown plastic PCT posts point your way straight ahead, contouring southwest across the dry creekbed, and below two water tanks. Easy, shaded descent carries you below the highway, soon reaching a small saddle atop which sits Camp Glenwood. **Water is available here.** Two minutes west of the camp's lodge, treading on the dirt access road, you pass a 14-foot-high, narrow steel water tank. Here the PCT drifts right, west-southwest, away from the road, onto a poor dirt road, indicated by plastic posts. In a moment, you dip across a culverted gully and walk up to a slightly better dirt road, which strikes left, south, for just a few yards to reach Highway 2 (6320-1.3). Now turn right, west, on the highway shoulder for 80 yards to a saddle with a large parking pull-out. Here we cross south to briefly ascend a dwindling dirt

road (still Road 10W15). After a few minutes, gentle descent resumes, this time above the highway, to emerge from big-cone spruce at Three Points (5885-1.9) on the Angeles Crest Highway.

The Chilao Flat/Waterman Mountain Trail here continues southwest, but the PCT goes north across the highway. In a moment it reaches Horse Flat Road 3N17 and a trailhead parking area with restrooms and seasonal water. This is just beyond the left-branching Silver Moccasin Trail, which continues west to Bandido Campground and Chilao Flat. Across gravel Horse Flat Road, the PCT, indicated by a signpost, continues north, climbing slightly onto a granite-sand hillside shaded by interior live oaks. A northward contour on this slope soon ends as the PCT swings west through a gap, then drops gently west under big-cone spruces to an unused dirt road (5760-1.5). Turn left along this track, descending to reach, in 200 yards, a continuation of the trail, which branches right from the track. This short leg drops to another dirt road (5655-0.2) which, like the one before it, leads left to populous Pasadena Camp. The PCT here follows the gently descending dirt road north just 130 yards down to a resumption of trail where the road ends. Winding in and out of small, sandy ravines, the trail descends easily out onto a chaparralled ridge on a more-or-less northward tack. This descent ends at a usually dry streambed, where the trail climbs for a moment to terminate on an old jeep road. Turn right, east, down the ravine for a moment to find a signed trail junction (5240-1.5). Here the hiker-only PCT branches left, while the signed equestrian PCT heads right, northeast, down to a dirt roadend and a stone water trough marking the horsemen's section of lovely Sulphur Springs Campground (5200-0.1).

**Water access:** Good water, lasting until summer, and adequate campsites

**See Maps D7, D8**

are available in the main campground, 0.2 mile east down the oiled access road.

The PCT leaves the environs of Sulphur Springs Campground via two different routes. From the trail junction southwest of the equestrian camp, the foot trail contours northwest on the shaded hillside above South Fork Little Rock Creek, then gently descends to step across that spring-flowing rivulet. A minute later, you merge with the signed equestrian trail. The horse route leaves the campground at its western entrance via its previously paved access, Road 5N40H. This ambles northwest, just north of South Fork Little Rock Creek, to a resumption of trail tread, which drops left, southwest, away from the road for a few yards to merge with the foot trail (5265-0.5). Now you wind up-canyon, generally west-northwest, through sagebrush and scattered pines to clamber to the shoulder of dirt Little Rock Creek Road 5N04 (5320-0.3), just a moment west of its junction with the road to Sulphur Springs Campground. Across the road, the tread steeply ascends a brushy ravine, then circles northwest. This section was recently rerouted away from its previous location in Pinyon Flats, the second place in Southern California where the PCT needed relocation to avoid gunfire from a shooting range—unfortunate reminders of our proximity to big-city violence. Continuing, you invisibly merge with the old alignment, and gently but relentlessly proceed up the brushy hillside.

Soon your path starts to zigzag in and out of numerous small ravines, sometimes shaded in their bottoms by interior live oaks, but usually a sunny mixture of ocean spray, hoary-leaved ceanothus, yellow-blossomed flannelbush, and pungent yerba santa. Eventually the PCT winds through a gap (5830-2.1) and turns southwest at the head of Bare Mountain Canyon, but not before you notice how easily the orange-rust-stained, rotting granite is quickly eroded by torrential rains into a badland of sharp-crested, barren ravines. Just below the level of a saddle at the head of Bare Mountain Canyon, the route turns northwest, then switchbacks briefly south, and ascends easily northwest to a grassy flat just shy of a shaded, seeping spring (6240-1.1) that emerges from the side of Pacifico Mountain. **An emergency camp may be made here, but be aware that the spring may be dry by early summer of drought years.**

Leaving the spring, your path climbs north to a notched ridge, then swings west to a chaparral-and-boulder-choked canyon dampened by Fountainhead Spring, 140 feet above you. Like the previous spring, it may be waterless by early summer of dry years. No camping is afforded here. Next your trail leads into and out of many small gulches clothed in 10-foot-high green-bark ceanothus, but these are soon left behind for a gentle amble up in an open forest of Jeffrey pine floored with rabbitbrush. After gaining Pacifico Mountain's north ridge, the trail swings southwest to a bare ridge-top vista point (6760-1.9), giving panoramas north down Santiago Canyon to Little Rock Reservoir, Soledad Pass, and the environs of Lancaster and Palmdale in the Antelope Valley.

From here the PCT begins a gentle descent southwest on steep, sparsely shaded slopes, passing above Sheep Camp Spring, where a planned side trail and camping area will eventually serve PCT users. Where the trail turns north in a shady gap (6645-0.8), trekkers may leave the PCT and walk south a few yards to a dirt road that can be ascended east to Pacifico Mountain Campground (no water) for outstanding sunrise views.

**Water access:** Here, too, you can descend south on the road and then east on Road 3N17 to a water fountain 0.9 mile from the PCT.

**See Maps D8, D9**

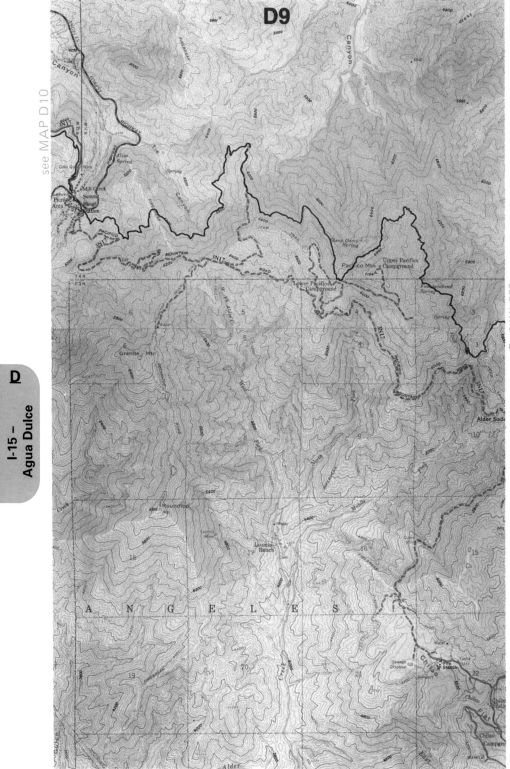

**D**

**I-15 –
Agua Dulce**

D9

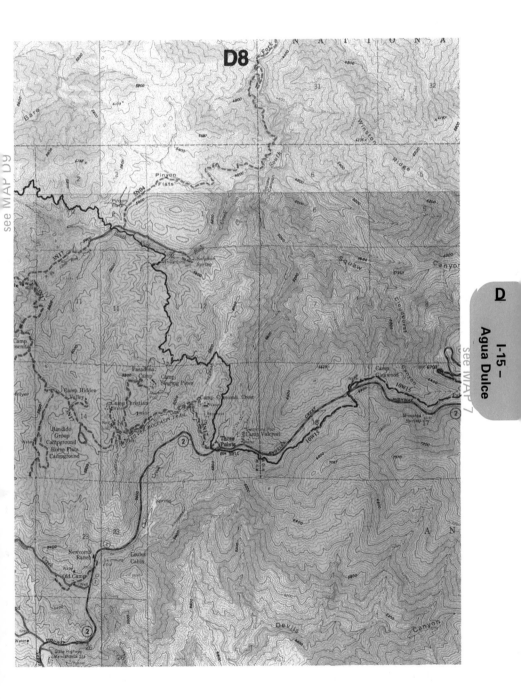

see MAP D9

see MAP 7

**D**

**I-15 –
Agua Dulce**

**D**

**I-15 – Agua Dulce**

Returning to the PCT, you descend gently northwest, then west under shading interior live oaks and big-cone spruces to a jeep road (6380-1.7), which is followed north down to its end and a resumption of trail (6210-0.5). Now the path gently descends the head of spruce-mottled Tie Canyon, named for the railroad ties that were lumbered here in the late 1800s. Lower, you swing west through a Forest Service tree nursery and under the first of a pair of high-tension powerlines, where you find a signed spur trail (4980-3.2). It climbs left, south, for just a few feet to Pacifico Mountain Road 3N17 and a paved PCT trailhead, with toilets, a water fountain and hitching rails. If the fountain is turned off, walk northwest down the paved road for just a minute to the Forest Service's Mill Creek Summit Ranger Station for water. Be sure to tank up here, since the next absolutely certain water on the northbound PCT is at North Fork Saddle, 17.5 miles away.

The PCT itself rounds down below the ranger station and a highway-maintenance yard, soon making tiny switchbacks to reach Angeles Forest Highway at Mill Creek Summit (4910-0.2).

Cut by the Mill Creek Fault, which is the cause of this saddle, the Mill Creek/Big Tujunga Wash area was the scene of a considerable mining rush in the 1880s, with men searching for the legendary Los Padres gold mines.

**Water access:** Aliso Spring, which is never dry, is found 0.7 mile east down Angeles Forest Highway, should no water be available around Mill Creek Summit.

North across Angeles Forest Highway, the PCT begins to climb close alongside paved Mt. Gleason Road 3N17, then leaves yerba-santa scrub as it turns west, just north of the ridgetop, in shading interior-live-oak stands. Frequent glimpses north include the shimmering Antelope Valley and the barren Sierra Pelona (Spanish for "a bald range—or ridge—devoid of trees"). The PCT dips to cross Mt. Gleason Road (5590-2.6), then keeps north of and below that road. An undulating traverse at about 5600 feet eventually turns south across the nose of a ridge. There it finds a very short, signed side trail (5640-3.1) that drops 80 feet down to cross dirt Road 4N24 and find the new, waterless location of Big Buck Trail Camp. It sits just off the road in a pine plantation. The PCT continues south, and soon switchbacks down to a narrow dirt road in a small northeast-trending canyon. Your route follows this track 0.1 mile southwest gently down to dirt Road 4N24 (5500-0.6). Across the road, trail resumes and interior live oaks, ponderosa and Coulter pines, brodiaea and lush grasses line the cooler parts of the way north of the Mt. Gleason Young Adult Conservation Corps Center—once an Army Nike missile base. **Here, in a deep, shady ravine, a flat just below the trail constitutes the best camp between Mill Creek Summit and Messenger Flats (5195-0.8). Water is available here only in earliest spring, but at any time the canopy of oaks, big-cone spruce and incense-cedar makes a nice stopover.** Beyond the camp, the way begins to climb easily, first north around a ridge, then south and west. Later, the PCT switchbacks up to black oaks and Jeffrey pines surrounding a junction with a south branching trail (6360-3.8).

Ignoring a north-branching trail which was part of an earlier, now defunct PCT route down to Acton, you start along the south trail, which climbs for a moment to top Mt. Gleason's north ridge and cross a narrow dirt road (6410-0.1). One could ascend southeast about 300 yards along this road to Mt. Gleason's viewful 6502-foot summit. The PCT, however, crosses the road and abruptly turns downhill into the

**See Maps D9, D10, D11**

head of Paloma Canyon, sadly burned in a Fall 1985 fire. Soon you are switchbacking down on poorly maintained, heavily eroded tread in a charred woodland of oak and manzanita. The trail then quickly makes a traverse just above Santa Clara Divide Road, but after a short while you leave the burned brush behind and, at the entrance to Messenger Flats Campground (5870-0.8), come to within a few feet of that road.

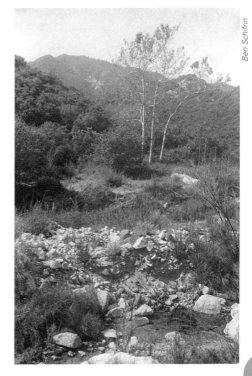

Ben Schifrin

Messenger Flats Campground a delightful area, nestled in a stand of ponderosa pines, has 10 campsites plus tables, toilets and a horse corral. Piped water is usually available during the spring and summer hiking seasons. **Contaminated water here has, occasionally in the past, sickened groups of PCT hikers, so you might be wise to filter it.**

*Mattox Canyon Ford, view southwest*

**Water access:** The next certain water is at North Fork Ranger Station, in 5.5 miles. Water is sometimes found in early spring just before the PCT crosses Moody Canyon Road—1.4 miles from Messenger Flats Campground.

Leaving the campground, the PCT descends northwest momentarily, staying on the road's northern shoulder. This gentle descent soon becomes moderate-to-steep, however, as the trail veers from the roadside to traverse under the north rim of the Santa Clara Divide. This 1980s trail segment is narrower and more tortuous than you have become used to. It was built by Forest Service crews, local Boy Scouts and service clubs after it had become apparent that the original PCT route, northward through Acton, had to be abandoned due to private-property considerations.

Initially you are shaded by the now familiar trio of big-cone spruce, live oak and ponderosa pine, but as the route drops, a low, chamise chaparral supervenes. The

otherwise monotonous scrub does, however, allow you excellent, if smog-shrouded, vistas north over Soledad Canyon and Acton, and northwest to ranks of low, seasonally green mountains, over which the PCT will pass on its way to the High Sierra. Soon you dip into a small ravine to strike Moody Canyon Road (5320-1.4). Seasonal water is available here, from the headwaters of Mill Canyon. Hikers desperately low on supplies could follow it north down to Acton, 11.6 miles away.

The PCT crosses west below Moody Canyon Road, and adopts a fairly level route, once again under open oak-and-spruce shade. This course eventually leads you to intersect a ridgeline gap and its Santa Clara Divide Road (5425-1.3). Here the PCT and the road coincide, descending gently west for just a moment to the next gap on the ridge, where PCT tread resumes (5395-0.1). Climbing west, initially beside

**D**

**I-15 – Agua Dulce**

**See Maps D11, D12**

see MAP D12

see MAP D10

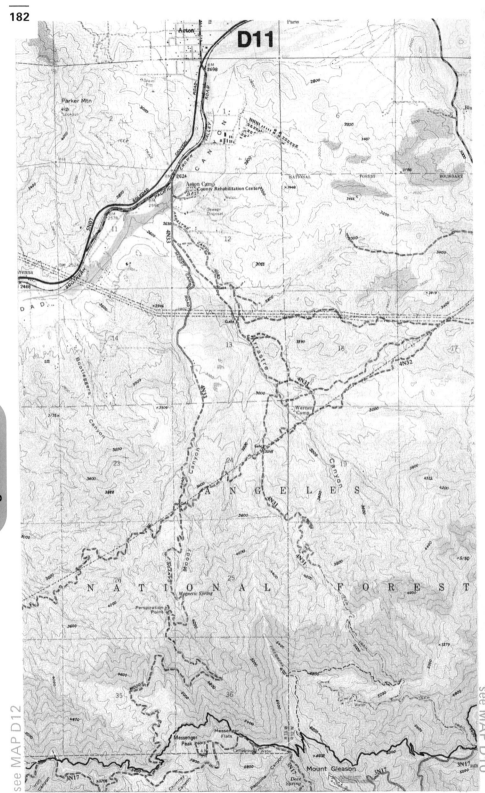

a poor jeep road, the trail now keeps on the sunnier south side of the divide, in low, dry chaparral. Beware of the multitudes of ticks residing on the brush hereabouts, and check your legs for them often. Presently, an easy ascent yields to a gentle descent, and you pass the scattered wreckage of an airplane—its pilot missed clearing the ridge by only a few feet. Soon after, the PCT reaches a firebreak atop the main divide, and descends from its steeply west-descending jeep track (5395-0.7). **Just a minute down the jeep track is a small flat, shaded by a single Coulter pine, which is the only nice, though waterless, campsite between Messenger Flats and North Fork Saddle.**

After an initial descent northeast, the PCT turns northwest to descend moderately across the forested head of Mill Canyon. A few short switchbacks lead to a more earnest descent on often rocky tread. You get frequent glimpses down into Soledad Canyon, and later, as the tree cover thins, you can look northwest to the fantastic, red Vasquez Rocks, this assemblage being the next major point of interest on your northward agenda. Another set of small switchbacks and further bone-jarring presently deposit you at North Fork Saddle, where you find BPL Road 4N32 (4210-2.0), under a crackling high-tension powerline. On the north side of the saddle is the Forest Service's North Fork Saddle Ranger Station, which has year-round water and a picnic

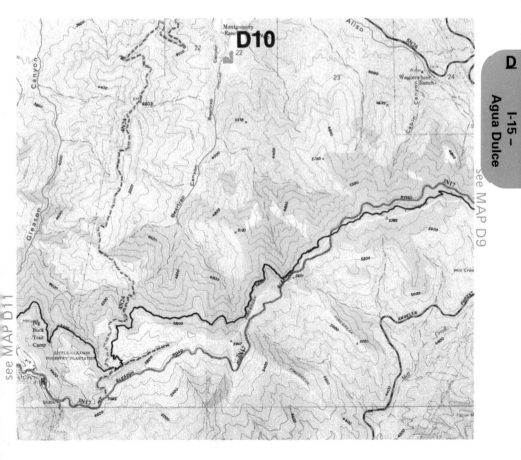

**See Maps D11, D12**

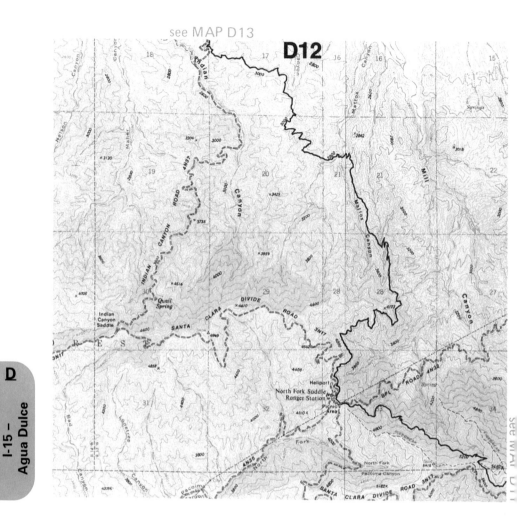

**D12**

area with tables and toilets. **No camping is allowed here, but hikers may camp anywhere along the nearby PCT.**

**Water access:** Northbound trekkers will find their next certain water in Soledad Canyon, 8.7 miles away, while southbound trekkers must carry water at least up to Messenger Flats Campground, 5.5 miles away, or possibly all the way to Mill Creek Summit, a long 17.5 miles away.

Bound for Soledad Canyon, the PCT descends northward from the BPL road, initially just under Santa Clara Divide Road, but soon far below it, on a diagonaling descent on steep, rocky hillsides above Mill Canyon. Soon you are clambering steeply up and down across narrow ravines. Later, the PCT drops at a gentler angle, but as it rounds the east side of point 4173, the path virtually plummets northward, into the head of Mattox Canyon. For the most part, your "economy model" PCT stretch steeply traces a ridgetop firebreak, but in one place, switchbacks do relieve the strain of your aching thigh muscles. When you can afford not to watch your footing, views east reveal a tree plantation in Mill Canyon.

Beside the trail in springtime, yerba santa bears fragrant blue blossoms, and chia and fiddleneck show small purple and white flowers, respectively.

Eventually, you encounter a second set of switchbacks, which deposit you at a step-across ford of Mattox Canyon Creek (2685-4.3). This small stream usually flows into May, but should not be relied on for water. Water access may be more certain a short way back up-canyon.

Some small flats next to the trail—and a pretty line of sycamores—make this the nicest camping area between North Fork Saddle and Soledad Canyon.

Pushing on, you ascend moderately west and north through dry chaparral to gain a 3000-foot ridgecrest. A short drop from its north end leads to a contouring traverse above Fryer Canyon. From here, you can identify the PCT route, under some large pink cliffs, climbing the north slopes of Soledad Canyon. About one mile later, your path starts a swoop down to a nearby saddle, just feet above Indian Canyon Road.

This pass is formed by the Magic Mountain Fault, one of a series of southwest-northeast trending faults that transect the PCT in the next few miles. Notice how the Precambrian feldspar-rich granitic rocks have here been crushed to a fine white powder by the fault's action.

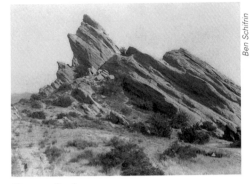

*Vasquez Rocks*

Ben Schifrin

Now the PCT makes a steep initial climb, paralleling Indian Canyon Road 4N37 and staying just above it. In a few minutes you reach a pass and dip to cross this dirt road (2640-3.3), which switchbacks steeply north down into Soledad Canyon. The PCT instead continues west, traversing gently down above the mouth of Indian Canyon before rounding back east to terminate on Indian Canyon Road at a point just 35 yards above that road's signed junction with 2-lane, paved Soledad Canyon Road (2237-1.1).

**Resupply access:** Congratulations are in order at this time, for you have now finished walking the length of the San Gabriel Mountains! Acton, with a post office, market, restaurants and a PCT register, lies 5.8 miles east up Soledad Canyon Road. Saugus, a larger town with complete facilities, is 12.5 miles west down the road. A number of RV parks are found in nearby Soledad Canyon. They all have water, and some offer hikers and equestrians use of their campground, showers, laundromats and small stores. Northbound, the next certain water is in Agua Dulce, 12.0 miles ahead. Southbound trekkers will next get water up at North Fork Saddle, a usually hot 8.7-mile ascent into the San Gabriel Mountains.

**D**

**I-15 –
Agua Dulce**

**See Maps D12, D13**

see MAP E2

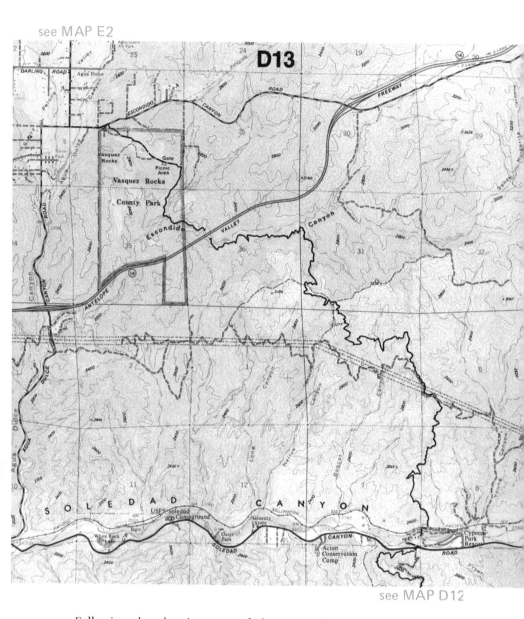

see MAP D12

Following the chaotic route of the northbound PCT across the Santa Clara River on the floor of Soledad Canyon can be very difficult since it is not properly signed. To achieve success, simply keep in mind that you want to attain the railroad tracks running along the north side of the canyon, and respect private property as you go.

From Indian Canyon Road 4N37, northbound PCT travelers amble east along the shoulder of Soledad Canyon Road for about 50 yards to a short, poor dirt-road spur that drops left, down-canyon, toward the riverside. Trail tread resumes from the eastern verge of this spur, marked by a brown metal PCT post. Two tiny switch-

**See Maps D12, D13**

backs drop 20 feet to the alluvial flat, where trail tread is often obscured by a growth of grasses and waist-high mustard. A line of half-buried oil barrels points the trail north, levelly across the sandy wash, which serves as an RV parking lot. (Here you can walk east 3 minutes along a fence around the RVs to the Cypress Park Resort, which welcomes hikers.) You pass a stand of Fremont cottonwoods to reach a ford of the Santa Clara River (2205-0.1). Usually, this ford is accomplished easily via a large log, amid false-willows and large ankle-high patches of watercress.

In the quiet of morning, one might disturb nesting mallards, or a great blue heron fishing in the clear shallow stream for a strange-looking fish, the endangered finger-long three-spine stickleback. This fish is now restricted in range primarily to Soledad and San Francisquito canyons.

Don't dismay if you lose the route as you emerge on the extensively bulldozed north banks of the river. Trail tread is washed away by every spring's floods, and hence the way is often confusing. Your indistinct path empties onto a flat alluvial maze of dirt roads, debris piles, and other assorted rubble. Head north toward the far valley wall via the easiest route. Find a dirt road adjacent to a barbed wire fence, just south of the Southern Pacific Railroad tracks. Now follow the road a short distance right, east, to a break in the fence marked with PCT emblems. It ushers you left, north, across another, better dirt road tracing the southern shoulder of the railroad tracks. This road may be followed east along a line of tables and water spigots to the main camp area of Cypress Park Resort, or a few minutes more to its entrance station, with a convenience store and snack bar. Alternatively, one might amble west into The Robin's Nest RV Park, which also accommodates hikers and equestrians. You step north, up to a stop sign marking your crossing of the Southern Pacific Railroad tracks (2243-0.1). A 3-foot-high cobble-and-concrete obelisk stands to the left of the trail, with a brass plaque embedded in its top that commemorates completion ceremonies for the PCT held here on June 5, 1993.

Leaving the shady canyon bottom to climb briskly back onto a brushy hillside, the trail quickly gains a saddle (2485-0.4), but hardly pauses before continuing upward. Soon you pass beneath strange, pinkish cliffs—our first encounter with the Vasquez Formation, which is a conglomerate of igneous and metamorphic cobbles set in a fine-grained pink siltstone. The sometimes steep ascent finally abates as the trail rounds the east side of a summit to cross Young Canyon Road (2960-1.5), which serves a trio of parallel, humming, high-voltage transmission lines. Across the good dirt road the way swings northwest, descending gently-to-moderately below the road, soon to cross a gap (2780-0.7) near the head of Bobcat Canyon. Around here you see, to the southwest, a spectacular formation of rock-candy pink Vasquez outcrops. Next the PCT climbs a bit, then drops into Bobcat Canyon's dry wash before climbing in earnest to cross a jeep road (3160-1.6) on the divide separating Soledad and Agua Dulce canyons.

Vistas south, east to Mt. Gleason, and north to the Sierra Pelona are obtained as you catch your breath, then you descend west, quickly recrossing the jeep road once, and then again at a saddle (2960-0.5), from where the trail leaves the ridgetop. In an unusual economy of PCT construction, the trail north from this saddle wastes no time—nor does it spare your knees—in a willy-nilly, steep descent north to a narrow branch of Escondido Canyon. After a bone-jarring half mile, the incline abates as the route hops to the ravine's west side, then levels out to turn west along a terrace above

**D**

**I-15 – Agua Dulce**

Escondido Canyon's seasonal creek. White-trunked sycamores in the canyon bottom contrast starkly with the surrounding red, rocky bluffs, dappled by yellow lichens, while yerba santa and white-flowered buckwheat dot the ruddy hillside.

Across the canyon to your north is an even greater contrast—four-lane Antelope Valley Freeway 14 climbing toward Palmdale.

A gradual descent carries you down to the level of the streambed at a side canyon and a use trail from the south (2400-2.0). Here a sunny, if often waterless and noisy, camp could be made. Now Escondido Canyon's trickling springtime stream, lined with watercress, bends more northward, and the PCT follows it, to abruptly enter a lengthy, 10-foot-high tunnel under Antelope Valley Freeway 14 (2370-0.1).

Emerging from the north end of the 500-foot passage, you find an abrupt change of scenery. Here the creekside is lined by thickets of willows and baccharis shrubs, while lush groves of squaw bush, flannelbush, and poison oak stand just back from the creek's edge. The air is noticeably cooler, and myriad birds call from the underbrush.

Your route proceeds directly down the shallow, sandy streambed for a few yards, then picks up a well-traveled path near the creek's north edge. You continue down-canyon and enter Vasquez Rocks County Park.

In the park, note how the canyon's south wall begins to steepen into pink and red cliffs of sandstone and conglomerate. These rocks are layered sediments of Oligocene and Miocene age, having a nonmarine origin.

Your path soon crosses to the canyon's south side, and then ascends slightly under a fantastic precipice of multilayered overhangs. Rounding north of this cliff, the route then drops to cross once again to the north bank (2335-0.6).

Here, at a major side canyon from the north, the southern cliff bulges into a huge, cobbled overhang. Just downstream, the northern canyon wall is also overhung by cliffs. Looking north, you can see the old PCT leading steeply up a hillside. However, the PCT continues to head southwest, downstream, between the purple walls of rock. You will cross the creek six more times, where it seasonally pools and trickles over a sandy bottom. Look for tadpoles, and beware of poison oak and nettles. For a lunch stop, find a delightfully cool cave under an overhang of the tallest southern cliff, or pick the shade of a checkerboard-barked sycamore tree.

Next, you climb easily northwest away from the streamside, up and over the southwest end of a low ridge. A few yards later, find a three-way signed junction with an equestrian trail (2315-0.9), which takes off to the left, southwest. Follow the PCT right, heading northeast up a very steep section of trail. This deposits you on a little-used dirt road on the north rim of Escondido Canyon, surrounded by a springtime profusion of Whipple's yucca. Once on the canyon's rim, you find a different world, an almost flat upland dotted with low buckwheat, sagebrush shrubs and head-high junipers. Lying in the northwest are the spectacular Vasquez Rocks, the 1850s hideout of famed badman Tiburcio Vasquez.

Now begin a very gentle ascent northeast as you parallel the western rim of the major tributary of Escondido Canyon, ignoring a north-branching track. Soon, across the canyon from some ridgetop homes, the route strikes a junction (2435-0.8) with another poor dirt road, descending west. This junction is marked by a yellow pipe post, and on the road, you follow a succession of similar posts west down past a cluster of picnic tables and across a large grassland to a gate (2485-0.1) at a large parking area.

**Water access:** Just before this gate is a green drinking fountain with year-round water, a horse hitching post with its own water supply, and the delightful shade of a large Brazilian pepper tree—perfect for lunch or camping.

From the drinking fountain, the treadless PCT veers right, north for a few yards, then, developing a discernable tread, heads northwest, just to the north of a 20-30-foot-high, overhanging, cobbly cliff band. Walking here may give you a sense of déjà vu—appropriately so, since these spectacular rock outcroppings have been made famous by dozens of cowboy movies and TV ads.

From a rocky gap below the summit of these rocks, you descend easily west. The path now serves dual-duty as a nature trail, and numerous signs teach you the names of many chaparral species that you encounter throughout the park. Soon, you wind near a number of homes just outside the park's north boundary, then amble northwest, around a half-dozen clifflets, to strike Escondido Canyon Road (2510-0.7) at the signed entrance to Vasquez Rocks County Park. The ranger station, where information concerning camping and water may be obtained, is just a minute's walk south down the entrance road.

For the next 2 miles, the PCT is temporarily sited along the shoulder of busy paved roads. Hopefully, this road walk will be eliminated in the next few years. Due in

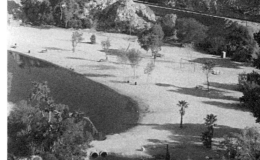

*Soledad Canyon, Bobcat Canyon cliffs*

Ben Schifrin

**D**

**I-15 – Agua Dulce**

large part to tireless lobbying by the PCTA, $1.5 million was appropriated in December 1999 for a 3-mile connector between trail in Vasquez Rocks and lower Mint Canyon. For the time being, though, here you turn left, west, along Escondido Canyon Road, soon coming to a stop sign at larger Agua Dulce Canyon Road (2470-0.3). Turn right, north, onto it, and head into the village of Agua Dulce. Passing a cafe, you soon reach "downtown" Agua Dulce at Darling Road (2530-0.5). Restaurants are nearby, as is a smaller grocery and a feed and supply store for equestrians. Host homes and showers for PCT trailers are available.

**See Map D13**

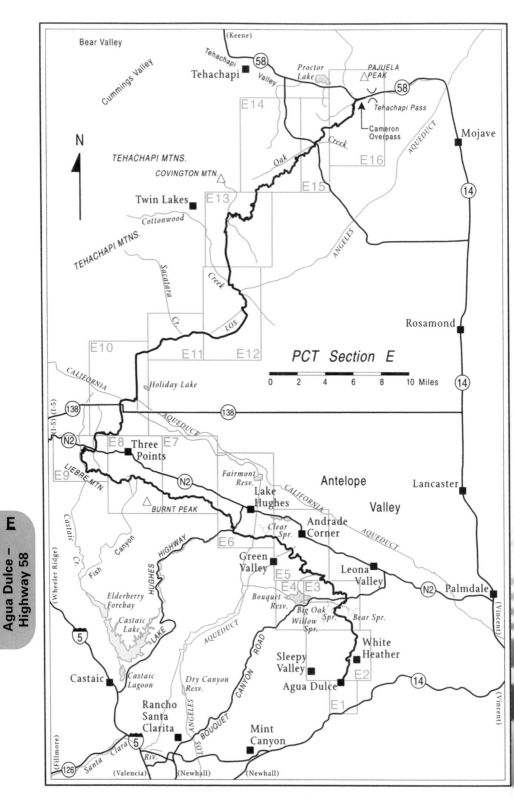

# Section E:

# Agua Dulce to Highway 58 near Mojave

The Mojave Desert is the arid setting for this short, least characteristic segment of the Pacific Crest Trail. Some of the route is not even really trail, but rather it follows dusty dirt roads along the Los Angeles Aqueduct. Congress's original intent was to align the PCT atop the ridge of Liebre Mountain, going all the way west to the vicinity of Quail Lake. (In fact, some of this trail was built by the Forest Service, and later abandoned.) There, it was to ascend into the western Tehachapi Mountains, the start of the Sierran chain, and follow their crest northeast. This route would have had all the necessary characteristics of the Pacific Crest Trail, including mountain vistas, cool black oak and pine forests, and numerous springs. The major snag in the government's plan to construct a true mountain-crest route was the refusal of the owners of the mammoth Tejon Ranch, which lies astride the Tehachapi Mountains, to allow right-of-way for the PCT. After years of wrangling and threatened litigation, the Forest Service surrendered in the contest of wills with so well-

heeled an adversary. Hence, no mountain path now connects the Southern California PCT with its Sierran continuation. A hot, waterless, dangerous, ugly and entirely un-Crest-like segment of trail now winds along a gerrymandered route that traces Tejon Ranch's boundaries, and entirely subverts Congress's vision of its greatest National Scenic Trail. Hopefully, future administrations will have the courage to relocate the PCT to its rightful course.

So for the time being, the PCT drops north from Liebre Mountain, abandoning any pretense of being a crest route, and strikes north across the heart of the Antelope Valley, which is the western arm of the immense Mojave Desert. The pronghorn antelopes seen by John C. Frémont when in 1844 he forced passage through Tejon Pass via this valley are gone, exterminated by hunters and later by encroaching alfalfa fields, but Antelope Valley's desert flavor remains.

Even in early spring, temperatures can soar over 100°F, and swirling dust devils can send unwary hikers sprawling or ducking for cover behind a grotesque Joshua tree. The temporary route strikes due north across the shrub-dotted desert, and then, at the alluvial stoop of the Tehachapi Mountains—a southern extension of the Sierra Nevada—you turn east beside the underground Los Angeles Aqueduct.

Beginning in the Owens Valley, on the east side of the Sierra, the Los Angeles Aqueduct was the brain child of William Mulholland, a former L.A. County Water Superintendent. It was constructed in 1913 and later extended northward to the Mono Lake basin. Bitter disputes, court battles, and even shooting wars raged when Owens Valley farmers realized that the water needs of a growing Los Angeles would turn their well-watered agricultural region into a dust bowl. Litigation continues today, as does resentment. But Mulholland is a hero to some Angelenos, for millions of Southern Californians drink Owens Valley water, and without this project Los Angeles might have remained a sleepy patchwork of orange groves.

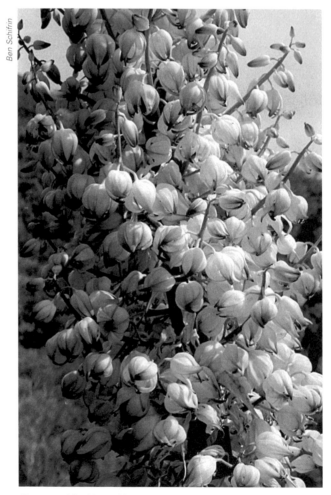

*Creamy white Yucca blossoms*

# Maps

Agua Dulce
Sleepy Valley
Green Valley
Del Sur
Lake Hughes
Burnt Peak
Liebre Mountain

La Liebre Ranch
Neenach School
Fairmont Butte
Tylerhorse Canyon
Tehachapi South
Monolith

# Declination

13¾°E

| Points on Route | S→N | Mi. Btwn. Pts. | N→S |
|---|---|---|---|
| Agua Dulce | 0.0 | 1.8 | 109.3 |
| Old Sierra Highway | 1.8 | 6.8 | 107.5 |
| Bear Spring | 8.6 | 2.2 | 100.7 |
| Bouquet Canyon Road | 10.8 | 6.1 | 98.5 |
| Road 6N09 in Spunky Canyon | 16.9 | 6.3 | 92.4 |
| San Francisquito Canyon Road Ảto Green Valley | 23.2 | 7.6 | 86.1 |
| Elizabeth Lake Canyon Road Ảto Lake Hughes | 30.8 | 7.0 | 78.5 |
| Upper Shake Campground Trail | 37.8 | 6.0 | 71.5 |
| Atmore Meadows Road 7N19 | 43.8 | 4.3 | 65.5 |
| Bear Campground | 48.1 | 6.8 | 61.2 |
| Pine Canyon Road to Three Points | 54.9 | 6.7 | 54.4 |
| Highway 138 | 61.6 | 1.8 | 47.7 |
| California Aqueduct crossing | 63.4 | 3.5 | 45.9 |
| Los Angeles Aqueduct; Ảnorth side Antelope Valley | 66.9 | 11.1 | 42.4 |
| Cottonwood Creek bridge and water | 78.0 | 6.6 | 31.3 |
| Tylerhorse Canyon | 84.7 | 3.9 | 24.7 |
| Gamble Spring Canyon | 88.5 | 12.2 | 20.8 |
| Tehachapi-Willow Springs Road: MOak Creek | 100.7 | 8.6 | 8.6 |
| Highway 58 at Tehachapi Pass | 109.3 | | 0.0 |

## Weather To Go

The second half of this section, north of the California Aqueduct, skirts the summer sunbaked Mojave Desert. Ideally, you'd walk here in April, after winter's incessant frosty winds and at the peak of wildflower displays, but before the 100+-degree days of June. Because most thru-hikers will come here in late May, expect hot, sunny days up to 100 degrees, tempered by cool evenings and pleasant spring conditions in the higher elevations.

## Supplies

The village of Agua Dulce has a small convenience store but, as of 2002, neither a full grocery store nor a post office (the closest is in Acton). It also has three great restaurants, a hardware store, a feed store, a veterinarian, and a hair salon. This area may also have the largest concentration of dedicated "trail angels" anywhere along the length of the PCT. Many hikers reaching this point choose to hitchhike southwest 14 miles on Highway 14 to Saugus, a large town with complete accommodations.

Later, the settlement of Green Valley is a short detour from the PCT where it drops into San Francisquito Canyon, 22.6 miles from Agua Dulce. It is reached by walking southwest 1.7 miles down San Francisquito Canyon Road to Spunky Canyon Road in quiet Green Valley, then heading southeast 0.9 mile to the combined post office, grocery store, and restaurant.

A 2.2-mile detour to Lake Hughes, 30.3 miles into your journey, is the last chance to reprovision before facing the Mojave Desert. This small village has a post office, restaurants, stores, motels, and a private campground with showers. Lake Hughes is the logical resupply point for those hikers opting to take the shorter alternate route across the Mojave.

Lancaster might seem an improbable choice for resupply: It lies in the middle of sweltering-hot Antelope Valley, fully 30 miles east of the PCT's crossing of Highway 138, some 61.1 miles into this section. However, access is surprisingly easy, since Highway 138 is very busy, and hitchhiking should not pose a problem. Also, Lancaster is the largest town in this section, and it boasts a complete array of needs for the PCT traveler, including shopping malls and specialty mountaineering and backpacking shops.

At Highway 138, the same point where you could detour east to Lancaster, instead you could walk west 1.3 miles to The Country Store. Seven days a week you'll find water, cold drinks and snacks, minimal groceries, medical items, and a phone. Also available are horse feed, a corral, and even a PCTA trail register. The Country Store will accept a PCT traveler's resupply boxes and hold them without charge. Send them to:

> c/o [Your Name]
> The Country Store
> Star Route 138 [mail]
> 28105 Hwy. 138 [UPS direct]
> Lancaster, CA 93536-9207
>
> Tel: (805) 724-9097

Tehachapi lies 9.2 miles west of the PCT route at the end of this section. It is more easily reached, as described later, by a 7.6-mile detour from Tehachapi-Willow Springs Road, at the 98.2-mile mark. Most hikers will make the detour, to minimize the need to carry heavy loads across the hot, dry Mojave Desert and Tehachapi Mountains segments. Tehachapi is a large and growing community, with many stores (including a K-Mart), restaurants, motels, and laundromats as well as a post office. Additionally, there are limited sporting goods available, as well as bus service and a small airport. Tehachapi has PCT host families who will help with travel to and from the trailhead—contact them via PCT

List on the Internet at: *PCT-L@mailman. backcountry.net.*

Mojave is a desert town, also 9 miles from the PCT at the end of this section, reached east along Highway 58. It is a fair-sized community, with services similar to Tehachapi. It now sports a large shopping center, with fast food, pharmacy, and groceries, and some chain motels, which sit right at the junction of Highway 58 and Highway 14. This makes a visit to Mojave quite convenient. Also in Mojave is a PCT-hiker's institution: White's Motel at 16100 Sierra Highway. Call (661) 824-2421, or (800) 762-4596 (for reservations only). The hiker -friendly managers offer inexpensive accommodations, a swimming pool, and a free shuttle service up to the PCT on Tehachapi Pass. The motel is, conveniently, only two blocks from the post office.

How to choose between Tehachapi and Mojave for resupply? Tehachapi is much cooler, prettier, and quieter. It has a somewhat greater depth of, if not a lot better, resources. For some, it will be a little harder to reach than Mojave. Mojave has the advantage of the services of White's Motel and a more-compact town plan—it is easier for walkers. For the ravenous, it has a superior mix of fast-food restaurants. On the minus side, it is usually blisteringly hot, always depressingly ugly, and constantly barraged by the noise of a stream of auto traffic and passing trains—the very antithesis of your ideal PCT experience.

## Water and Desert Survival

The Mojave Desert was a formidable barrier to early travelers, causing much hardship and greatly slowing Southern California's growth. That part of the Mojave traversed by the PCT is now tamed by criss-crossing roads and dotted with homes and ranches, eliminating any dangers—as imagined by the uninformed—of dying like French Legionnaires, with parched throats and watery dreams. Still,

the Mojave Desert stretch of the PCT can broil your mind, blister your feet, and turn your mouth to dust—in all, an unpleasant experience—if you are not adequately prepared. With a little forethought, enough water, and the right equipment this hike can be a tolerable variation from the PCT's usual crestline surroundings.

Water is the key to all life, and enough of it will make yours more enjoyable. While planning your nightly stops or possible side hikes to water sources, you might consider the following government figures, arrived at by subjects operating under optimal experimental conditions. (They weren't carrying heavy packs!) Without water you can survive only 2 days at 120°F if you stay in one spot, 5 days at 100°F, and 9 days at 80°F. If you walk during the day, you will survive only one third as long. If you rest during the day and hike at night, then these figures become 1, 3 and 7 days, with 12, 33 and 110 miles being covered. At 100°F, the mid-figure, you would be able to hike 20 miles for every gallon of water you carried, though you would become hopelessly dehydrated in so doing, and eventually incapacitated. Actual hiking conditions require at least 2 gallons a day while hiking in 100° heat with a backpack, and most persons will function better with 2.5 gallons.

Be aware that humans are the only mammal that does not drink automatically to replace the body's lost water stores, when water is available. Even when water is plentiful, exercising humans tend to become dehydrated, since most people drink only enough to keep their mouths and throats wet! Unfortunately, however, only a small degree of dehydration will exact a considerable toll on performance and endurance, and possibly result in health problems. Hence, you must force yourself to drink enough water while exercising, and drink at frequent intervals. It is much better to drink a cup of water every

15 minutes or so, than to stop every few hours and force down 2 quarts of water.

When drinking, pick the most palatable liquid (although most hikers will have little more than plain water). The addition of a small amount of flavoring helps the chore of forced hydration, and some salts and a bit of sugar may actually help absorption of water from the stomach. Beware, though, that most instant drink mixes, including many specialty athletic drinks, contain enough sugar and salts to actually delay stomach absorption, and may lead to nausea during heavy exercise. Diluting commercial drinks to twice their volume usually prevents this problem. Otherwise, all that is necessary to make sure that vital body electrolytes are replaced during prolonged exertion is to eat a balanced diet while drinking plain water. Most hiking foods contain more than enough salts to maintain body stores.

The best way to conserve water is to hike at night, and night-hiking has added bonuses in the Mojave Desert: astounding star-filled skies, fewer passing cars, and the chance to observe some little-seen desert wildlife—inquisitive kit foxes sometimes play tag with hikers. Yucca night-lizards, which spend their days under fallen Joshua trees, also scurry about at night. But use a flashlight, even on moonlit nights, because rattlesnakes like to lie on the warm roads.

If you prefer to hike in daylight, start early, before sunrise, say at 5 in the morning during spring. Hike about 4 hours, perhaps getting in 12 miles, rest until evening, and then hike about another 2 hours. By day, walkers should ignore their desire to shed sweaty shirts or pants, since clothing prevents excessive moisture loss and overheating, and it also forestalls an excruciating high-desert sunburn.

It is no secret that water is a critical issue throughout arid Section E, and especially so in drought years. After about May 1, don't count on water at any sites away from human improvement. Even before then, most streams are small seasonal trickles, and likely to be polluted. Note, too, that all campground water in the Saugus District of Angeles National Forest (north of Agua Dulce) has been turned off due to possible water-supply contamination with *Giardia* and *Cryptosporidium* parasites. This should not overly inconvenience PCT travelers, since the (untreated) streams and springs that supply the campgrounds are still as accessible as ever. Treat all water with iodine, or use a filter before drinking water from any natural sources. In an emergency, you may be forced to try to obtain water from springs or creekbeds that are barely flowing. A trick for tapping these seeps, without the frustration of scooping up mud and debris as well, is offered by PCT expert Alice Krueper: carry a 6″ length of narrow-gauge aluminum tubing. It weighs next to nothing, and makes a fine straw with which to lead a trickle of clean water to your canteen.

## Permits

Day-hikers and section-hikers, but not thru-hikers, will be affected by the National Forest Adventure Pass system now in effect for all parked cars within Southern California's national forests. This pass is required for all vehicles, while parked along any road or even at a designated trailhead, in Angeles, Cleveland, Los Padres and San Bernardino National Forests. It is not required for PCT travelers, per se. Cost is $5 per visit to one forest, or $30 per year (good for all four forests). Plans are to return 85% of collected monies to the individual forest for human-use enhancing projects. Passes can be purchased from the USFS, from Southern California outdoor shops and multiple vendors near or in the forests.

No wilderness permits are required for overnight PCT campers.

## Special Problems

### Fires

No campfires of any kind are allowed in Angeles National Forest, outside of designated campgrounds. Use gas stoves only.

# THE ROUTE

Agua Dulce is reached via Highway 14, 18 miles east of its junction with Interstate 5 in Sylmar or 21 miles south of Palmdale. Take Highway 14's Agua Dulce Canyon Road exit, then head north 2.5 miles up that road to east-west Darling Road, in Agua Dulce. Your first chance for camping and water north of town, discounting homes, is at Bear Spring, 8.1 miles. However, in recent drought years, Bear Spring has been quite unreliable, so plan to carry water until the next certain water, at San Francisquito Ranger Station, a long 22.7 miles away.

Leave Agua Dulce by walking northward on Agua Dulce Canyon Road very gently up grassy Sierra Pelona Valley. You pass numerous homes and side roads, a few businesses, an airfield, and finally a church before your road ends at wide, paved Old Sierra Highway (2725-1.8). Turn left and go west along its north shoulder for just a bit to paved Mint Canyon Road (2730-0.1). Follow that road up and right, west, shortly to a low gap where paved Petersen Road (2755-0.1) branches north. Turn right on Petersen Road and descend gently to the southern edge of a ranch-dotted bench in Mint Canyon. Here a dirt road (2750-0.1) servicing a line of high-tension electric wires, branches right.

The PCT route begins by climbing momentarily northeast up this road, ignoring a right-branching spur, then descends for a short while. The road then ascends moderately again, on exposed slopes of withered chamise on the east flank of Mint Canyon. Pass a second right-branching spur. Walk up past a chain-link fence and reenter Angeles National Forest, where you resume trail tread (2905-0.4) some 50 yards beyond a large steel electrical tower. Follow the tread left, northward, as it contours around a nose, then makes a long, easily descending traverse to the shadeless southeast banks of Mint Canyon's infrequently flowing stream. At a step-across ford of the creek (2865-1.3) you pass a horse trail that continues up-canyon. The PCT, however, clambers west up onto a low bench with an equestrian trail register. Beyond, you walk straight uphill on an old jeep road, passing another that runs down-canyon. You now see evidence of a brush fire that burned here in 1985. Where a jeep road climbs left along an old barbed-wire fence, you follow the obvious PCT right, ascending north. A promontory overlooking large Annan Ranch is soon reached, after which the path climbs moderately northwest to survey more blackened chaparral on the headwall of Mint Canyon. By walking a few minutes more, you reach Big Tree Trail 14W02 (3330-1.1) astride a saddle.

Leaving the saddle, you see the old Big Tree Trail heading steeply up the spine of the ridge. The PCT, however, starts a traverse to the left of the ridge, gaining elevation gradually at first, on cobbly schist tread. You climb more rapidly as the path drifts northwest, presenting excellent over-the-shoulder vistas south to the bizarre Vasquez Rocks, purported refuge of bandit Tiburcio Vasquez, and farther east to Mts. Gleason, Williamson, and Baden–Powell. You now switchback steeply up almost to the ridge, where you switchback again, back to the north. When the climb moderates, you soon reach Sierra Pelona Ridge Road 6N07 (4500-2.7). Now turn right (east) and walk gently up to a low saddle (4555-0.3). Here, atop Sierra Pelona Ridge, wind gusts have been measured in excess of 100 miles per hour. Now, PCT posts lead your way northeast via a disused jeep road,

E

Agua Dulce –
Highway 58

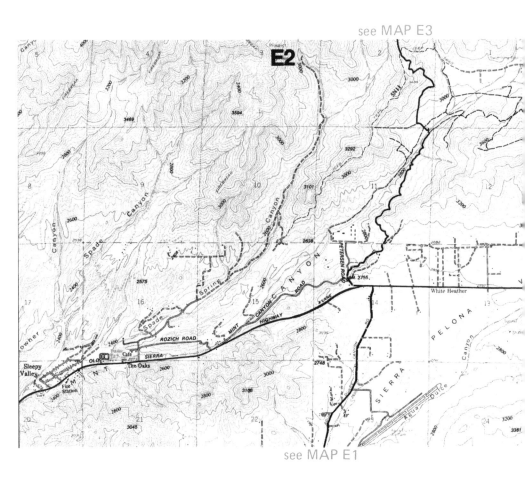

through a white pipe gate, then steeply down the hillside at the head of Martindale Canyon. The little-used path soon crisscrosses the even more steeply descending jeep track multiple times, and is easily lost on sloping hillside meadows of foxtails and grasses. Presently, you circle just above the levelest such flat, grown waist-high in yellow mustard. Hidden in a tangle of wild grape vines at its foot is Bear Spring (4350-0.7). The spring's dripping pipe is about 35 feet uphill from the trail, while a metal trough is just below the trail. **This waterhole often runs late into springtime, but should not be relied upon.** Camping hereabouts is suboptimal. Continuing down

**See Maps E1, E2**

E

**Agua Dulce – Highway 58**

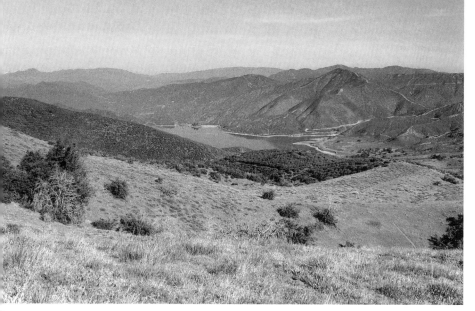

*Ben Schifrin*

*Bouquet Reservoir*

with vistas north across Antelope Valley to Owens Peak in the southern Sierra, you circle the upper reaches of fault-aligned Martindale Canyon, soon reaching a ridgetop-firebreak jeep trail (3995-0.7). This you descend, continuing west, down to a junction (3785-0.6) with the old PCT trail alignment, which formerly climbed south up to Big Oak Spring. Now you turn right for a more gradual descent on chaparral-choked trail, leading northeast to paved Bouquet Canyon Road 6N05 (3340-0.9).

Merging under Bouquet Reservoir, 2½ miles to the west, the San Francisquito and Clearwater faults run Bouquet Canyon's length and separate southern Pelona schists from granites on the canyon's north wall.

The PCT drops across the dry wash draining Bouquet Canyon, then arcs easily up, northwest, to cross a jeep road near a water tank in a small canyon. Now the trail ascends moderately on coarse granitic sand to just north of a powerline, where the PCT branches northwest from the old CRHT (California Riding and Hiking Trail) (3985-2.7), which continues north up to Leona Divide Truck Road 6N04.

The PCT climbs along the steep south-facing slope through sickly, low chamise, crosses a descending firebreak, and then veers more northward, just under the Leona Divide Road, to gain a pass (4300-1.4) with another firebreak, which tops a ridge dividing Spunky and Bouquet canyons. A gentle switchback in now-denser chaparral and occasional shading oaks drops you to the head of Spunky Canyon, where you turn west down-canyon, then climb slightly to strike Road 6N09 (3725-2.0).

**Resupply access:** If you're thirsty, seeking a campsite, or needing supplies, then first walk west 1.7 miles down this dirt road to paved Spunky Canyon Road

**See Maps E3, E4, E5**

6N11. On it, wind northwest 1.1 miles to Spunky Campground or 0.8 mile farther to Green Valley, with a post office, grocery store and restaurant.

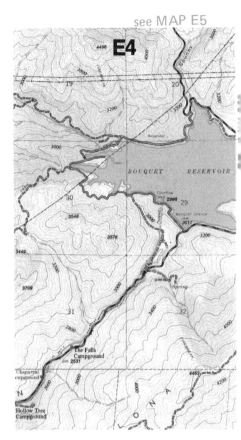

see MAP E5

   The PCT climbs gently away from Road 6N09, winding in and out of small ravines on a westward bearing. Eventually the path tops a small ridge, again with a firebreak (3815-2.1), and then the trail angles northeast, through a gap and down into the upper end of Dowd Canyon. Seen from here, Jupiter Mountain looms impressively across the valley. You reach a low point of 3475 feet in Dowd Canyon, in a gully where native bunchgrasses grow, then you amble first north-northwest before heading southwest around Peak 4087 over to a ridgetop separating Dowd and San Francisquito canyons. From here a final northeastward swoop under shady interior live oaks brings the PCT to paved San Francisquito Canyon Road (3385-4.2). Green Valley Ranger Station, with water, is 250 yards southwest. San Francisquito Campground no longer exists, but there is a trail camp near the ranger station, under shady canyon live oaks. A restaurant is now found at the junction of San Francisquito Canyon Road and Spunky Canyon Road, 1.7 miles southwest of the ranger station. Green Valley, which has a combined post office, grocery store, and restaurant, as well as phones and a fire station, is just beyond that road junction.

   Across San Francisquito Canyon Road the PCT begins its climb of Grass Mountain by ascending northwest into a nearby side canyon, above which it strikes a dirt road (3520-0.3) serving two powerlines. The trail follows the road north momentarily, then switchbacks west and progresses unremittingly up chaparralled slopes to Grass Mountain Road (4275-1.3), striking this dirt road just above its junction with Leona Divide Truck Trail.

**E**

**Agua Dulce – Highway 58**

   Panoramas unfold northward over Elizabeth Lake—a sag pond on the San Andreas Fault—to distant Antelope Valley and the Tehachapi Mountains, and if one is enjoying a smogless spring day, Owens Peak in the southern Sierra Nevada may be seen.

   You enjoy this scenery as the path contours, then descends the north slopes of Grass Mountain to a saddle (3900-1.3), where four dirt roads converge at the head of South Portal and Munz canyons.

   Keeping on a steep hillside south of the ridge, the PCT contours from this gap over to another saddle, where it crosses dirt

see MAP E5

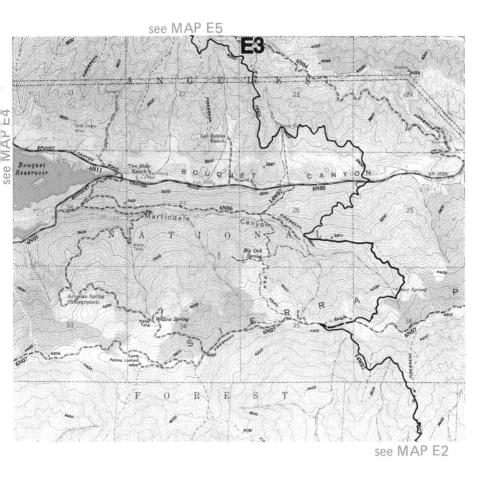

see MAP E2

Tule Canyon Road 7N01 (3900-1.2) by its junction with Lake Hughes Truck Trail. Onward the route rolls across dry ravines in dense chaparral, switchbacks once to pass through a gap, and then descends unhesitatingly toward Elizabeth Lake Canyon by crossing an interminable array of narrow, rocky gulches. At the bottom of this unpleasant segment, your path bursts from brush cover to traverse the broad, sandy wash of Elizabeth Lake Canyon. Southbound trekkers may lose their way here in a welter of game trails; they should head straight for the ridge's shoulder, where it strikes the canyon's bottom. Northbound

hikers head for nearby, paved Elizabeth Lake Canyon Road 7N09 (3050-3.5).

The next permanent on-route water hole along the PCT is a distant 32.6 miles northwest, at the California Aqueduct, so be sure that you know which of the less-reliable sources ahead are truly available before you leave this point. The next usually reliable water source near the northbound PCT is at Upper Shake Campground, a 0.6-mile detour that leaves the PCT in 7.0 miles.

**Resupply access:** If you need water or supplies, you should detour north, 1.5 miles up-canyon along Elizabeth Lake Road to Newvale Drive, which is on the

**See Map E6**

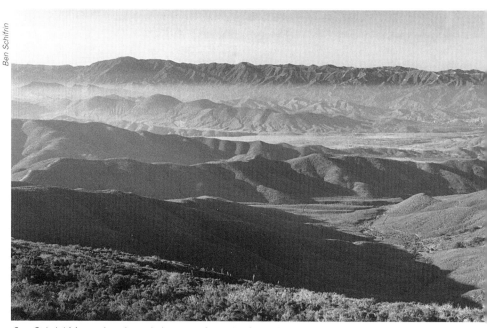

*San Gabriel Mountains above L.A. smog, from the Sierra Pelona crest*

Ben Schifrin

west side of the small resort community of Lake Hughes. A small convenience store sits at the intersection of Elizabeth Lake Canyon Road and Newvale Drive. Other very small stores, a hotel, a cafe and the entrance to a private campground and picnic area are on the east shore of small Hughes Lake (great for your blistered feet!). These are reached by following Newvale Drive east 0.3 mile to Elizabeth Lake Road, then walking 0.4 mile farther east along Elizabeth Lake Road, just across from another nice campground. The next chance to resupply on the northbound PCT is at Tehachapi, which lies west of the PCT at the end of Section E. The Lake Hughes Post Office is another 0.5 mile east along the highway.

**Alternate route:** Travelers who do not want to walk along the sunny, frequently very hot, permanent PCT route along the Los Angeles Aqueduct might

consider the following alternate. It follows a temporary PCT route, used during the 1970's, past Lake Hughes, north across Portal Ridge, then down past Fairmont Reservoir to 170th Street West. Follow this road arrow-straight across the western arm of Antelope Valley, to restrike the PCT at the mouth of Cottonwood Canyon, where there is a permanent water source. Overall, it subtracts 26.0 miles from the distance between Elizabeth Lake Canyon Road and Highway 58 at Tehachapi Pass. It also makes Lake Hughes a logical resupply point. (Despite these attractions, the author does not recommend this route over the permanent PCT alignment. Though it cuts one day's worth of arguably uninteresting walk alongside the Los Angeles Aqueduct, it has little else to offer. By taking the alternate, you will miss the gorgeous, open, black-oak forests along crests of the Sawmill and Liebre mountains, and many terrific vistas over Ante-

**See Map E6**

lope Valley to the Tehachapis. Most of all, you will miss the true Pacific crest, which is accurately traversed by the next stretch of trail.)

Begin the alternate route by following directions in the Resupply Access (above) to Newvale Drive (3225-1.5-1.5). Turn right, east, on Newvale Drive, passing homes, to reach busy Elizabeth Lake Road (3245- 0.3-1.8). You walk levelly right, southeast, to left-branching Lakeview Road (3235-0.3-2.1). "Downtown" Lake Hughes is five blocks east. Your next chance for water is at Fairmont Reservoir in 3.8 miles, and your next supplies are found at the end of this section, in Tehachapi or Mojave.

Ascend north on Lakeview Road past a few residences, and then follow the twisting dirt road up to the top of grassy, viewful Portal Ridge, which is a mass of granite thrust up by the powerful San Andreas fault to the south. Pass a few more ridgetop homes on dirt Road 7N03, as it winds east to splendid vistas over western Antelope Valley, then turn north on Road 7N16 at the entrance to Sky Haven Ranch (3790-1.4-3.5). Go through a gate and descend a ridge along the head of Myrick Canyon to a welter of dirt and paved roads at the south end of the dam of breezy, barren Fairmont Reservoir (3045-2.4-5.9), storage for the Los Angeles Aqueduct. Walk north, eventually arcing west atop the dam, then leave it at dirt Aqueduct Road (3045-0.8-6.7). This road heads north to dirt Avenue H (3040-0.4-7.1), which you follow briefly right, east, to its intersection in a weedy field with wide, dirt 170th Street West (3001-0.2-7.3).

The PCT temporary route now goes north, soon crossing the tempting California Aqueduct (2960-0.3-7.6) where hikers must tank up—the next certain drinking water on-route is clear across desertic Antelope Valley, at the Los Angeles Aqueduct in 13.6 miles. Continue north down 170th Street West, past a horse ranch to busy, paved Lancaster Road (2805-1.1-8.7), where the road you're on is signed 167TH STREET WEST. Turn left, trekking first north then west, to a continuation of 170th Street West (2785-0.6-9.3), now paved.

Head due north, arrow-straight across windswept Antelope Valley, which is dotted here and there with alfalfa, onion, barley, and sugar-beet plantations. **Irrigation sprinklers at these farms might be a source of emergency water.**

You also see diminishing stands of Joshua trees. At one time Joshua trees, or tree yuccas, were more widely distributed, as evidenced by fossils of an extinct, giant, yucca-feeding ground sloth, found in southern Nevada where you no longer find Joshua trees. These giant members of the lily family, with their unusually branched, sometimes human-like form, were likened by Mormon pioneers to the figure of Joshua, pointing the route to the Great Salt Lake. Botanists now know that Joshua trees will not branch at all unless their trunk-tip flowers are damaged by wind or boring beetles. Each time a Joshua tree blossoms, an event determined by rainfall or temperature, it sprouts a foot-long panicle of densely clustered greenish-white blooms that produce football-shaped fruits later in the year. Like other yuccas, Joshua-tree pollen is too heavy to reach another plant, even in strong desert winds. Because they cannot pollinate themselves, they rely on a symbiotic relationship with the little, white Pronuba yucca moth. Unlike other insects, which might unwittingly carry pollen from one plant to another, the Pronuba moth makes a separate trip to carry pollen, which it stuffs deep into a Joshua tree blossom. It then drills a hole in the base of the flower, where it lays an egg. When the Pronuba moth grub hatches, it has fruit to feed upon. Another ani-

**See Map E6**

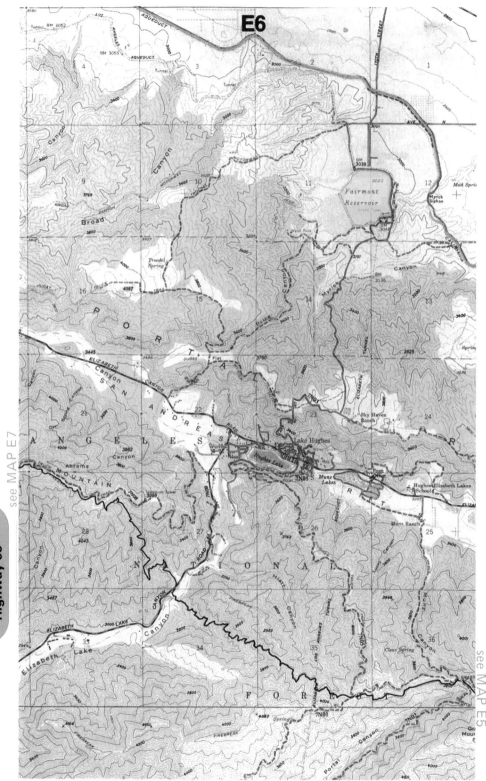

see MAP E7

see MAP E5

mal that apparently can't live without Joshua trees or other yuccas is the small, mottled night-lizard, which hides under fallen Joshua trees, feeding on termites, spiders, and ants.

Halfway across Antelope Valley, you're walking on sediments eroded from the Tehachapi and San Gabriel Mountains that geologists estimate are up to 5000 feet thick.

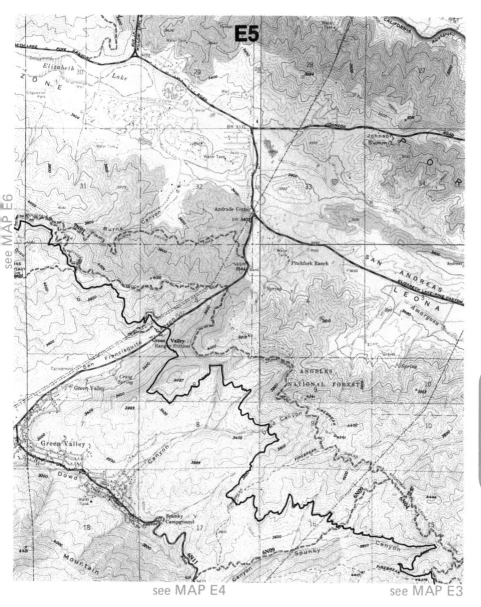

see MAP E6

see MAP E4          see MAP E3

**E**

**Agua Dulce –
Highway 58**

**See Map E6**

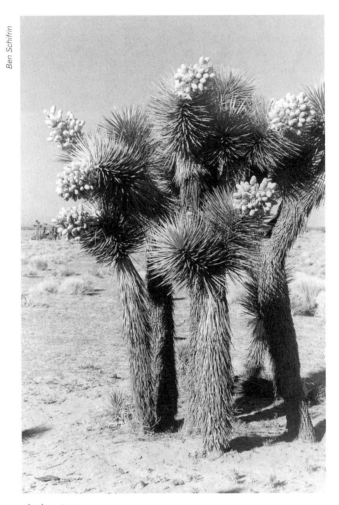

*Joshua trees*

   Pavement on 170th Street West ends at Rosamond Boulevard (2761-8.5-17.8), near Antelope Valley's north margin. Continue straight ahead, north, on sandy dirt road. Soon, your route takes the form of two, closely parallel roads—take whichever is easiest on your feet. Cross numerous sandy washes amid scattered Joshua trees, junipers, ubiquitous low gray bur-sage and green creosote bushes.

   Note how evenly spaced the glossy-leaved creosote shrubs are. They secrete a toxin, washed to the ground by rain, that poisons nearby plant growth and provides them root space to collect sufficient water. Observant walkers may note some of the creosote bushes growing in clustered rings, up to a few yards apart. Botanists have discovered that root-crown branching by those shrubs results in rings of plants, each one an identical genetic clone of the colonizing plant. By

**See Maps E6, E7**

radiocarbon dating and growth-rate measurements, scientists have dated some creosote bush clonal rings in the Mojave Desert back an estimated 11,000 years—far older than the bristlecone pine!

Eventually, you strike dirt Broken Arrow Road (2914-1.6-19.4), which branches left, northwest, sandily up the low, open, alluvial mouth of Cottonwood Creek canyon. Ascend it easily, passing numerous smaller spur roads, often abuzz with motorcycles. You finally rejoin the permanent PCT route at the subterranean Los Angeles Aqueduct (3120-1.8-21.2) and its parallel roads, just 0.1 mile east of the shade and permanent water at the Cottonwood Creek bridge.

Across Elizabeth Lake Canyon Road 7N09, the PCT attacks Sawmill Mountain's east flank. The trail climbs quickly northwest into a small valley, which has a sycamore-shaded flat that could serve as an adequate, though waterless, campsite. Soon the route, now back in chamise-and-oak chaparral, passes the mouth of an old graphite mine tunnel, then switchbacks to climb more steeply southwest past two more tunnels. After reaching a ridge, the trail again swings northwest to ascend moderately through yerba santa and chamise back into the canyon. Here you find some shade in the form of interior live oaks and a cluster of disheveled big-cone spruces surrounding a trailside wet-season spring (3710-1.2). No camping is possible on the steep slope here. Continuing on, the path leads up the now-narrow ravine, then veers southwest at its head to reach a viewful intersection with the Sawmill-Liebre Firebreak (4190-0.6), just above a wide dirt road, Maxwell Truck Trail 7N08.

Now-familiar vistas north over the western part of Antelope Valley to the Tehachapi Mountains are presented here and accompany you as the PCT adopts a leisurely, traversing ascent of Sawmill Moun-

tain's spine, always keeping just a stone's throw south of Maxwell Truck Trail. Repeated crossings of the ridge and its firebreak in a mix of chaparral eventually lead you to Maxwell Truck Trail 7N08 (4505-1.9) in an open glade of black oaks.

A few yards down a gully south of the road is signed FISH CREEK CANYON PCT TRAIL CAMP, constructed by Boy Scouts in 1984. In a hillside field of pentstemon and mariposa lilies, it has a table and a fire pit but, unfortunately, the nearby water tank is firmly shuttered, so the camp is waterless.

Back on the trail, you walk 35 yards northwest along the road to where trail tread resumes. The PCT drops slightly, then assumes an undulating traverse in and out of gullies on the north slope of Sawmill Mountain. After a short while the PCT becomes situated just below moderately ascending Maxwell Truck Trail and maintains that arrangement through chaparral sprinkled with Coulter pines. Eventually the PCT turns south into a larger ravine to cross two dirt roads (4680-2.9) in quick succession. These rough access roads mark the site of a small plantation of trees, whose young Coulter pines and incense-cedars shade pleasant Maxwell Trail Camp, which is just 100 feet north, down the first road. **It has a unique "guzzler" self-filling water tank, where green algae-stained water is available to wildlife and hikers alike.** Even nicer camping lies just a minute before you strike the old road down to the trail camp. Pushing on, you ascend a shadier hillside and soon reach a trail intersection (4805-0.4).

**Water access:** The poorer branch climbs steeply southeast to strike Maxwell Truck Trail, while a good branch, descending northwest, drops via switchbacks 0.6 mile to Upper Shake Campground, which has tables, fire rings, and toilets. A small, usually flowing stream can be found in Shake Canyon, just north of the campground.

The northbound PCT heads southwest gently up from the Upper Shake Campground trail junction, traversing the hillside first under shady oaks and big-cone spruces as it ducks into and then heads out of a small canyon. This pleasant segment crosses an abandoned jeep road dropping

into the head of Shake Canyon, then continues to a ridgetop road junction (5245-2.6). From here Maxwell Truck Trail 7N08 starts south on a generally eastward traverse, Burnt Peak Road 7N23A traverses west, and Sawmill Mountain Truck Trail 7N23 traverses northwest and also descends northeast to Pine Canyon Road.

**Water access:** Just west of this intersection, 200 feet up the hillside, lies a 10,000-gallon, buried, concrete water tank, used by firefighters. Its rectangular steel

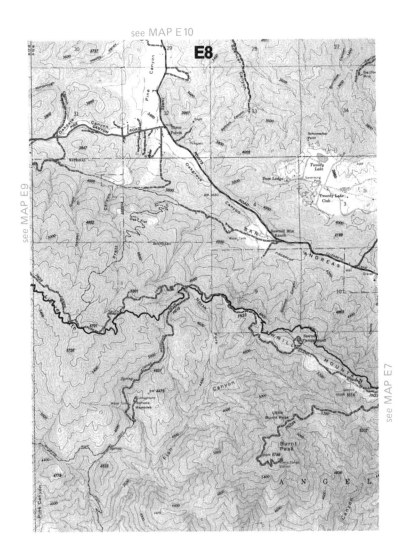

**Agua Dulce – Highway 58**

**E**

lid is usually unlocked, making it a good prospect for resupply. **Adequate, if sunny, camping is nearby.**

The PCT descends gently north under the upper branch of Sawmill Mountain Truck Trail, now in even shadier mixed forest and chaparral. Next a long, descending traverse leads across a broad black-oak-clothed ridge nose to a junction (5015-1.8). From here a spur trail ascends southeast 0.2 mile to small Sawmill Campground, which is pretty but waterless.

You first contour and then switchback twice to resume a position just north of and below Sawmill Mountain Truck Trail. Presently, you cross that road (4790-1.1) at a large turnout. Across the road, your trail drops indistinctly southwest, through a corridor of Coulter pines, then winds west around the head of wild, rugged North Fork Fish Canyon. Soon you reach a saddle junction of Sawmill Mountain Truck Trail and Atmore Meadows Spur Road 7N19 (4705-0.5). The PCT follows the latter road southwest for 80 yards to a resumption of trail tread in a steep ravine.

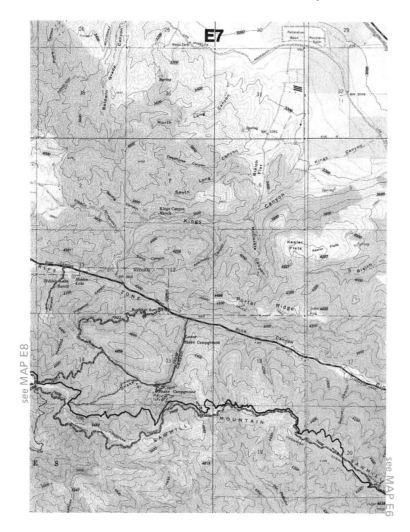

**See Maps E8, E9**

see MAP E10

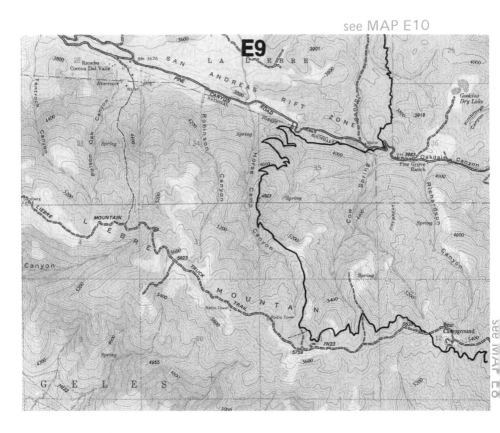

see MAP E8

**Water access:** Before continuing, however, hikers may wish to detour 1.7 miles farther along Atmore Meadows Spur Road to a fair spring, or another 1.0 mile beyond it down to a series of shaded glens, the site of Atmore Meadows Campground, which has water, tables and toilets.

Next on the PCT's agenda of chaparral-cloaked summits is Liebre Mountain, and the steep, seasonally hot trail that climbs from Atmore Meadows Spur Road quickly dispels any thoughts of a sedate ascent. After an effort you are high on brushy slopes, panting toward a grassy saddle (5655-2.1), which marks an end to the unpleasant grind. Step across a jeep road that crosses the saddle, then descend easily northwest, still just under the truck trail.

**Water access:** Soon after beginning your descent, look north, just across the road, for another water tank—the 10,000-gallon Red Rock Water Tank, with a usually removable, yellow, iron lid. Wind 50 feet through low brush to reach it. Camping nearby will be shadeless and hot.

Now descending easily, zigzags lead northwest first close to Liebre Mountain Truck Trail, then into and out of interminable dry washes that alternate with brushy ridgelets. Sometimes you have good views south to the wildlands of deep Cienaga Canyon. Eventually the undulating descent ceases and the grade becomes a moderate ascent. Moments later, you encounter a junction with a spur trail (5370-2.2) that climbs north a few yards to waterless Bear Campground. An additional three minutes' climb along the PCT leads to a crossing of Liebre Mountain Truck Trail 7N23 (5545-0.2).

**Water access:** Another water tank can be reached from this point. Walk back right, east, 100 yards down the road. Look north down a shallow gully, under an open grove of black oaks, where a fiberglass water tank for the use of wildlife and hikers lies under a low, white, corrugated aluminum roof. The best camping is three minutes back down the road, at Bear Campground.

Now on the cooler north slopes of Liebre Mountain, your way becomes much nicer, winding almost level along hillsides shaded by open groves of black oaks. In spring the grassy turf underfoot is a green sea dotted with brodiaea, baby blue-eyes and miner's lettuce. Soon you cross a north-descending dirt road (5580-0.9) on a ridge nose as the PCT winds west close to the gentle summit of Liebre Mountain. You

wind over two more small, delightfully oak-clothed ridgetops, then merge with a poor jeep track, still traversing more or less levelly, for just a minute to reach another jeep road (5745-1.2) on the crest of a broad, open ridge. Here a sign points out the new alignment of the PCT, branching right, northwest, down the ridgetop on the jeep road. You ignore the older, abandoned trail alignment, which continued straight ahead along the summit of Liebre Mountain and has now been overrun by four-wheel vehicles. Either jeep track, however, continues only a minute before striking a fair dirt road (5720-0.1).

Here, take a few minutes' detour, and walk left, south, back up to the top of Liebre Mountain's ridge for its expansive vistas south to the Santa Monica Mountains, the Pacific Ocean, and the highrises of Hollywood looming over the white rollercoasters of Magic Mountain amusement park. Possibly more interesting is an eastward inventory of terrain

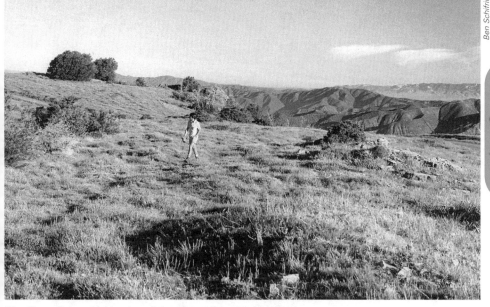

*Ben Schifrin*

*The Sierra Pelona highlands and the distant Tehachapi Mountains*

**E**

**Agua Dulce – Highway 58**

**See Maps E9, E10**

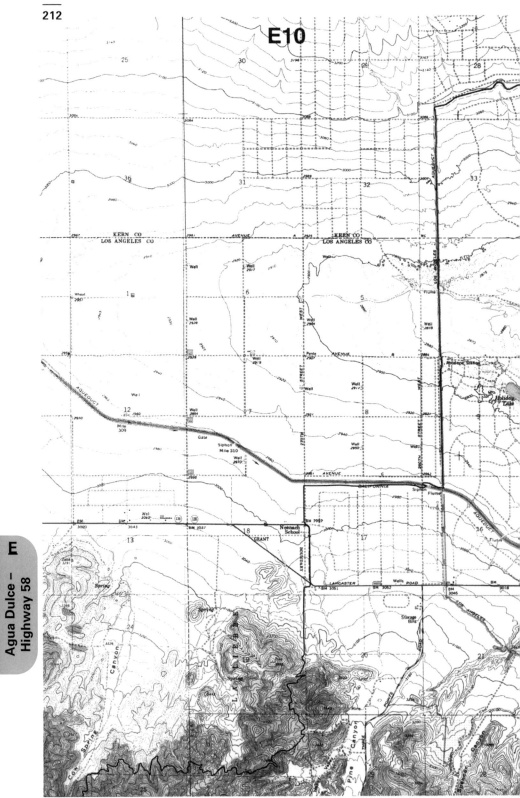

see MAP E9

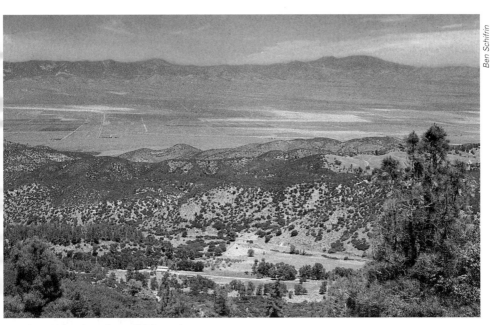

*Antelope Valley from Sawmill Mountain*

conquered: beyond Vasquez Rocks, the San Gabriel Mountains, from Mts. Wilson and Gleason on the west, to towering Mount Baden–Powell and Mount Baldy on the east, are all there for inspection.

The newer PCT heads north, downhill, on this closed ridgetop road, passing through a plantation of young black oaks and their older in-laws. Soon the downgrade steepens and sagebrush replaces much of the understory. Windswept panoramas over the westernmost corner of Antelope Valley remind you that you have now ended a sweeping 250-mile skirting of the southwestern border of the Mojave Desert, which has led you west from Whitewater along the summits of the San Bernardinos, the San Gabriels, and Sawmill and Liebre mountains—a job well done!

Continuing your descent, you lose these views as you re-enter big-cone spruce, pine and oak cover below 5200 feet in elevation. Soon thereafter, the road, which has diminished to a rough jeep track, ends

(5140-1.0). Switchbacks lower you gently from just beyond this point into a saddle—a good but dry camp—just short of a conifer-clad 4923-foot knob. If you choose to camp here in early season, you may find water 100-200 feet down the gully to the east. Beyond, the enjoyable trail enters thick chaparral, descends moderately via switchbacks, and presently levels out at a dirt road spur (3995-2.5) atop a minor pass just south of paved Pine Canyon Road.

The very last segment of permanent Pacific Crest Trail was finally constructed north from here, in Summer 1993. After years of legal wrangling with the Forest Service, the massive Tejon Ranch finally allowed construction of a part of the PCT around the border of their lands. Unfortunately, the final route was clearly designed by lawyers intent on inconveniencing hikers, rather than by trail planners trying to accommodate them. The trail's actual construction was

**See Map E10**

likewise amateurishly undertaken with a small bulldozer, which resulted in a road-wide, poorly laid rut which will be quickly destroyed by erosion.

This new trail segment heads right, south, away from the road spur, descending easily in a hillside stand of Coulter pines and black and scrub oaks. The trail finds a sandy traverse eastward and eventually comes upon the south banks of a small sag pond (3810-0.6) which lies on the San Andreas Fault. Here, under huge black oaks, dozens of migrating waterfowl hide in the rush-rimmed shallows. **No formal campsites are found here, and the water certainly requires treating before drinking, but this locale is the last nice camping spot before the Tehachapi Mountains.** It is commonly dry by fall. The PCT continues east from the pond, ascending gently past a sign notifying you that you have passed out of Angeles National Forest and onto private property. A moment later, you step across seasonally trickling Cow Spring Canyon creek, which runs into late May of all but the driest years. Next, the path swings close to and then crosses paved Pine Canyon Road (3845-0.3).

**Water access:** If desperately low on water, you could continue east along Pine Canyon Road, over a low saddle and down to the hamlet of Three Points, which has a convenience store and a campground, 2.7 miles from the PCT.

A brown signpost marks the road crossing, which leads to a gentle ascent right alongside the switchbacking road, soon to reach a large sign diagramming the PCT's course through the Tejon Ranch's property. **The sign asks that hikers not leave the path for any reason for the next 7 miles, and expresses a prohibition against camping and fires.**

Now commences a tiring and annoying stretch of trail designed to keep hikers

as close to the boundary of Tejon Ranch lands as possible. Up and down you march, north across hillsides of hot, dry, low chamise and manzanita scrub on shaly, loose trail tread, marked by frequent tiny, reverse-banked switchbacks. Eventually, you drop steeply down a ridge nose to the verge of a dry grassland in Cow Spring Canyon. Here the ranch boundary, marked by a four-strand barbed-wire fence, turns abruptly east, so you do, as well.

The next leg continues on an eastward bearing, ascending up and across a number of small, sunny ridges. In due time, you descend 100 feet from one of the ridges to cross a jeep road (3522-3.8) in a sandy, buckwheat-dotted wash. Beyond, you climb eastward steeply out of the wash, through a gap, then traverse a hillside with an overlook of Pine Canyon. Steep, then gentle, descent soon ensues, now turning north to bisect a broad wash. Now heading north again, you amble over a broad saddle, then descend via over-engineered switchbacks to merge with a good jeep road (3175-2.1) in a small, narrow valley. Turn right, northeast, along the gently descending road, which passes above a small ranch at the canyon's mouth. Beyond, the road descends north, arrow-straight out onto the alluvial verge of the Antelope Valley. Pass some branching fence-line jeep roads, but continue straight ahead, soon reaching a new alignment of busy, paved Highway 138 (3040-0.8), just west of its intersection with signed 269th street west. Green metal gates now allow horse and foot traffic access to the pavement. Hurry across—the highway is very busy.

Leave Highway 138, passing through a green gate to regain your fence-side dirt road/trail, still descending easily on a due north bearing. In less than a half mile you find another sign announcing the special restrictions for using the PCT in the Tejon Ranch. Beyond it, you pass through two sty-gates to reach Barnes Ranch Road at its

**See Map E10**

E

Agua Dulce – Highway 58

junction with paved Neenach School Road (2992-0.5).

**Water and resupply access:** Water is available just north of this point, during school hours, from Neenach Elementary School. Alternatively, "The Country Store" is about 1.1 miles west on Barnes Ranch Road, which merges with Highway 138 in about ½ mile. Use the store for resupply, if needed, instead of going to Tehachapi or Lancaster. Seven days a week, you'll find water, cold drinks, snacks, minimal groceries, medical items, and a phone. Also available are horse feed, a corral, and even a PCTA trail register. The Country Store will accept PCT travelers' resupply boxes and hold them for no charge. Send them to:

> c/o [Your Name]
> The Country Store
> Star Route 138 [mail]
> 28105 Hwy. 138 [UPS direct]
> Lancaster, CA 93536-9207
>
> Tel: (805) 724-9097

Back on the PCT, walk north along Neenach School Road, near the elementary school. A moment north of the school, pavement ends (2970-0.3), and arrows point the PCT right, east, through a gate and onto a sandy dirt road. This road parallels the behemoth California Aqueduct, a veritable concrete-lined river flowing in a channel hidden behind a massive earthen berm to our north. Follow the PCT-marked path or either of two firmer, more-used roads, just south of the aqueduct, levelly east to a pair of roads. The first of this pair, 260th Street West, is paved, and bridges the aqueduct at a siphon (2965-1.0). Cross north over the aqueduct, then walk a short distance right, east, through a gate along its northern bank to the historic Los Angeles Aqueduct (2965-0.3).

Here, the Los Angeles Aqueduct is a huge, buried pipe, and engineers were faced with the rather bizarre problem of routing the larger California Aqueduct under the smaller waterway. **For the northbound, the next certain water lies in Cottonwood Canyon, 13.3 miles ahead. If you're heading south on the PCT, the next water is at Upper Shake Campground, a long 25.9 miles up on Liebre Mountain.**

Now the northbound PCT does just that: turns left, due north, on a sandy tack just east of the buried Los Angeles Aqueduct. Indestructible, 3-foot-tall, brown-painted iron posts, each emblazoned with a large white PCT emblem, redundantly indicate the route at numerous intersections with other dirt roads.

You pass a few habitations, all built in the peculiarly eccentric style of California desert residents. Later you descend to your lowest Antelope Valley point, 2865 feet, to cross the sandy wash of a seasonal creek bed. Here the shade of a wooden trestle supporting the massive, black-tarred, 8-foot-diameter aqueduct pipe offers a rest spot amid another quintessentially California desert feature, an ad-hoc garbage dump of cans, household appliances and auto carcasses, all riddled with bullet holes.

Now the route north leads into a low, scraggly "woodland" of Joshua trees, the hallmarks of the Mojave Desert.

You amble into Kern County, your unimproved way occasionally signed as AQUEDUCT ROAD, and then just over a mile later, your straight-north course turns east (3090-3.2) as the Los Angeles Aqueduct itself bends east, transforming from a black-tarred pipe to an underground channel with a broad, flat, concrete roof. (Contrary to a USGS topo, the aqueduct actually lies just north of the main dirt access-road that the PCT route follows.) Your way leads east, climbing imperceptibly alongside the aqueduct as it traces a scalloped, contouring route across a succession of broad alluvial fans footing the Tehachapi Mountains. In the first mile, you pass through a nice grove of Joshua trees—a possible, but waterless, place to camp. Unfortunately, barbed-

**See Maps E10, E11**

E

Agua Dulce – Highway 58

wire fences make it difficult to stray from the aqueduct. Even more unfortunate is the fact that, although one is walking alongside a buried river of cool, pristine High Sierra water, there is no way to get at it! The Los Angeles Department of Water and Power has undertaken a series of repairs to the roof of the aqueduct which have resulted in the cementing-over of all of the "water holes" that PCT travelers previously relied on, along this otherwise waterless stretch. **The next reliable water for northbound hikers is in Cottonwood Canyon, a hot 11.1 miles away!**

Forging ahead, you soon find a long stretch of aqueduct that was recently resurfaced. It winds across the broad fan of Sacatara Creek, passing innumerable branching dirt roads bound for everywhere and nowhere.

The route now turns across Little Oak Canyon Creek's wide, dry wash, then winds

monotonously across a gentle alluvial hillside to an intersection (3110-5.5) with a good dirt road that crosses the aqueduct via a concrete bridge, marked #1731-92. Here the PCT is signed to branch right, southeast, via brown metal posts with emblems. This junction is just a short distance before the Los Angeles Aqueduct disappears altogether at the western foot of a rugged hillside. Now you amble gently down, soon curving east-northeast, then northeast, at the pediment of a fascinating badland of steep-sided ravines and ridges. Flash floods have carved the firm red and yellow sediments into a complex of narrow gullies, which has a sparse flora of low juniper trees and rabbitbrush that give color contrast. Eventually, you come to a trio of high-tension electric lines marching uphill from the southeast. Ignore the dirt road (2893-3.0) that runs along their route and instead continue straight ahead, northeast, on the better

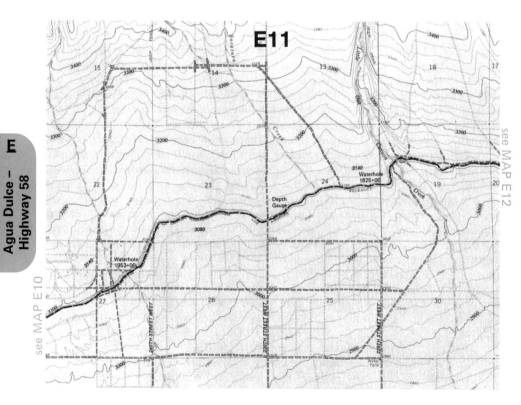

**E12**

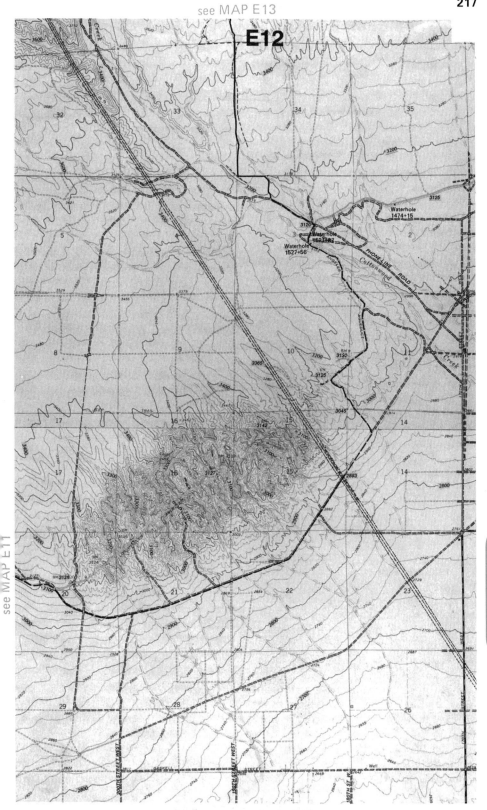

**E**

**Agua Dulce – Highway 58**

road. Very soon you strike a poorer dirt road, your first left turn, at a triangular junction (2915-0.4). It takes you gently but directly up-slope, soon coming along the southwest side of a small, shallow canyon. Quickly you once again rejoin the Los Angeles Aqueduct (3105-0.6), here underground, and turn right, northeast, along its road.

You climb over a low rise, then descend momentarily to resume a nearly level amble, curving north and then northwest into the massive, broad valley of Cottonwood Creek. There are no cottonwoods in evidence along the usually dry creek bed, but there is a nice stand of Joshua trees.

**Water access:** Here you finally find a reliable summer-long water hole: a reinforced concrete horse trough, which is fed continuously by a pipe from the aqueduct. It sits below the southwest end of concrete Cottonwood Creek bridge (3120-1.6), just north of a small concrete maintenance structure with a walkway that overlooks the wash, and below the level of the aqueduct road. (Be aware, however, that water may not be available here year-round—Los Angeles Department of Water and Power may have drained the aqueduct for maintenance at any time between October 1 and May 1).

Beyond the trough, the bridge carries you across the main wash. **A nice flat north of the wash makes a logical campsite before you tackle the waterless Tehachapi Mountains,** but most springtime hikers camp like trolls under the bridge—the only significant shade in this scorching locale. Wherever you bed down, be aware that this has become a noisy staging area for dirt-bikers and ATV enthusiasts. Be sure to get an early morning start, and load up with water before leaving the aqueduct—the next reliable water, discounting its infrequent presence in Tylerhorse Canyon 6.6 miles away, is at the bottom of Oak Creek

Canyon, a long 22.7 miles away. An alternative to getting water from the sometimes-dirty-and-bee-infested horse trough southwest of the bridge is Waterhole 1521-66, at the immediate east end of the bridge. Via a 3″ plastic pipe, it provides water to a small pool in a cluster of shrubs about 50 feet below the road.

Walk briefly along the aqueduct to the next dirt road (3120-0.1) branching left, northwest, up Cottonwood Creek. It is frequently signed by 4-foot-high brown plastic posts topped with PCT emblems; they are just as frequently blown to smithereens by thoughtless target-shooters. Follow it gently up through a sunny Joshua tree grove to a resumption of PCT trail tread (3160-0.4) branching right, north, up the first ravine that cuts the 50-foot-high alluvial embankment above your road. This junction and all others in the next few miles were also originally marked by brown PCT posts, but some dirt-bikers have made a project of uprooting them. Ascend to the top of the slope, emerging on the bajada—a formation consisting of alluvial fans—up through them your route will wind into the Tehachapis. **Be aware that dirt-bikers have also heavily used the trail to access the Tehachapis, creating many diverging and sometimes confusing paths.** At first, you walk north to the lip of another ravine, where posts indicate your turn across two prominent dirt-bike paths to head due west along the Section 3/34 line, soon finding another good bike path (3250-0.5) right on a lip overlooking Cottonwood Creek. Here is a pipe benchmark locating the adjacent corners of Sections 3, 4, 33 and 34. Now, as indicated by a brown plastic post, turn right, due north, following wooden stakes through the open desert. Soon you parallel and then leap-frog a jeep track on a hot, gentle ascent. Cross an east-west jeep road (3465-1.0), then turn a bit west of north to continue up, now with increasing numbers of low junipers and decreasing Joshua trees beside your shadeless path.

**E**

Agua Dulce –
Highway 58

**See Maps E12, E13**

see MAP E14

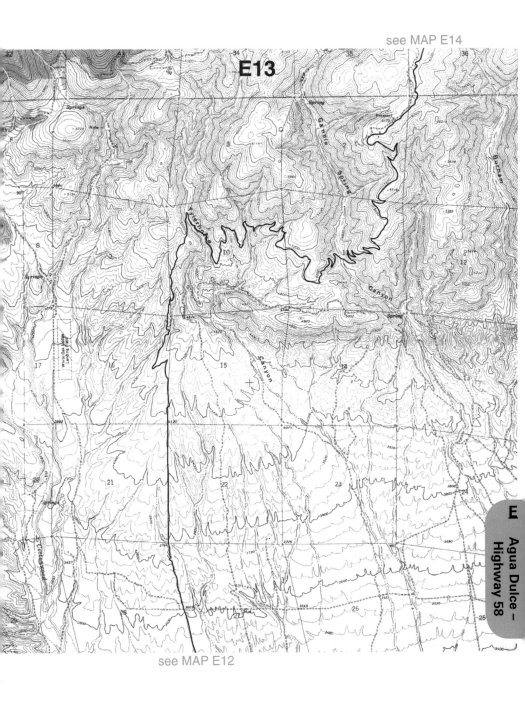

**E13**

see MAP E12

Strike more poor dirt roads at a T-junction (3609-0.5), after which the trail is quite indistinct, but continues on the same bearing up to a viewful and breezy knoll (3800-0.4), where you take note of your progress and survey the southern flanks of the Tehachapis. Next, descend briefly across a pair of ravines to cross a poor jeep road (3790-0.2) that traces the south boundary of a barbed-wire fence. The PCT parallels the 4-strand fence, with its steel and wooden posts, as it marches due north up along the Section 21/22 boundary, in sandy, open grassland. Approaching the west side of a large ravine, you join with a good jeep road (4070-0.7), walk along it for 0.1 mile, then resume your fence-line position to soon find a perpendicular jeep road and the end of the fence (4120-0.3).

From here, the path takes a more logical line, and a slightly steeper one, northward to the head of the ravine, then over two low ridge noses and across a dry streambed, now in much denser cover of sagebrush, rabbitbrush and low junipers. A brisk ascent follows, eventually reaching a wide, rough jeep/dirtbike path (4960-2.2) which climbs the ridge west of Tylerhorse Canyon. Climb momentarily north along that path to find a post marking PCT tread, which drops steeply down into often cool and shady Tylerhorse Canyon (4840-0.3). Often, within a week or two of spring rains, a trickle of water will run here, and tall junipers and Coulter pines will afford a nice quiet camp. **Beware of flash floods during and after storms.**

The PCT continues up into the Tehachapis by now turning generally east, making a hot but well-graded ascent across three major ravines, then descends a bit to a saddle (4960-3.2) overlooking Gamble Spring Canyon. Here you ignore the now-familiar plethora of dirtbike trails, and instead descend almost 400 feet, via sandy switchbacks, to the dry floor of Gamble Spring Canyon (4625-0.7). **There is often water here in springtime, but it cannot be relied upon,** especially in drier than average years. Above, the final 1600-foot leg of our 3000-foot climb into the Tehachapis awaits: First, eight hot switchbacks, badly abused by motocross riders, lead up to a brief respite where you traverse around a 5716-foot knob. Two more switchbacks attack the next slope, but not nearly as viciously as the dirtbikers have—a huge, rutted swath cuts directly up the ridge, obliterating the PCT in places. Near the top, you round clockwise across a breezy nose that is cut by a jeep road (6070-3.0) and pocked with prospect pits in a small outcropping of Paleozoic marine metasediments. Here, the trail swings northeast, keeping just below the ridgetop and its jeep track, soon finding the welcome shade of stands of junipers and pinyon pines which frame vistas south over Antelope Valley.

On a clear morning, Mt. San Antonio, San Gorgonio Peak and San Jacinto Peak can all be seen, as well as the massive buildings of the NASA space shuttle center in Palmdale.

Soon the PCT begins to undulate up and down between groves of fragrant pinyon and Coulter pines and large junipers, which clothe slopes between dry flats of sagebrush scrub and mountain mahogany brush. You stay close to, but rarely see, a good dirt road that serves a scattering of vacation cabins. Without fanfare, you reach the PCT's 6280-foot highpoint in the Tehachapi Mountains, then descend easily, winding along the pinyon-forested ridge that forms the south side of Oak Creek Canyon. Beyond a gap at the heads of Burnham and Pitney canyons (5980-2.6) you climb for a few minutes, then resume your easy descent.

**See Maps E13, E14, E15**

Frequent vistas are had over mead-ow-bottomed Oak Creek Canyon, which is carved along the active Garlock Fault, whence the southern Sierra Nevada rises. Oak Creek Canyon is home to one of the last herds of wild dark brown horses that once roamed the Antelope Valley area, having descended from horses lost by Spanish explorers.

The canyon, like these slopes above, is private property, so no camping is allowed, and hikers must stay on the trail. Anyone who drops into the canyon bottom for any reason will be prosecuted.

Continue winding easily down the ridge, in open groves of juniper, occasion-ally making well-marked crossings of vague, branching jeep trails.

Presently, the hum of electric gen-erators and the whoosh of blades are heard, and the way descends to the edge of a vast array of wind turbines. These harvest electrical energy from the nearly incessant breezes that blow across the Tehachapis, spawned by temperature gra-dients between cool coastal air and the hot Mojave Desert. You will grow used to these mammoth windmills, since you will walk among them all of the way to Highway 58, but initially their incongru-ous presence reminds one of an enor-mous flock of squeaking, flapping sea-gulls.

The wind farms force our route to trace the lip of the canyon wall, then to switchback sandily down it, eventually reaching the streamside of Oak Creek, in a delightful open stand of white oaks. In a minute you step through a pipe gate, then cross Oak Creek (4075-6.4) via a small steel bridge at the dam of a stream-flow gauging pond, where water is almost always available through early summer. Unfor-tunately, this is private land and camping is not permitted.

Now, parallel the stream on its north bank for a moment, then turn northwest up across a gentle ridgetop. Soon, pass under a double-pole powerline, step across a poor dirt road, and drop a few feet to two-lane, paved Tehachapi-Willow Springs Road (4150-0.2), at its junction with paved Cameron Road.

**Resupply access:** Here, most Trailers will veer from the PCT to head 9.4 miles into Tehachapi for resupply. Access to Tehachapi is much easier from here than via Highway 58, at the end of this section. Go carefully up Tehachapi-Willow Springs Road 1.8 miles to 4834-foot Oak Creek Pass, then descend north through fields of California poppies to paved Highline Road (3.6 miles). Here, one has two equi-distant options—walk left, west, on High-line Road 3.0 miles to Summit Road, then right, north, 1.0 mile into the center of Tehachapi; or continue north on Teha-chapi-Willow Springs Road, over High-way 58 via an overpass, 1.0 mile to Teha-chapi Boulevard. Now turn left, west, 1.0 mile to cross under Highway 58 and find a very good hotel, restaurant, bar, gas sta-tion and mini-mart at Steuber Road. Continue 2.0 miles farther west on Teha-chapi Boulevard to reach the center of Tehachapi, with numerous motels, large markets, laundry, restaurants, banks, pharmacies, hardware, and a hospital.

Back on the PCT in Oak Creek Can-yon, cross Tehachapi-Willow Springs Road and pick up slightly indistinct tread head-ing east, marked by a 4x4 post with a PCT emblem. Turn northward across three dirt roads in quick succession, the first two sub-serving polelines. Then gently ascend across a broad, dry, sandy ravine, in open grass-

E

Agua Dulce –
Highway 58

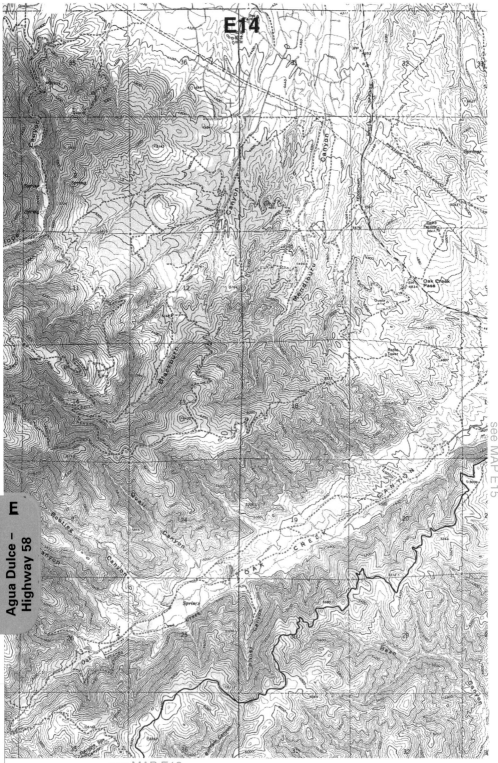

see MAP E15

**E**

**Agua Dulce – Highway 58**

see MAP E13

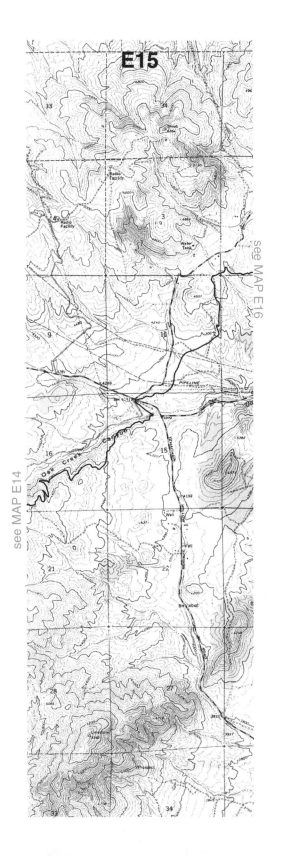

see MAP E16

see MAP E14

E
Agua Dulce –
Highway 58

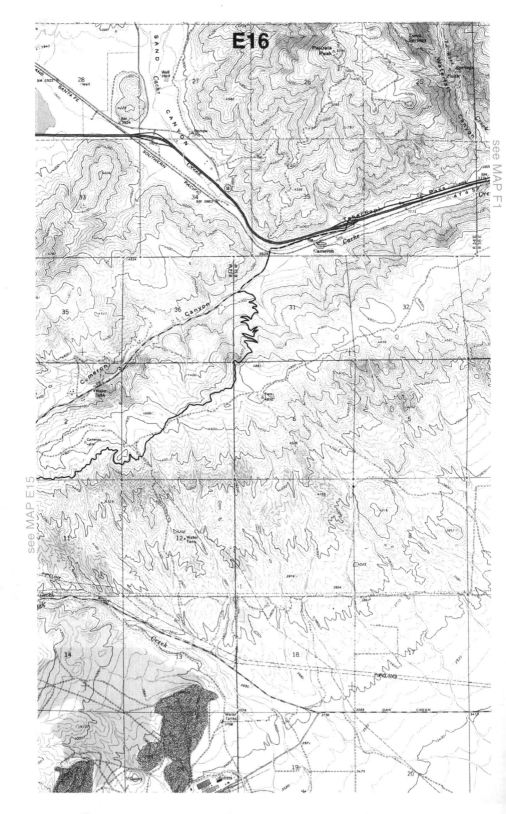

E16

see MAP F1

see MAP E15

and dotted with sagebrush and a few low junipers, to the melodious calls of flocks of meadowlarks. Reaching a hillside, you might lose trail tread momentarily where bulldozers have cut a wide swath, but plastic marker-posts show the way across one good dirt road (4165-0.8) to a second (4160-0.2), just below another large windmill plantation. Now you turn north, attacking the hillside at a moderate angle, soon crossing numerous dirt roads of varying quality which serve the wind farm and the double-pole powerline that runs along its western boundary.

The climb eventually abates at a small saddle (4495-0.6). Here you drop north for a few yards, step across a dirt road, and bend eastward. Open two pipe gates in a barbed-wire fence, drop into a gully, then climb steeply east to another gate and again gain a viewful ridgetop (4560-0.6). Wide vistas extend south over wind farms, Joshua trees and desert to the San Gabriel and San Bernardino mountains.

For the next leg, you undulate eastward under the propeller-bedecked crest of the Tehachapis on sunny, sandy trail which three times crosses dirt access roads. At a fourth, good dirt road (4485-1.6), you note a guardhouse for one of the wind farming corporations at a road junction just to your north. You pass south of that road, then cross it and ascend gently over the ridgecrest and down to a saddle, also with a poor dirt road (4600-0.5). The path from here makes its way onto the steeper northern slopes of the ridge, with sweeping panoramas over Cameron Canyon to the Tehachapi Valley and beyond to the southern Sierra. An easy ascent eventually finds a narrow ridge, where you step across a dirt road (4765-0.9) just below a heavy steel gate, then pass through a barbed-wire gate in a cluster of junipers. A single switchback leads to a steep hillside, heavily eroded by wild horses. Below, a dozen well-graded switchbacks lower you to the floor of Cameron Canyon. Reaching the bottom, you turn west

momentarily to strike two-lane paved Cameron Road (3905-2.1) at a pipe gate. Now follow brown plastic PCT markers along that road's south shoulder, easily down to cross Atchison Topeka and Santa Fe and Southern Pacific Railroad tracks (3824-0.5). From here, the PCT, unmarked, follows Cameron Road east to its overpass of busy four-lane Highway 58 at Tehachapi Pass (3830-0.8). Welcome to the Sierra Nevada!

**Resupply access:** Tehachapi, with its extensive facilities described previously, lies 9.2 miles west on Highway 58, but is difficult to reach from this spot, due to the rarity of traffic that exits or enters via the Cameron Road off-ramp. Rather than hitchhiking from here, consider a walk partway into Tehachapi. Avoid Highway 58. Instead, turn left, west, along the aforementioned railroad tracks. Walk the roadbed that parallels the railroad, keeping well away from the heavily used tracks. Cross under Highway 58 in 1.5 miles, and then at the first opportunity walk north over to paved, frequently used Tehachapi Road, which parallels the tracks and the freeway. You should be able to hitch a ride here. Continue west on that road 7.5 miles more to the downtown area. You pass a Travelodge with a gas station, a restaurant, a bar, and a mini-mart at the Steuber Road intersection, 2.0 miles before you reach the center of town.

Tehachapi Post Office is now north of Hwy. 58 on North Mill Street, across from the AM/PM Mini Market. This location is, unfortunately, less convenient to hikers, though less than ½ mile from downtown.

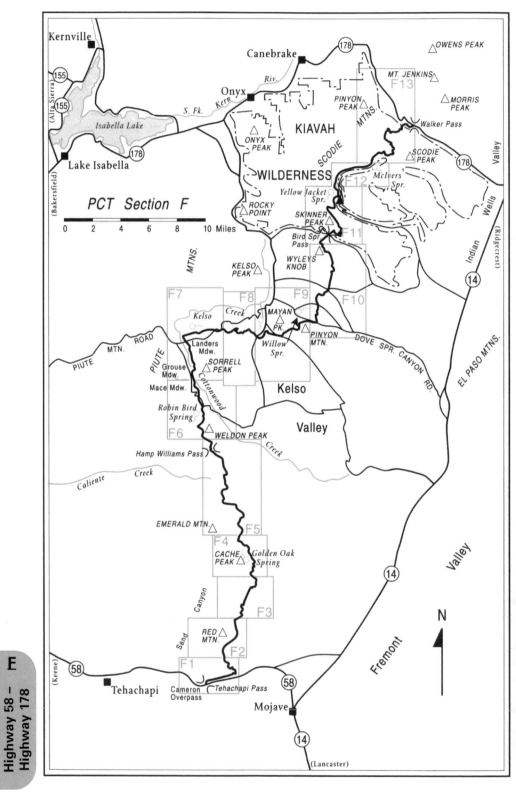

PCT Section F

0   2   4   6   8   10 Miles

## Section F:

# Highway 58 near Tehachapi Pass to Highway 178 at Walker Pass

Surprisingly to many people, most geographers include the Tehachapi Mountains as part of the mighty Sierra Nevada, calling the range the "Sierran Tail" or the "Sierran Hook." The Sierra's southernmost tip, then, is the southwest point of the Tehachapi Mountains below the junction of the San Andreas and Garlock faults.

In the Sierra north of the Tehachapi range, the PCT immediately climbs onto the Sierra crest, where it remains for most of this section, traversing the granitic Sierra Nevada batholith, which is exposed so widely. It quickly climbs from a Joshua/juniper woodland to a pinyon pine/oak woodland, with five species of oak along the route. A cool Jeffrey-pine forest in the Piute Mountains offers a refreshing midsection change for the hiker before you drop to a desert community of plants, then progress again to a pinyon-pine woodland.

The charm of this section lies not only in its diversity of flora, but also in the unobstructed views of rows of sharp ridges and deep valleys, of sprawling desert lands and distant peak silhouettes, of faraway pockets of populated, sometimes historic enclaves, of evidence of the human quest for riches and energy to power our lifestyles.

# Maps

Monolith                          Claraville
Tehachapi NE                      Pinyon Mountain
Cache Peak                        Cane Canyon
Cross Mountain                    Horse Canyon
Emerald Mountain                  Walker Pass

# Declination

13¾°E throughout this section.

| Points on Route | S→N | Mi. Btwn. Pts. | N→S |
|---|---|---|---|
| Cameron Overpass at Highway 58 | 0.0 | | 84.1 |
| | | 16.1 | |
| Golden Oak Spring | 16.1 | | 68.0 |
| | | 18.2 | |
| road to Robin Bird Spring | 34.3 | | 49.8 |
| | | 0.4 | |
| Jawbone Canyon Road in Piute Mountains | 34.7 | | 49.4 |
| | | 5.6 | |
| Piute Mountain Road, first crossing | 40.3 | | 43.8 |
| | | 3.0 | |
| Piute Mountain Road, second crossing | 43.3 | | 40.8 |
| | | 4.8 | |
| Kelso Valley Road | 48.1 | | 36.0 |
| | | 2.1 | |
| Butterbredt Canyon Road | 50.2 | | 33.9 |
| | | 4.1 | |
| road to Willow Spring | 54.3 | | 29.8 |
| | | 9.2 | |
| Bird Spring Pass | 63.5 | | 20.6 |
| | | 6.0 | |
| road to Yellow Jacket Spring | 69.5 | | 14.6 |
| | | 6.7 | |
| road to McIvers Spring | 76.2 | | 7.9 |
| | | 7.3 | |
| Walker Pass Campground spur trail | 83.5 | | 0.6 |
| | | 0.6 | |
| Highway 178 at Walker Pass | 84.1 | | 0.0 |

E

Highway 58 –
Highway 178

## Weather To Go

Because much of this section is exposed, it can be hot; the beginning can be very windy. The terrain you cover receives snow in winter, with the higher elevations blanketed. Early-to-mid spring and mid-to-late fall are optimal times to enjoy your trek here. Most thru-hikers arrive at the best time.

## Supplies

You have a choice between the rapidly growing town of Tehachapi, 9.6 miles west, and the desert town of Mojave, 9.6 miles east, both off Highway 58. Of the two, Tehachapi is the better choice. To walk to Techachapi, avoid Highway 58. Instead, turn left (west) along the railroad tracks. Walk along the parallel roadbed, keeping well away from the heavily used tracks. Cross under Highway 58 in 1.5 miles and then, at the first opportunity, walk north over to paved Techachapi Road, which parallels the tracks and the freeway. You may be able to hitch a ride here. Continue west on that road 7.5 miles more to town. You pass a Travelodge with a gas station, restaurant, bar, and minimart at the Steuber Road intersection, 2.0 miles before you reach the center of town. From town the post office is 1.2 miles: north on Green St., left on West H St., right on North Mill/Capital Hill St., across Highway 58, and left (1085 Voyager Dr. 93561).

At the end of this section, Onyx has limited groceries and supplies and a post office 16.5 miles west of Walker Pass Campground off Highway 178. Also regional transit for towns around Isabella Lake and Bakersfield reach as far east as Onyx P.O. A KOA Campground is 7.0 miles farther west off Highway 178. Kernville is 36 miles northwest of Walker Pass Campground: take Highway 178 and Sierra Way. It has a post office, supplies, motels, etc., and for your rest and relaxation days, kayak rentals

and one-hour to multiday raft trips on the tumultuous Kern River during adequate water flow.

## Water

Available year-round water sources are sparse in this section. During periods of extended drought, even usually reliable springs dry up. A series of springs in this section were upgraded in the 1990s to remove cattle contaminants, but you still need to boil, filter, or add iodine tablets to render the water suitable for you. Both the BLM and the Forest Service continue to upgrade the springs. Although there is usually a breeze on this mostly shadeless trail section, days can be hot and humidity can be low. It is advisable to hydrate yourself well at every water source and to carry a minimum of two quarts per waterless 10 miles.

## Permits

The required fire permit can be obtained from the Bureau of Land Management or Sequoia National Forest. No wilderness permit is needed for this section.

## Special Problems

### Rattlesnakes

See this section of Chapter 2.

### Ticks

These bugs rank as the most sinister and sneaky of the nuisance bugs encountered in the Southern Sierra. Ticks can cause serious diseases that, fortunately, are uncommon in this area: most notably Lyme disease and Rocky Mountain spotted fever. Lyme disease usually presents a ring-like red rash around the bite; spotted fever causes reddish-black spots. Both diseases involve flu-like symptoms. Specific antibiotics offer a cure, and should be given early in the illness.

Ticks seem most prevalent in late winter and spring. They neither jump nor fly, but transfer from grass or brush to animals or you. You hardly see them and often do not feel their bite. This eight-legged creature can be as tiny as a dot of this *i* (larvae) or up to ¼ inch (adult). To remove the tick secure it with tweezers next to the skin and pull gently upward and outward. Try not to crush it, as doing that releases its fluid into the bite. Inspect your clothes frequently when in brushy, grassy areas.

### Off-highway Vehicles (OHVs)

Be forewarned that the seemingly unlimited open space along some stretches in this section attracts weekend OHVs, but very few during the week. They are prohibited on the PCT.

# THE ROUTE

The closest source of water north on the trail is Golden Oaks Spring, 16.1 miles ahead. Before starting this often windy, exposed section north of Tehachapi Pass, you should hydrate yourself well and carry at the very minimum three quarts of water. The trail passes through a crazy quilt of private and BLM lands. Because of private lands, you are asked not to stray from the trail, even for peakbagging.

You begin your trek at the south end of Cameron Overpass (3800-0.0), then cross busy Highway 58 on the overpass to the trail on the north side. There is often litter here and a strong stench of human waste. Hikers have been blamed, but truckers are at fault. Hurry past. Here you descend, pass through a gate, and then parallel the highway east-northeast along a fenced corridor and through another gate (3780-1.2): this one opposite the CAMERON ROAD EXIT 1 MILE sign. Next you dip through the large wash of Waterfall Canyon and turn northeast to ascend to the right of the flood-control berm next to the wash.

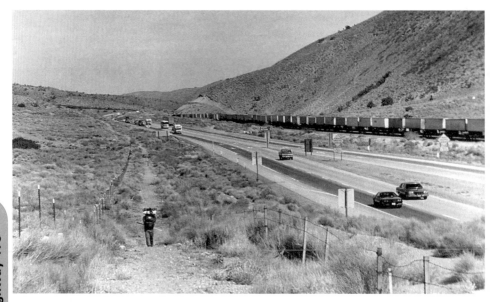

*The PCT briefly parallels Highway 58*

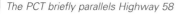

**See Map F1**

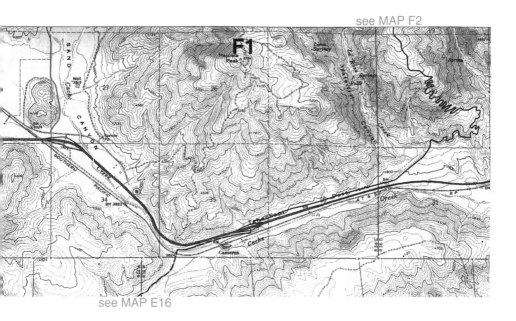

see MAP F2

see MAP E16

Leaving the berm, you progress east while passing groves of juniper trees interspersed with Joshua trees and a few yuccas. Along the foothills you will find that a dirt road briefly usurps the PCT trail; hike on it.

While in the Tehachapi Pass area, you cross over the northeast-southwest Garlock fault, the second largest fault in California. Movement along the fault here is approximately 7–8 millimeters per year. To the north there is no movement; the fault is locked. Seismologists expect a major earthquake in the locked area. These hills show the fault-zone mishmash of granitics and metamorphics. Geologists identify the rocks as mafic and ultramafic plutonic rocks and associated amphibolite, gneiss and granulite.

Climbing north via three switchbacks and some curves, you arrive on a broad slope among scrubby junipers 3.0 miles into your trip—a level place for a camp if needed.

From below you hear the distant chug of locomotives pulling a long chain of freight cars to and from the 17 tunnels and the famous loop at Walong, just west of the town of Tehachapi. Built in 1875–76, the loop is one of the most photographed railroad sections in the world. It is composed of a tunnel and an ascending circle where a gain of 77 feet elevation puts the locomotives over the caboose if the train is more than 4000 feet long.

Usually you feel the prevailing winds that race through Tehachapi Pass. They activate the forests of windmills

**E**

**Highway 58 – Highway 178**

strung on ridges seen from here. The winds are the result of cool air rushing in from the coastal west to replace hot air rising from the desert east. The flow of air increases as it compresses against the ridges, resulting in wind speeds recorded here of up to 80 miles per hour.

The wind farms you see were developed as an alternative to energy generated by air-polluting fossil fuels. Wind-energy people estimate that each turbine displaces approximately 1100 barrels of oil annually, which, in turn, reduces air pollutants by 1900 pounds. But the windmills, some claim, are esthetically polluting, the terrain disturbed during construction is subject to erosion, and the ridges become gouged with roads. The possible expansion of the Sky River wind farm ahead, and the introduction of other wind farms, has heightened concern in neighboring communities and among PCT users.

Moving on, you climb a long, tight series of switchbacks that on the map resemble a recorded earthquake on a seismograph. At length you reach gentler slopes along a broad ridge where camping is possible.

Viewing clockwise from the ridge you see the Mojave Desert to the east, and the isolated features of Soledad Mountain and Elephant Butte rising south of the town of Mojave. Those low volcanic mountains produced millions of dollars worth of gold and silver extracted from contacts between rhyolite and granitic rock along 100 miles of tunnel. Farther southeast you view the barren expanse of Edwards Air Force Base with Rogers Dry Lake air strips, which is home base for experimental aircraft and occasionally

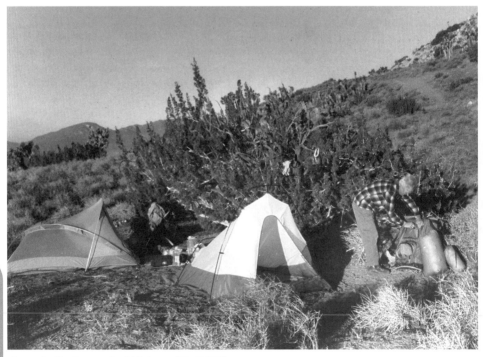

*Campsite 3 miles north of Highway 58 off PCT*

**See Map F1**

see MAP F3

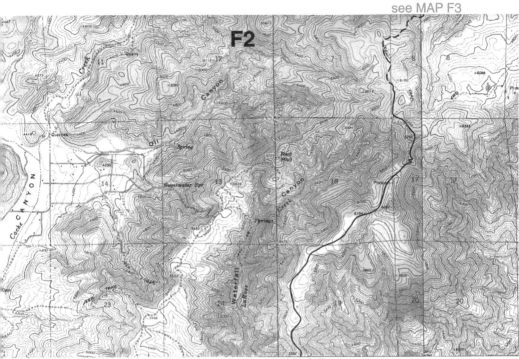

F2

see MAP F1

the landing for space shuttles. To the south loom the Tehachapi Mountains, and west, their namesake town. The large scar on the north side of Tehachapi Pass resulted from excavations by Monolith Cement Company. Their product was used in the construction of the Los Angeles aqueduct, which runs along the east side of the Sierra.

The PCT descends slightly to straddle a narrow ridge between steep canyons, resumes its ascent, and shortly crosses from east-facing to west-facing slopes. In time it encounters pinyon-pine trees.

From these trees, in days of yore, the Kawaiisu Native Americans gathered pinyon nuts. They gathered and hunted from the Tehachapi Mountains north through this area to the South Fork Kern River Valley. To preserve their culture, in 1994 the State of California purchased land surrounding a former village in Sand Canyon, 2.5 air miles west, for a historical park.

Now your trail seeks the crest on ascending slopes. To the right on the crest before a descent, a river of sand hidden amid pinyon pines offers wind-protected campsites. To the left colorful Waterfall Canyon dominates views. The trail next crosses a jeep road that leads to a prospect, then climbs a ridge via three switchbacks and passes a chalky white hill of tuff protruding at the head of an east-facing canyon. Soon the PCT parallels the jeep road, crosses it again, and curves around the head of Waterfall Canyon. Abruptly, the trail ends and the route joins that jeep road (6120-7.1).

E

Highway 58 – Highway 178

**See Map F2**

see MAP F5

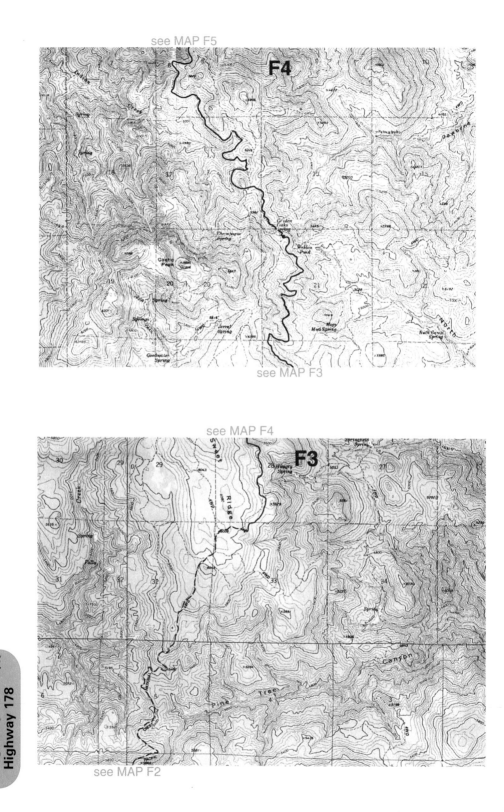

see MAP F3

see MAP F4

see MAP F2

You turn left on the seldom-used jeep road, which heads generally north, descends to the east, and then heads north again. At the bottom of the descent, 2.0 miles along the road, you curve around a huge gray pine tree on a flat offering several sites for camping. Again you climb a ridge, perhaps serenaded by a mountain chickadee's clear three-note "How-are you" —the "How" a whole note, the "are you" two eighth notes at a lower pitch.

Ahead, as the route eventually descends into a sagebrush swale, you see the first of the 90- and 140-foot wind-turbine towers perched over 5 miles of ridgeline.

The Vestas V-27 three-blade turbines, used here in the early 1990s Sky River project, are far more efficient than the earlier versions you saw previously on ridges. Total output of Sky River exceeds 600 million kilowatt hours per year— enough to supply electricity for a residential population of 300,000. Now the twirling giant pinwheels produce a mechanical hum to accompany the chickadee's serenades.

In this hollow the course crosses a dirt road, passes a road that is returning to nature, and forks right where the sign on the locked, gated road to the left declares SKY RIVER RANCH—PRIVATE PROPERTY. In 0.2 mile from the gated road, the PCT branches right (6000-4.3), leaving the jeep road where it becomes closed and abruptly descends.

Your route ahead crosses several roads to turbines; most are mentioned in the text; none are mapped. The company asks that you not venture near the machines.

The PCT, a trail again, zigzags, turns sharply left, and crosses both a wide road to turbines and the ragged jeep road you just left.

Here you see your first view of Olancha Peak far to the north over waves of ridges. Mount Whitney beyond, the highest mountain in the lower 48 states, barely reaches above the waves. Pointy Owens Peak rises southeast of Olancha Peak, with Mt. Jenkins at its right. The PCT eventually passes near all of these peaks, and long-distance hikers on the trail are given many opportunities to view this scene as they progress.

Your path, cut on very steep slopes, begins a long, descending traverse around the east side of turbine-bristled Sweet Ridge. It then rounds the flanks of 6698-foot Cache Peak, the highest peak in the southernmost Sierra north of Tehachapi Pass. In time, the trail, passing slender snowmelt streamlets, descends to cross a jeep road at an offset junction, and arrives at a resurfaced stone-and-cement trough catching a piped-in, year-round flow from Golden Oaks Spring (5480-3.5). In 1994 the BLM constructed a new spring box, fenced the spring to protect it from cattle contaminants, and installed a new pipe from the box to the trough. This important water source is now easily accessible to hikers and still serves the cattle and wild life in the area. The level cul-de-sac on G.E. Wind Energy's private property above the spring and off the adjacent jeep road is no longer posted with NO TRESPASSING signs.

Springs are important to wildlife, of course, as well as hikers. The area's mule deer, bobcats, mountain lions and black bears will shy away from this water source while people are near. Bighorn sheep frequented this spring as well as other springs in these mountains as recently as the early 1900s. At that time domestic sheep infected with scabies were released in the area. The scabies spread to the native bighorns, resulting in their demise. In 1978 tule elk were transplanted here from Owens Valley, but most of the elk migrated to lower elevations and found their way to the alfalfa fields in Fremont Valley.

With full water containers to last until Robin Bird Spring, 18.3 miles, you head generally northwest, crossing a closed road, then paralleling a wide road to turbines before crossing it. You resume on trail a few paces up the road and on it traverse steep slopes to eventually round prominent Point 5683. Next, on a pair of switchbacks, you descend below an old jeep road now used to access turbines; where the descent eases you find camping possibilities. You then cross a ravine and climb up its west side. Beyond a switchback, a turbine road and a saddle, you arc west around the extensive drainage of Indian Creek, providing good views of Cache Peak to the south. In time, after noting a white plastic pipe marking a miner's border, you reach an east-west ridge, which you cross via a green gate (5102-6.5) in a cattle fence.

Beyond the gate, the route heads generally west in shade, then swings north to follow a sunny crest, the watershed divide between Caliente Creek to the west and Jawbone Canyon to the east.

This crest affords comprehensive views of multicolored Jawbone Canyon and, to the north-northeast, of Kelso Valley and Mayan Peak. (The PCT eventually curves alongside distant Mayan Peak.)

The trail undulates near or on the crest, then descends a north-facing ridge to a blue-oak savannah with a large grassy area to the left nicely suited for camping. Several gleaming quartz rocks form fire rings here. Your route is crossed below the campsite by an east-west road (5010-3.0).

This road connects with other roads to offer passage from Highway 14 on the east to Highway 58 on the south, but it is a private, gated and locked road, and extremely rough to the west.

Traveling north, you ascend easily across a grassy ridge with a springtime wildflower sparkle of baby blue eyes, curve around a minor eastward extension, and then hike along a narrow saddle. The path north of the saddle looks ominous, and it is a steep climb by PCT standards. The curious upslope swath cut through scrub oak followed the original trail design. Grateful you are not panting up that route, you ascend north through a scrub-oak aisle.

Scrub oak resembles live oak in miniature: its growth is dense; its branches are ridged; its forest is impenetrable without the help of cutting tools.

Upon turning northwest, you leave the chaparral oak for the domain of lofty Jeffrey pines and spreading black oaks, the first appearance of these pines and oaks on this section of the PCT. **If looking for campsites, you will find a shaded area off the path at the north end of the forest.** Just beyond the forest you descend to traverse below Hamp Williams Pass (5530-3.3).

Once again you are faced with a steep climb by PCT standards, lined with scrub oak and relieved slightly by four switchbacks. Breaks in the oak cover offer vignettes of Jawbone Canyon Road below. You will cross that road where it winds in the mountains ahead. Here you make a traverse, a zig and a zag, and climb over a saddle to west-facing slopes, again among welcome Jeffrey pines and black oaks. Just

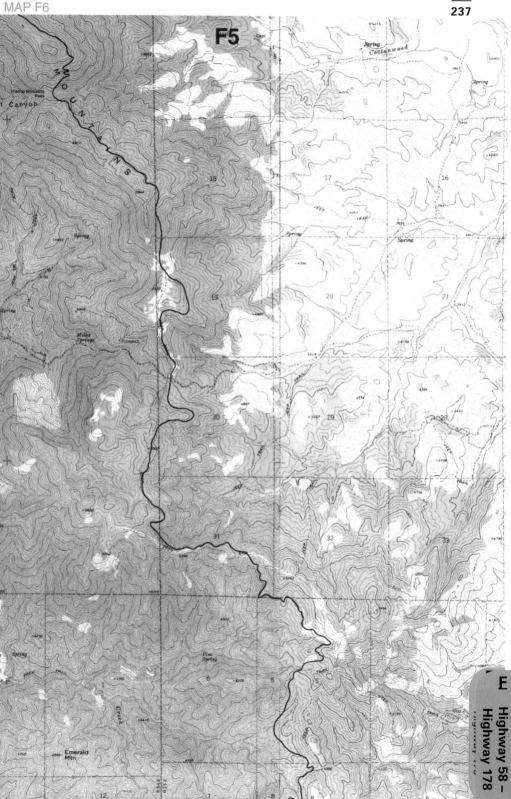

F5

E

see MAP F7

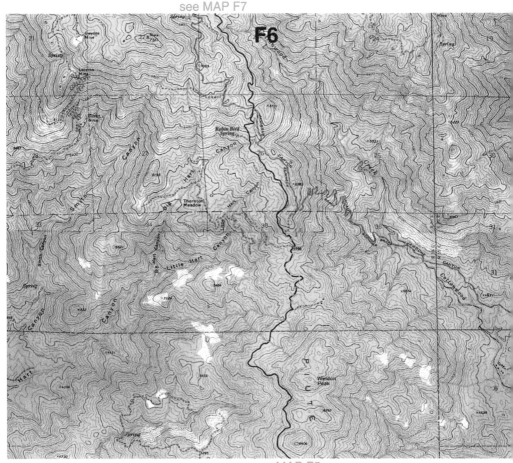

see MAP F5

where the Piute Mountains begin in the south is uncertain, but you are surely in the Piutes now. You descend on a traverse past two peaks and part way around Weldon Peak before the descent increases down a west-facing ridge, then decreases as you turn northeast to enter a cluster of privately owned small parcels. **No camping allowed.** Much of the land you crossed in this section was large blocks of privately owned land or BLM-governed land. Your PCT path ends on a curve of a private dirt road (5620-3.2).

Turning right, you proceed up the main private road, permitted for PCT use. You turn left at the first fork at 0.1 mile, pass several spur roads, ease around a locked cable crossing the road, and then meet a T-junction (5996-0.8) with a west-descending, prominent unpaved road. Here you keep right, then ascend along a tight right curve, and find the PCT path resuming to the left (6160-0.4). (The road continues to Jawbone Canyon Road 0.2 mile beyond.)

**E**

**Highway 58 – Highway 178**

**See Map F6**

Walking north, on the PCT path again, below and parallel to Jawbone Canyon Road, you enter Forest Service land in 0.2 mile and soon angle across a dirt road (6360-1.0).

**Water access:** Your first water source since Golden Oaks Spring is 0.1 mile down this road. In 1994 the Forest Service developed this flowing spring, freed it from cattle contaminants, and piped the water, making it easily accessible to you. They then cleared the enormous amount of rubble of a dilapidated two-story house, leaving a flat area for camping. With a deserved sense of pride, they named this lovely area Robin Bird Spring.

Beyond the spring access road, the PCT switchbacks up to unpaved Jawbone Canyon Road (6620-0.4).

**PCT access route:** This lightly traveled PCT access route, Jawbone Canyon Road, leaves east down the Piute Mountains, crosses Kelso Valley, winds among low, exposed hills, and reaches State Highway 14, 26.4 miles later. The BLM OHV visitor center is located at the junction. To the west of the PCT, Jawbone Canyon Road curves north to connect with roads that continue north to Highway 178, 32.0 miles later.

North of Jawbone Canyon Road the PCT descends among scattered Jeffrey pines, white firs and mistletoe-trimmed black and live oaks. It drops down a few switchbacks and winds along east-facing slopes where cascades of white-flowered spreading phlox perk up the early-season wayside scenery. In 0.5 mile the trail passes above a seasonal spring hidden by willows; a use path descends next to the spring, but easier water sources are at Cottonwood Creek ahead. The path gently undulates now, passes a magnificent golden oak to your

left—a tree climber's delight—then adds gravel to the dirt tread as boulders surrounded by manzanitas appear.

In a short time the trail crosses a willow-lined branch of **Cottonwood Creek with possible camping nearby: a good source of water until late summer. The stream, coming from Mace and Grouse meadows on this multi-use mountain, may be water that cows have enjoyed as well.** The path briefly parallels another willow-hemmed branch of the slender creek, crosses it on a log footbridge (6480-1.8), and then proceeds above it.

The well-defined path continues to wind and dip, generally heading north. Strips of Jawbone Canyon Road appear to the west before the PCT turns up a canyon, crosses a logging road (6720-1.0) and climbs over a saddle, the watershed divide of Cottonwood and Landers creeks. Within ½ mile, watch for a spring above the trail whose water is caught by a crude cement structure.

Below the trail squat the roofless remains of a crumbling log cabin with an upright chimney. Apple trees and lilac bushes soften the clutter. This area and its short mine shaft tunneled into a creekbed are worth investigating.

Back on the trail, you walk above, then switchback down to the headwaters of Landers Creek: a trickle through a pocket meadow with nearby camping potential. In minutes you see an old sluice box sitting among the willows by the creek. Later you switchback down to cross Landers Creek (6300-1.9) and quickly cross back to the east side again.

Before recrossing the creek, you can hike 0.2 mile along the west bank where a dirt road leads to creekside Waterhole Trail Camp. (The dirt road con-

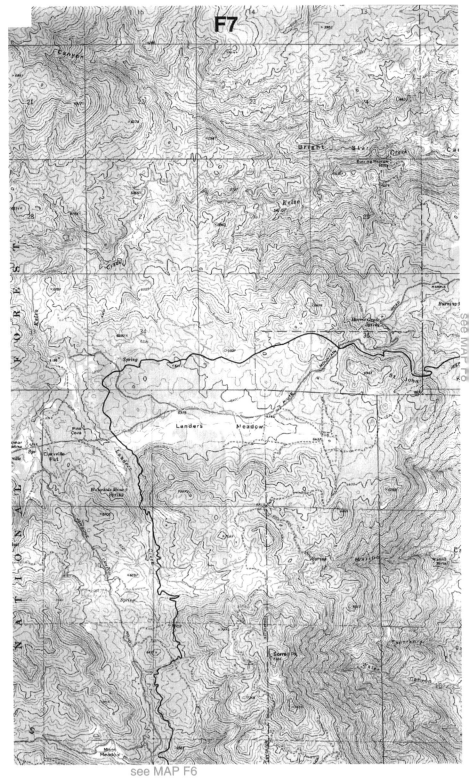

**F7**

tinues to Piute Mountain Road.) The camp has a table and piped-in spring water. Since this is one of the Fire Safe areas in the Piutes, you can usually have a campfire here even during periods of restricted fire use. You can easily cross Landers Creek here to pick up the PCT again on the east bank.

Heading north, the trail remains in the little canyon until the canyon flares near Landers Meadow, spreading to the east. After crossing the meadow's outlet stream, the path bridges a trench and crosses Piute Mountain Road (6220-0.9). The PCT crosses this road again in 3.0 miles.

On the north side of Piute Mountain Road, the Forest Service has installed an ingenious gate across the PCT, flanked by fences. This discourages motorcyclists, but hikers and horses can easily step over it. The trail beyond gently weaves along a rolling, selectively logged pine flat inland from the creek, then meets graded, unpaved SNF Road 29S05 (6300-0.7), unsigned at the junction.

**Water access:** This road leads left to a tree-shaded Fire Safe Area primitive campground in 0.3 mile. A spring above the campground is captured in a tank and piped to splash into a cattle trough, the last source of water for 8.8 miles. A curious mortarless stone hut sans roof sits near the spring.

Returning to the PCT, you head east while aloof wallflowers, standing straight and single, display clusters of bright orange blossoms in season, and blue-purple lupines add a dash of contrasting color. Pinyon pines signal your approach to drier climes, and a logging road crosses your path. In time lichen-splashed boulders appear, along with golden oaks and a few dramatic yuccas.

Yuccas grow tough, daggerlike leaves a foot or more long, with sharp tips that puncture the unwary. The stalks, with massive creamy white blossoms that seem to explode in spring, reach 8–14 feet tall.

Soon you enter BLM land and meet Piute Mountain Road (6620-2.3) again, this time at the summit of Harris Grade, Piute Mountains' best access. Here you cross both the trail-protecting gate and the road.

In 0.1 mile, as you begin a descent along the north and then east slopes of St. John Ridge, you again see far off to the north majestic Olancha Peak, reigning over the Kern Plateau.

To the northeast, pointed Owens Peak with curved, serrated Mt. Jenkins next to it, divides the desert from the mountains, and all three peaks delineate the Sierra crest.

While gradually losing elevation, you eventually descend by switchbacks and a long traverse across the slopes of St. John Ridge, passing en route a motorcycle path occupying a gully.

In time, and after two more switchbacks, you spot a post just below the path near a large fremontia bush. It marks the boundary of a mining claim. Fremontias especially attract attention when frocked in large, waxlike yellow flowers.

Farther below, a jeep road climbs up a steep grade. Soon in the east the serpentine sliver of paved Kelso Valley Road appears. Mayan Peak is in the east, and, to its right, the Butterbredt Canyon road winds up to the Sierra crest. Your exposed trail descends through colonies of bitterbrush and its companion plants to meet Kelso Valley Road at a pass (4953-4.8).

**See Maps F7, F8**

**Resupply access:** Lightly traveled Kelso Valley Road leads north 19.7 miles to Highway 178, which crosses the lower Sierra from Highway 99 in Bakersfield on the west to Highway 14 on the east, along the desert. Emergency supplies are available in towns around Isabella Lake, west on 178. (A short cut to the water source described next leads 1.7 miles to the left down this road, to the stream beyond the large cottonwoods and willows. Return 0.5 mile to the Butterbredt Canyon road, SC123; hike up it 0.7 mile to pick up the PCT—total 2.9 miles.)

After crossing the summit of Kelso Valley Road where it loses its pavement, you approach two distinct paths: an OHV path and the PCT. The OHV path climbs the ridge ahead, becoming one in a web of trails that covers the transitional range you are about to hike: an OHV playground on weekends. These OHV paths cut erosively across your trail, and new ones are added periodically. Although the BLM posts signs that clearly indicate the path of the PCT and forbid OHV use of it, it nevertheless receives their heavy traffic. This use has led to ruts in the trail, to layers of loose dirt on it, and to tight, annoying undulations along its entire length in the transitional range.

Take the trail to the left that heads in a southeast direction on a crenulated course across slopes mantled with bitterbrush, sagebrush and Mormon tea—all dominant brush throughout the range. Next curve across a gully where, downslope to the left, pepper-colored debris excavated from several claims collectively known as the St. John Mine becomes visible.

Beginning in 1867, miners extracted gold here for over 70 years. Most of them lived in the now-vanished settlement of Sageland, just a few miles north.

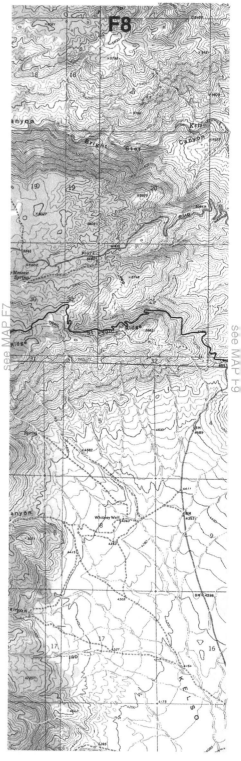

**See Maps F8, F9**

**E**

**Highway 58 –
Highway 178**

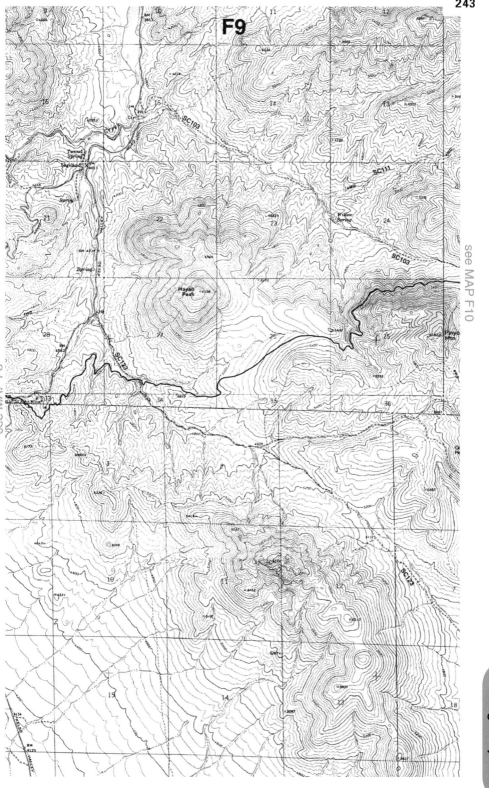

F9

see MAP F10

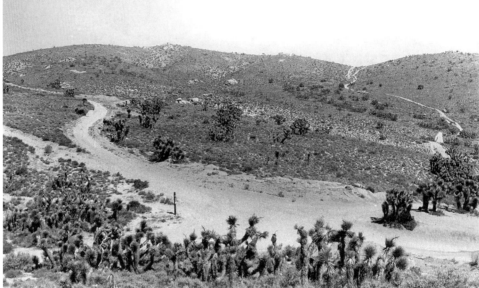

*Multi-road, cycle path, and PCT junction on the Sierra crest saddle*

The route turns northeast to descend on a prominent ridge, curves across a ravine with lines of OHV tracks, traverses north-facing slopes while crossing a band of Joshua trees, and eventually meets the Butterbredt Canyon road, SC123, near the mouth of its canyon (4540-2.1).

**Water access:** Before continuing, check your water supply. At this intersection, year-round water is available at a spring-fed stream 0.7 mile down the Butterbredt Canyon road, then 0.5 mile down paved Kelso Valley Road; a 500-foot elevation loss. A group of cotton-wood and willow trees just west of the paved road marks the spring, but the water flows freer just beyond. An unused cement cow trough lies hidden by brush near the road in this private grazing land that abounds with cows. The next depend-able water is at Willow Spring, 4.1 miles from the Butterbredt Canyon road junc-tion, then 1.8 miles down-canyon with 760 feet elevation drop.

The shadeless, often hot and windy PCT ahead continues from this offset junc-tion at the unpaved road by climbing switchbacks up the ridge between Butter-bredt Canyon to the right and an east-trending gulch to the left, then ascending on an easy-to-moderate grade just south of the gulch. The slopes of the gulch eventually flatten as the path traces the valley's elon-gated curve to the east.

The temple of 6108-foot Mayan Peak to your left rules out northwestward views of the Piute Mountains, but it can-not block out the ribbon of Kelso Valley Road draped on a shoulder of the Sierra crest.

The trail crosses a bike path on a south saddle of barely discernable Point

**See Map F9**

5402; the path west could confuse south-bound hikers. The PCT descends to wind around two canyons, then ascends gently to contour past many lesser ravines cut in the north slope of Pinyon Mountain. The impounded waters of Willow Spring glisten like a distant mirage far below while around you a moderately dense stand of pinyon pines cloaks the north slopes, the only forest for miles.

Long-eared owls have been seen on the eastern edge of this forest. Look under the trees by the trail for their pellets, composed of bone and fur regurgitated by the bird.

As you proceed east, the ranks of the forest dwindle and trees are replaced by xerophytic brush. Still on the slopes of Pinyon Mountain, you reach a multi-road-and-path junction on a Sierra crest saddle (5283-4.1). Pinyon Mountain, a steep 0.8-mile climb of 900 feet to the southeast, has a camping area protected by boulders and pinyon trees, and offers a full view that is especially enticing when the sun hangs low in the southern sky and the shadows stretch long on the desert floor.

**Water access:** If you need water, Willow Spring is 1.8 miles left, down-canyon, on Road SC103 to the northwest. The BLM has upgraded this spring and installed a special pump-action faucet for hikers. To find the pond, where there are no willows but plenty of cows, look for a fence above the road to the right and the outlet stream that flows on the road from the spring. Road SC103 continues to Kelso Valley Road. The next reliable water is at lower Yellow Jacket Spring, 15.9 miles from the Willow Spring road junction, and 0.7 mile down-canyon with 400 feet elevation loss. Road SC103 east of the junction passes Dove Spring in 3.3 miles

on its way to Red Rock Canyon State Park (no supplies) and State Highway 14.

You leave the saddle to wind north around gullied, east-facing slopes, climbing a little at first and then contouring. Along the way Indian Wells Valley, the El Paso Mountains and Fremont Valley intercept your gaze as it sweeps the eastern horizon from north to south. Presently you arrive at another multi-road-and-trail junction (5382-1.6) on a saddle with flats for camping. Road SC111 leads west past the Sunset Mine road to connect with the Willow Spring road just below the spring and pond, and east to connect with the Dove Spring road just above its spring.

You diagonal northwest across the junction saddle, then wind gently upward, staying west of the crest.

Glancing downslope you can see the rubble of Sunset Mine. Upon closer inspection, you find two shafts about 35 feet and 70 feet deep covered with ply-wood held in place by iron belt-driven flywheels, patented 1916; a hulk of a rusted bus; and rails from the mine to the chute. Then you see below the litter around two more prospects.

Again you climb the slopes beside, and then across a road before reaching a ridgecrest saddle (5700-1.1).

To the west, prospect digs, a prominent ore chute and, next to parallel concrete slabs that slash the slope, an overturned Ford, all of which indicate the past activity here at Danny Boy Gold Mine.

Wyleys Knob, the 6465-foot radio-tower-crowned summit to the north, now stands as a gauge of your progress. From the saddle, the wide PCT path to the right makes a moderate descent northeast via

E

Highway 58 – Highway 178

two rounded switchbacks to intersect Road SC328 on a crestline saddle (5300-0.8). Ahead the austere journey takes you generally north over a low hill to another crestline saddle (5380-0.2), where Road SC47 crosses.

**The path gains a low east-west ridge 0.2 mile beyond the saddle, where there are good campsites among the boulders to the right.** Next the PCT dips to a Joshua-tree-covered gap, climbs north on a moderate grade while paralleling a gully, and then curves along a ridge. The gradient eases and the trail first winds around spur ridges emanating from the Sierra crest, then crosses a gap in the crest itself. The Scodie Mountains and the granitic outcrop of Wyleys Knob loom to the north. The trail traverses just east of the crest and passes three rounded, weathered crestline boulders that form a barely balanced stack. Below Hill 5940 a switchback, cut across by cyclists, leads you to skirt a hill on the crest, then to diagonal across an intersection (5740-3.0) with Road SC42.

Now your moderately ascending route curves west, passes granite bluffs and, below Wyleys Knob, begins a gentle-to-moderate descent. It first drops among pinyon pines but later crosses exposed northeast-facing slopes. The path travels just downslope from the Wyleys Knob road, SC24, and quickly reaches a junction (5355-2.5) at Bird Spring Pass, where camping is possible.

This pass was first crossed by Caucasians when in March 1854 John Charles Fremont, on his fifth expedition west, led his party through this passage.

**PCT access route:** Unpaved but maintained, the Bird Spring Road, SC120, is the most used access road to the Pacific Crest Trail in the transitional mountain range. From the saddle it drops west to paved Kelso Valley Road and east to the aqueduct road, north to SC65 and east to State Highway 14.

Thanks to the sweeping California Desert Protection Act signed into law by President Clinton in 1994, you now enter an unbroken network of Congressionally mandated wildernesses that take you through the Sierra. Ahead lies the Kiavah Wilderness. Unlike the "rock and ice" areas of remarkable beauty first encompassed in the National Wilderness Preservation System established in 1964, this 88,290-acre area is designated to preserve the biota of a semiarid land. You know the area as Scodie Mountain, but the Native Americans called it Kiavah.

Leaving Bird Spring Pass, you ascend on the PCT northeast into a side canyon along a sandy path ornamented with nosegays of blue penstemons—showy tubular flowers—and enter into Sequoia National Forest and Kiavah Wilderness. Ahead you pass a trail-register box and a spur road, then climb south from the canyon's wash.

The curious fenced-in square seen below is a quail guzzler constructed to catch rainwater for the local fauna—at this point you could use a PCT guzzler! An occasional Joshua tree and some straggly pinyon pines dot the slopes that abruptly slant away to the vast alluvium of Bird Spring Canyon, spreading far below.

Southwest across the pass the radio tower, its road, and the PCT slowly recede as you climb moderately up long-legged, then short-legged switchbacks, and cross over a ridge with a westward orientation (6460-2.4). You can find small flats to

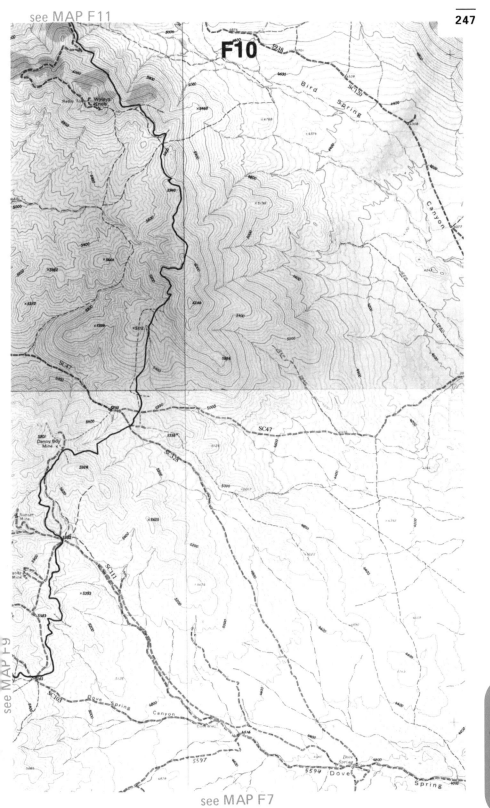

F10

sleep on here. After a long ascending traverse and several short, steep switchbacks, you hike over a ridge, also with room for possible waterless camping, above the Horse Canyon watershed.

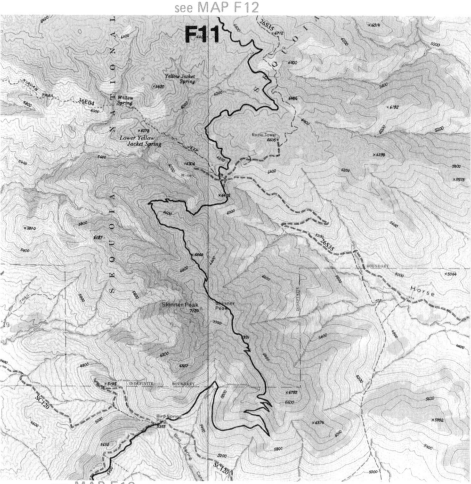

To the north, the High Sierra rises above the crests of east-west Scodie Mountain ridges, while around you manzanitas and golden oaks join the scattered pinyon pines and numerous spring wildflowers.

The PCT soon reaches its highest point (6940-1.3) in this section, then drops along a switchback and descends northwest close to the ridgecrest above a drainage of Cane Canyon.

Across the canyon the northern extension of the Piute Mountains borders the valley of Kelso Creek.

Following two quick switchbacks, your trail turns east across north-facing slopes, allowing glimpses of the eastern

**See Map F11**

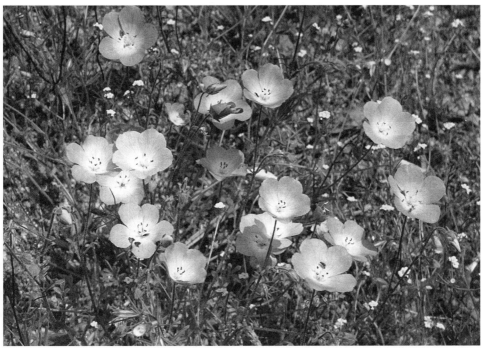

*The PCT cuts across a grassy slope with springtime baby blue eyes*

reaches of Isabella Lake. Lower on the path you see a mining scar gouged in creamy quartz rock across the ravine, and a telephone microwave relay tower perched on a point to the northeast. The route's descent eases at a saddle, then traverses 1⅓ mile across the grassy slopes of minor Peak 6455, above sprawling Horse Canyon. Heading north, the PCT cuts across a road that reaches the mine you just saw, and seconds later crosses another road (6260-2.3), both branching from the Horse Canyon road.

**Side route:** The maintained Horse Canyon road, SC65, also a PCT access road, serves the relay station and descends east to Highway 14. It is not a part of the wilderness, and the rutted northward extension of the road, which the PCT later uses for its route, is outside the wilderness as well.

**Water access:** There is usually water seeping at Lower Yellow Jacket Spring. Dig a hole below a seep, let the soil settle, and then filter the water directly from the hole. To get there, hike down the second branching road to the first broad intersecting canyon, 0.7 mile. The seeps are on the slope to the left. Upper Yellow Jacket Spring, 0.7 mile up-canyon, is unreliable. The next water source near the PCT is McIvers Spring, 7.0 miles from the second branching road junction.

Back on the PCT, abundant pinyon pines, the dominant tree on Scodie Mountain, supply ample shade. The distinguishing characteristics of the pinyon, which grows in high desert ranges, are the single, gray-green needle, the blackish-barked trunk, the much-branched crown

**See Map F11**

*Ruby Johnson Jenkins*

E

Highway 58 – Highway 178

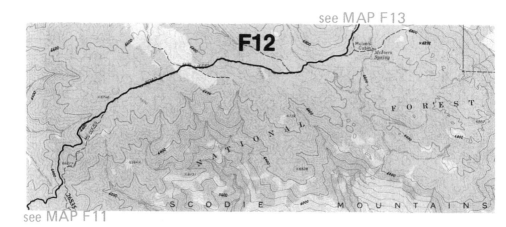

see MAP F13

see MAP F11

and the 2x3-inch cones. You are allowed to gather the nuts of this tree for non-commercial use.

Pinyon nuts tucked beneath the scales of the pitchy pine cones ripen in early autumn. To gather pinyon nuts, collect closed cones in a brown paper bag; then, to open them, place the bag in an oven and set the heat on low. After the cones open and the nuts have been loosened, shell them, and eat them raw or roast them again in oil and a little salt.

The fall gathering season of protein-rich pinyon nuts was one of reverence and fellowship for Native American families. After a solemn ritual, the men shook the trees or loosened the cones with hooks fashioned on willow poles. Children gathered the cones in woven willow baskets for the women to roast. Some nuts were eaten whole, but most were ground into flour. The grinding action created the many holes (mortars) in boulders you find scattered about the mountains. These nuts are still gathered by Native American descendants as part of their diet. Continuing this gathering binds today's Native Americans to this important aspect of their past.

Below the tower, the PCT gradually gains elevation as it undulates and weaves in and around scalloped slopes, and then below the road to McIvers Spring. At length it reaches and joins that road (6670-4.5), arcing east.

The "Ichabod Crane" forest of pinyon pines continues to surround you as you walk northeast along the road. The naturally denuded lower branches, gnarled and twisted, make contorted figurations that awaken your imagination. But the forest from here to north of (not including) McIvers cabin was severely burned in a 1997 lightning-caused fire. In the fire's wake, Poodle Dog Bush *(Turricula parri)* largely replaced the burned brush, and may still be here. Its 3- to 8-foot height has numerous long, slender leaves and clusters of purplish, funnel-shaped flowers. DO NOT TOUCH. This bush can cause severe contact dermatitis.

Abruptly, the trees give way to a sagebrush/buckbrush expanse, and then forest reappears. In less than a mile after the PCT left the path, a short road forks sharply left off your route, and then within the next mile two spur roads fork right. Some rills cross your road that have early-spring water

**See Maps F11, F12**

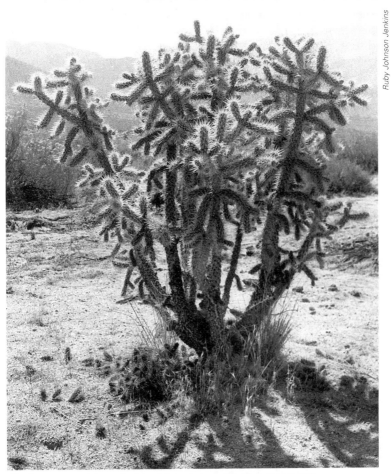

*Ruby Johnson Jenkins*

*Cholla cactus, spiniest of all cacti found along this high desert trek*

and late-spring puddles of lavender-flow-ered, inch-high "belly" plants; and, 0.3 mile before the PCT route returns to path, a seasonal brook flows across it.

At a fork (6680-2.2) the PCT route leaves the road and resumes as trail head-ing northeast.

**Water access:** If you need water or a campsite, you can stay on the road for 0.3 mile to reach McIvers Spring. The next water is 7.4 miles ahead at Walker Pass Campground.

Snuggled among picturesque slabs at the spring is a batten-board hut with porch and outhouse once owned by McIvers and Weldon, who equipped it with the bare necessities of a 1938 rustic retreat. Although run down, it remains today. Hunters, motorcyclists and OHVers have used it over the years. Barring a drought, some water issues from this spring year-round, and good campsites abound here in this bright green oasis among the gray-green pinyons.

**E**

**Highway 58 – Highway 178**

**See Map F12**

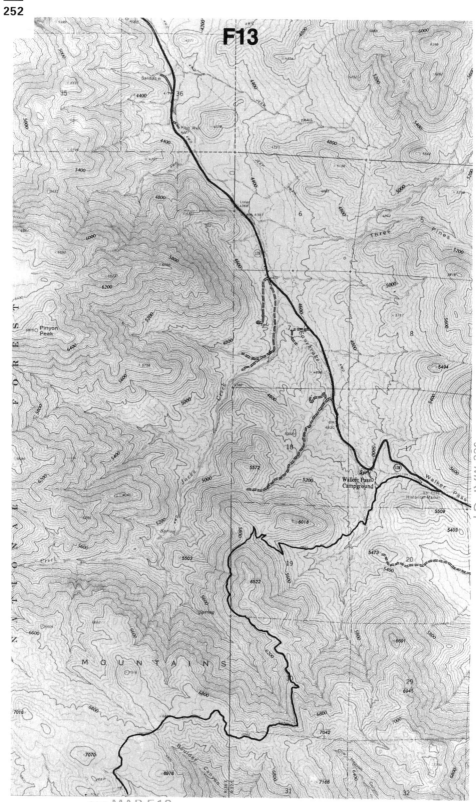

## F13

Highway 58 –
Highway 178

**F**

At the junction where trail resumes, you hike on an ascending, undulating path. Manzanita appears along with a few stands of Jeffrey pine and black oak.

The declivitous slopes of Boulder Canyon fall away to the southeast, and vistas of the Mojave Desert and the ethereal San Gabriel-San Bernardino mountains appear through the haze.

Soon you round some three-story boulders, dashed with rust and chartreuse lichen, supporting a pinyon pine tenaciously growing from a slight crack. Leaving the gentle tableland, you descend on north-facing slopes, with views of the Mt. Whitney group in the distant north and, in the northeast, the top of Olancha Peak.

Next the trail curves around a sharp canyon crease (6680-3.0). Beyond, the PCT briefly reaches over the ridgetop at a switchback where you catch a fleeting glimpse of the Owens Peak group and the hairpin curve of Highway 178, with Walker Pass Campground at the south end of that curve. Far to the north, the slash of Canebrake Road cuts across slopes, and to the northeast the PCT rises above Walker Pass. The trail continues on a long descent across steep west-facing slopes high above Jacks Creek Canyon. In time it passes a use trail angling down the slope to Jacks Creek, crosses a slight ridgeline saddle (5860-2.2), and descends on the mountain's northeast-facing slopes.

After the second switchback down the mountainside, you round just below a ridgetop where, obscured from your view but easily reached, the Forest Service has placed a substantial guzzler for small animals. You then skirt along the lower slopes of Peak 6018.

Among other plants along this section of the PCT, you may see an occasional large, tissue-paper-thin, white flower of a prickly poppy—resembling a fried egg, sunny side up.

Quite soon the trail crosses the usually dry bed of Canebrake Creek, leaves Kiavah Wilderness, and crosses a path (5100-2.1) leading 0.1 mile to the comfortable Walker Pass Trailhead Campground, built especially for PCT trekkers. If the camp faucets are turned off, spring water flows from a pipe into a 9-foot-square cement-enclosed "cattail garden" cow trough, to the left of Highway 178, 0.1 mile down, next to the 30 MILES PER HOUR sign.

The PCT continues to Walker Pass winding northeast and exiting at a historical marker (5246-0.6).

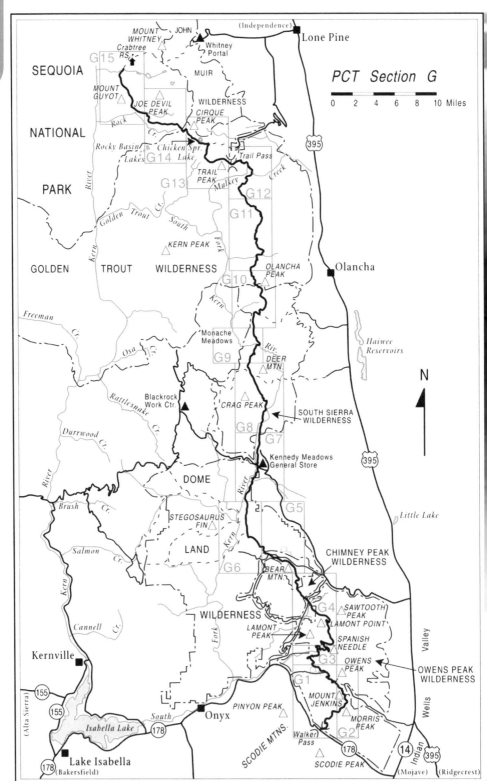

PCT Section G

0  2  4  6  8  10 Miles

SEQUOIA

NATIONAL

PARK

GOLDEN     TROUT     WILDERNESS

MOUNT WHITNEY
Crabtree RS.
JOHN
Whitney Portal
(Independence)
Lone Pine

MUIR

WILDERNESS

MOUNT GUYOT
JOE DEVIL PEAK
CIRQUE PEAK

Rock Cr.

Rocky Basin Lakes
Chicken Spr. Lake
G14
G15
G13
TRAIL PEAK
Trail Pass
Mulkey Creek

River

Golden Trout Cr.
South Fork

KERN PEAK

G12
G11
G10

395

Kern

OLANCHA PEAK

Olancha

Monache Meadows

Osa Cr.

Freeman Cr.

Rattlesnake Cr.

DEER MTN.

Riv.

Haiwee Reservoirs

G9

Blackrock Work Ctr.
CRAG PEAK

SOUTH SIERRA WILDERNESS

Durrwood Cr.

G8
G7

N

Kennedy Meadows General Store

River

DOME

395

Brush Cr.

STEGOSAURUS FIN

G5

Little Lake

Salmon Cr.

LAND

Kern

G6

CHIMNEY PEAK WILDERNESS

BEAR MTN.

SAWTOOTH PEAK
LAMONT POINT
G4

WILDERNESS

LAMONT PEAK
SPANISH NEEDLE

Cannell Cr.

Kernville

Fork

G3
OWENS PEAK

OWENS PEAK WILDERNESS

Valley

155
155

MOUNT JENKINS

PINYON PEAK

(Alta Sierra)

South

178
Onyx

G1

MORRIS PEAK

G2

Wells

Isabella Lake

Walker Pass

14

395

Indian

178
Lake Isabella
(Bakersfield)

SCODIE MTNS.

SCODIE PEAK

(Mojave)  (Ridgecrest)

*Section G:*

# Highway 178 to Mt. Whitney

Near the end of this section PCT hikers reach the celebrated High Sierra, with its 14,491-foot Mt. Whitney, the highest point in the contiguous United States. Your journey there passes entirely within federally designated wildernesses on the Southern Sierra's Kern Plateau, a land of meadows and mountains. Hikers in this nearly pristine country can enjoy the sinuous South Fork Kern River, included in the prestigious National Wild and Scenic Rivers System; sprawling Monache Meadows, the largest meadow in the Sierra; groves of high-elevation, twisted, foxtail-pine trees; and vast lands of solitude where the only sounds are the serenades of nature.

As always, the PCT seeks the high crest whenever possible, and hence it traces the semiarid eastern heights of the Southern Sierra. This often-exposed country offers a series of expansive, panoramic views.

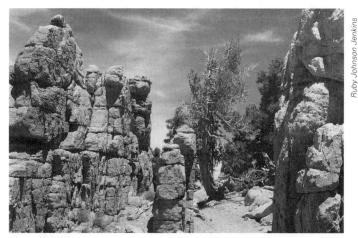

*Ruby Johnson Jenkins*

*Foxtail pines and craggy outcrops line the PCT above Death Canyon*

# Maps

Walker Pass
Owens Peak
Lamont Peak
Sacatar Canyon
Rockhouse Basin
Crag Peak
Long Canyon

Monache Mountain
Haiwee Pass
Templeton Mountain
Olancha
Cirque Peak
Johnson Peak
Mount Whitney

# Declination

14¼°E throughout this section.

| Points on Route | S→N | Mi. Btwn. Pts. | N→S |
|---|---|---|---|
| Walker Pass at Highway 178 | 0.0 | | 113.5 |
| | | 11.5 | |
| Joshua Tree Spring | 11.5 | | 102.0 |
| | | 16.8 | |
| Canebrake Road near Chimney Creek Campground | 28.3 | | 85.2 |
| | | 7.9 | |
| Long Valley Loop Road | 36.2 | | 77.3 |
| | | 13.0 | |
| Sherman Pass/Kennedy Mdws. Rd. near general store | 49.2 | | 64.3 |
| | | 2.4 | |
| Kennedy Meadows Campground | 51.6 | | 61.9 |
| | | 11.5 | |
| South Fork Kern River bridge in Monache Mdws. | 63.1 | | 50.4 |
| | | 4.4 | |
| Olancha Pass Trail | 67.5 | | 46.0 |
| | | 3.6 | |
| saddle west of Olancha Peak | 71.1 | | 42.4 |
| | | 6.1 | |
| Death Canyon creek | 77.2 | | 36.3 |
| | | 14.0 | |
| Trail Pass Trail | 91.2 | | 22.3 |
| | | 4.8 | |
| Cottonwood Pass Trail | 96.0 | | 17.5 |
| | | 0.6 | |
| Chicken Spring Lake's outlet | 96.6 | | 16.9 |
| | | 10.1 | |
| Rock Creek crossing | 106.7 | | 6.8 |
| | | 6.0 | |
| Mt. Whitney lateral/Crabtree Meadows | 112.7 | | 0.8 |
| | | 0.8 | |
| John Muir Trail junction | 113.5 | | 0.0 |

## Weather To Go

Though you begin this section a mile high in elevation, your start is on the desert (east) side of the Sierra and, therefore, very warm in summer. Summer temperatures moderate after Kennedy Meadows, and can be cool (even snowy) as you climb to higher elevations. Mid spring (or late fall) is best for the first part of this section, and summer, after snowmelt, is ideal from Kennedy Meadows north. Afternoon thundershowers are common in the Mount Whitney area. Thru-hikers should refer to "Snow" under Special Problems, below.

## Supplies

The closest post office and groceries to Walker Pass are in Onyx, 17.6 miles west off Highway 178. Also regional transit for towns around Isabella Lake and Bakersfield reach as far east as Onyx P.O. area. The next provisions are at Kennedy Meadows General Store, 49.9 trail miles north of Walker Pass, where there are groceries, gas, and usually a Saturday night movie. For small fees the owners will hold your food packages and furnish material for your return packaging. To confirm, call (559) 850-KMGS.

For major resupplying at the north end of the Kern Plateau, descend 2.1 miles north from Trail Pass to the parking lot at the end of Horseshoe Meadow Road and hitchhike 22.8 miles down it and the Whitney Portal Road to Lone Pine.

## Water

Each source of water and the mileage to the next water is mentioned in the text. Since this is a high, near-crest trail and, in this section, is on the Sierra's drier east side, it is wise to take advantage of each source, especially during drought years. A spring, where you usually obtain water, is, after all, an accumulation of rain

and snowmelt that was prevented from penetrating deeper into the ground. It follows, then, that during a drought even the dependable springs, and the creeks that flow from them, could be in trouble. For assurance, you may want to carry extra water from source to source.

## Permits

Short-trip hikers will need a wilderness permit and a fire permit for Golden Trout Wilderness and Sequoia National Park. They will need only a fire permit, good for one calendar year, for the other wildernesses and for nonwilderness areas. A special permit is required if you plan a climb up Mount Whitney. Obtain these permits before your trip.

## Special Problems

### Bears

They're present but usually not a problem until Sequoia National Park, if you keep a clean camp and use bear canisters. See Chapter 2.

### Mountain Lions

Also known as cougars, mountain lions are so infrequently seen that you are fortunate if you catch a glimpse of one. See Chapter 2.

### Snow

At any time of year, be prepared for unexpected snowstorms in the Sierra. In some years, thru-hikers will find ice and deep snow when they arrive in the high country. Hiking through the snow-covered Sierra with its wondrous scenery can be an incredible adventure, but it should be attempted only by very competent, strong hikers. In snow conditions an ice axe is highly recommended. It has many uses: as a walking stick for balance in snow, as a tool to chop steps in ice or hard snow, as a brake to stop a slide after a fall. Skill with a compass is also recommended: few markers or signs indicate a snow-obscured trail. Proper clothing is essential, of course, and knowledge of hypothermia symptoms and treatment is a must. Snow travel is fatiguing and slow; hiking early in the day when the snowpack is firm may be helpful.

Some hikers take the bus through Owens Valley to bypass the Sierra snow, then return to travel the high country last, before the next winter's storms set in. One alternative is to experience the snow until you reach Trail Pass, and there decide whether or not to exit. If exiting, descend to Horseshoe Meadow and hope to hitchhike to Lone Pine to catch a bus. Rides may be scarce before snowmelt. However, the 22.8-mile distance down the road offers breathtaking views of Owens Valley and the distant snow-capped mountains. This plan also helps avoid crossing Sierra streams when they are swift and swollen with snowmelt, and avoids emerging swarms of mosquitoes too. Anticlimactic? Maybe, but think of finishing your PCT odyssey in the High Sierra during its most accommodating season.

## The Route

You need to hydrate yourself well before starting your hike. The next water is at Joshua Tree Spring, 11.5 miles. Since the California Clean Water Act passed in 1988, the standard for healthful drinking water has become so stringent that agencies who test their backcountry piped water seldom find it meets the high level of purity the California Act requires. At the spring in 1993 and at the Chimney Creek Campground, slightly higher than acceptable levels of uranium were found. (It is reasonable to assume that the free-flowing, untested stream water would show the same result.) The end product of uranium

is lead, and it is cumulative in the body; you would not want to drink this chemical element every day of your life. However, you are just passing through, and the minimal amount of impurities you would swallow seems negligible.

Because of the propensity for winter rock slides on the steep slopes of Mt. Jenkins, equestrians are urged to contact the BLM in Bakersfield for current conditions.

The PCT resumes north of Highway 178 opposite the Walker Pass historical marker (5246′). The trail soon enters 74,640-acre Owens Peak Wilderness.

It and Chimney Peak Wilderness ahead were mandated by Congress in 1994 by the California Desert Protection Act, designed to keep the area in its natural state and to protect its diversity of plant and animal life.

You ascend moderately northeast, where the trail makes a highly visible line across steep, sandy slopes of medium-grained granodiorite, then becomes gentle as it winds above a canyon.

A look back showcases pine-clad Scodie Mountain. Below, your gaze follows Highway 178 east to the distant El Paso Mountains. Around you in early spring of some years, the slopes are carpeted with blue chia, a sage that has two and sometimes three pompons ringing one stem. Chia seeds were roasted by Native Americans for food and used by Spaniards for medicinal purposes. Here, too, are lupines and tiny white forget-me-nots that perfume the air.

You veer gradually north on the path, and then negotiate six switchbacks in the welcome shade of pinyon-pine trees. Shortly you cross the crest at a saddle and note a few golden oaks added to the pinyon forest.

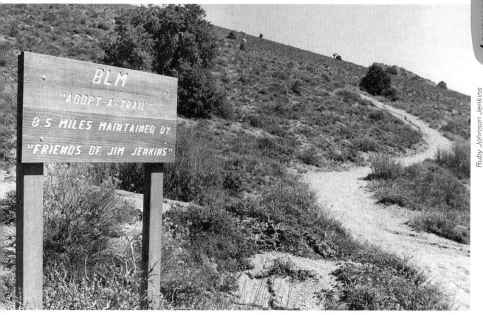

Ruby Johnson Jenkins

*PCT north of Walker Pass*

The trail, now an easy grade near the crestline, crosses a south-facing slope, then regains the crest amid forest near a trailside medium-sized campsite (6190-2.1). The path proceeds on a long traverse across northwest-facing slopes, over a crestline gap and then across west- and north-facing slopes to a saddle (6585-1.8) with a medium campsite southwest of Morris Peak.

After rounding Morris Peak you attain the Morris/Jenkins saddle (6500-0.8), where a campsite to the south of the small hill on the crest can accommodate several tents. Beyond the hill you cross the crest to the east side of Mt. Jenkins. Now you ascend slightly to the commemorative plaque (6580-0.3) cemented to a granite boulder, which has a small seat formed during trail construction blasting. Here you may rest, reflect and view.

Indian Wells Canyon spreads to the desert below, where the towns of Inyokern and, farther away, Ridgecrest waver in the desert sun. Vast China Lake's Naval Air Weapons Station, where many sophisticated weapons have been conceived and developed, occupies the land north of Ridgecrest.

In December 1984 the United States Board on Geographic Names officially named this mountain Mt. Jenkins. This sprawling, serrated 7921-foot mountain on the Sierra crest commemorates James (Jim) Charles Jenkins, who as a teenager hiked across its steep slopes while helping scout a route for this trail. He had been assigned to write the section of the PCT from the town of Mojave to Mt. Whitney for this guidebook.

Jim soon expanded his interest. In the following years he hiked over all the

**See Maps G1, G2**

CANEBRAKE ROAD  3.8 MI.

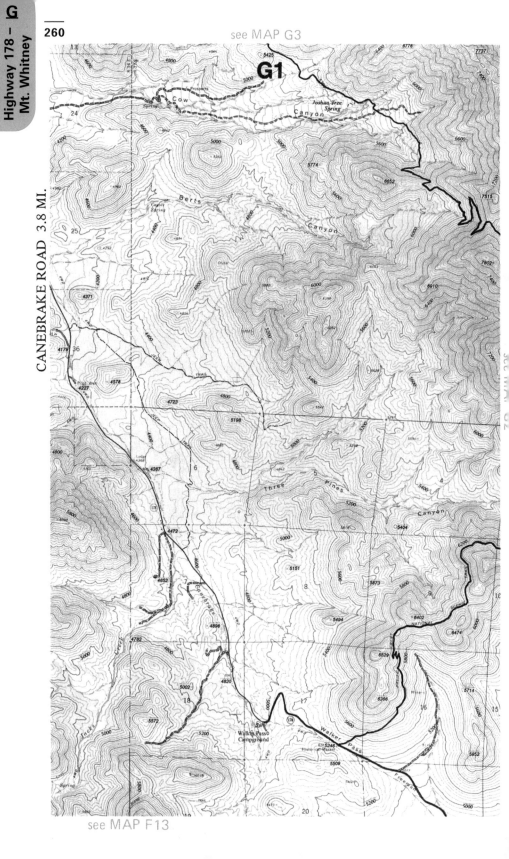

**G1**

trails in the whole Southern Sierra, some several times, no matter how obscure; climbed most of the peaks; covered miles of cross-country; and drove on every bumpy, rutted ribbon of dirt that passed for a road. He gathered information about plants, animals, geology, weather, and the lore of gold miners, cattle ranchers, and the Native Americans who preceded them. While doing fieldwork and research, he developed a deep appreciation for these mountains, which is reflected in his guidebooks: *Self Propelled in the Southern Sierra* (2 volumes), now revised with a name change: *Exploring the Southern Sierra* (2 volumes).

He also became greatly involved in promoting conservation and protection for the Southern Sierra. For his contributions to this area Mt. Jenkins was named in his honor, the culmination of a five-year, grassroots effort by his friends. The official record in the archives of the United States Department of Interior reads, ". . . named for James Charles Jenkins (1952–1979), noted authority on the flora, fauna and history of the southern Sierra Nevada who wrote guidebooks on the area."

While you hike along the PCT, you may see vivid deep-blue Charlotte's phacelia. This exquisite flower, found beside the plaque when the mountain was dedicated, is uncommon and should be left to propagate. In contrast to the less-than-foot-high velvety phacelia is *Nolina parryi*, reaching 10 or more feet high. This plant is indigenous in the Sierra to only this small corner. Nolina's pliant leaves are sharp-edged but not sharply tipped. Its trunk is broad, and its blossoms when dry resemble creamy parchment paper, lingering until late autumn and sometimes into the following year. Nolinas are often mistaken for yuccas.

**See Maps G1, G2**

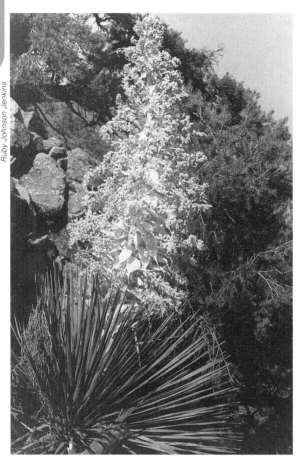

*Ruby Johnson Jenkins*

Nolina parryi, *rarely found elsewhere in the Sierra*

where another, similar commemorative plaque rests. The views are spectacular, and the register pad in a metal box placed by Sierra Club members is fun to read and sign. Registers are found on most named peaks above 5000 feet in the Southern Sierra and on selected peaks in the High Sierra.

Striding along the PCT, you hike over chunks of metamorphic rocks, negotiate minor rock slides, observe Jeffrey pines, sugar pines and white firs—uncommon in this high-desert environment—and proceed around another ridge where you see ahead the ragged light granites of Owens Peak. You then gradually descend while crossing more mountain creases.

Above the trail, one of these creases marked by a duck, 2.9 miles north of the trail plaque and 0.6 mile south of the Jenkins/Owens saddle, conceals scattered pieces of a Navy C-45 twin engine Beechcraft. The 1948 crash took the lives of five scientists and two pilots from China Lake's Naval Air Weapons Station who were on their way to a classified symposium on the Manhattan Project in Oakland. This secret project dealt with the building of the first atomic bomb.

The path, weaving around the extensions and recesses of Mt. Jenkins, undulates slightly, passes a prominent ridge, which supports a few exposed campsites, curves deeply into the mountain scarred with slides of quartz diorite rocks, and then rounds another ridge. At the rounded point of that ridge (6950-1.3), ducks flanking the trail indicate the start of the best route to climb Mt. Jenkins.

**Side trip:** Climbers turn west to scramble up the ridge and follow the ducked use path to and over the sky-scraping, nontechnical Class 2+ summit rocks to the highest point, 7921 feet,

Moving on, you reach the Jenkins/Owens saddle (7020-2.2). A small campsite is upslope on Mt. Jenkins and more space is available on the windy Sierra crest, the jumping-off point for 8453-foot Owens Peak, the highest peak fully within Kern County.

**See Maps G2, G1**

see MAP G4

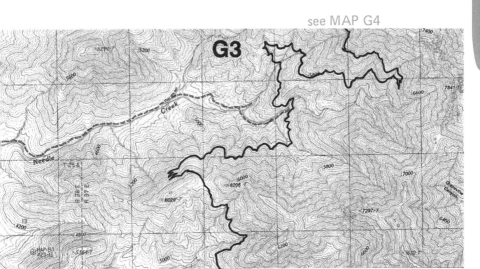

**G3**

see MAP G1

The PCT descends west from the saddle, and you see Highway 178, distant Isabella Lake, Canebrake Road, which you will cross, and the Dome Lands. Beyond four switchbacks and several small slides of diorite rock, the path contours northwest, skirts a minor knob, and reaches a lesser saddle (6300-1.3) east of conical Peak 6652. After another set of four switchbacks the trail curves around the Cow Canyon watershed. In this canyon it crosses a rough dirt road (5500-1.3), which the Civilian Conservation Corps work crews, who built much of this section of PCT, used for access.

**Side route:** This rutted road reaches Highway 178 in 3.9 miles, at a point 6.7 miles west of Walker Pass. This unsigned road is closed to vehicles since becoming part of Owens Peak Wilderness.

**Water access:** Beyond the rutted road, you cross a seasonal creek, then reach a ¼-mile spur trail (5360-0.4) to year-round Joshua Tree Spring, whose water quality was mentioned above.

At the spring, boughs of golden oak arch over several places for campsites near an elongated cattle trough. A pipe brings water from a spring box, affording easy access for hikers. The seasonal creek flows below the spring. Volunteers from the American Hiking Society helped the BLM develop the spur trail and lay the spring box. The next seasonal water is 4.4 miles ahead at Spanish Needle Creek, the next nonseasonal water 16.8 miles ahead at Chimney Creek.

The PCT loses elevation as it tracks a northwest route around a major ridge from Owens Peak, the approximate epicenter of a 6.0 earthquake in 1946, and later by a decade of smaller quakes in the 1990s. Then after ascending to cross this ridge at a saddle (5240-1.1), it climbs, sometimes steeply, northeast up a draw before again resuming a northwest direction to still another saddle (5860-1.1). Leaving views of Highway 178 and the South Fork Valley behind, the path continues in pinyon forest and its associated understory brush. The wide, smooth PCT again loses elevation now by a series of five switches, while below and off to the west the prominent slash of Canebrake Road gains elevation via one lengthy switchback.

**See Maps G1, G3**

A summit block of Lamont Peak looms directly north of you, hiding its sheer, jagged north ridge, and Spanish Needle soon shows to your right. At your feet, sometimes in the middle of the path, arrowleaf balsam root's big yellow flowers bloom—everything is big about this sometimes 32-inch-tall plant.

Beyond the switchbacks the trail nearly levels before again descending east along the steep slopes. Within your view below, a private, gated road hugs the path of Spanish Needle Creek. After crossing a canyon with early-season runoff, your path bends north and its gradient eases. A half mile later it crosses a headwaters branch of Spanish Needle Creek (5160-2.2). A large shelf just off the trail before the creek crossing makes an ideal campsite for weary PCTers.

Usually some water trickles along the Spanish Needle Creek drainage, which is shaded by willows and cottonwoods.

While in the drainage you may look for a recently discovered species— the Spanish Needle onion, *Allium she-vockii*—the tipped-back flower petals are bright maroon above and lime green below.

Leaving the trees momentarily, the trail climbs out of the canyon around exposed slopes and again enters a forest, here with a few alders added, well-watered by a spring-fed finger of **Spanish Needle Creek** (5300-0.7), **your best source of water in this canyon.**

Because water is so scarce along the crest, the PCT was routed to drop into Spanish Needle Creek canyon in order to take advantage of this series of springs.

The trail's circuitous routing added several extra miles of hiking.

You next climb in a pinyon-pine woodland along a minor ridge where you are likely to startle coveys of mountain quail, seemingly abundant in these mountains. You negotiate a sharp turn in a side canyon which points you generally east to cross a spring-fed streamlet, this one frocked with wild roses (5560-0.6). Then you clamber briefly along a blasted area, cross a seep and again enter a shady canyon adorned with occasional bracken ferns. Once more you cross a finger of Spanish Needle Creek (5620-0.2); this and the previous streamlet join to form the creek you crossed below. The next reliable water is 10.9 miles away at Chimney Creek.

After a brief stretch south, the trail climbs east across the south-facing slopes of Spanish Needle Creek canyon, then contours around another ridge. Here the first of several white marbleized veins was blasted to carve the path.

On this stretch you are treated to open views of jagged peaks bracketing Spanish Needle, which looks like a rounded, protruding thumb on a clenched fist.

The trail again turns southeast, abruptly turns back, climbs a switchback and ascends out of the canyon. A pair of short switchbacks, 0.3 mile apart, helps you gain elevation to reach the ridge between the Spanish Needle group and Lamont Peak (6800-3.0). Campsites were developed along the divide, to the left of the trail, to accommodate trail crews, and more have been added above the trail by PCTers.

While looking north and east at the BLM's Chimney Peak Recreation Area below, you see land favored by the Tubatulabal Native Americans and prob-

**See Maps G3, G4**

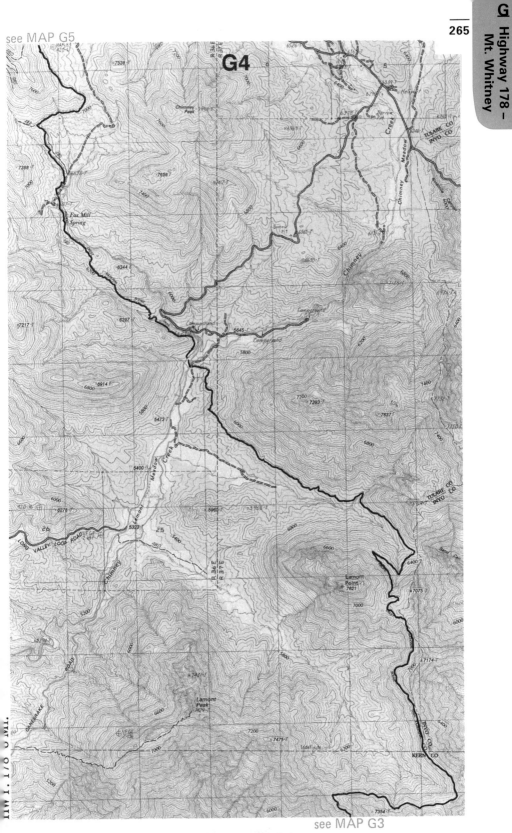

G4

ably by prehistoric tribes before them. The area is rich in archeological sites; for instance, some bedrock mortars are within easy access of the trail. An act of Congress made it illegal to remove or disturb anything pertaining to Native American culture; even pocketing an obsidian chip is unlawful.

The PCT once again curves above a canyon, but this eastward leg takes you through another break from pinyons and live oaks to north-facing slopes of Jeffrey and sugar pines, white firs and black oaks—a mix of trees found in abundance on the west side of the Kern Plateau. After gaining some elevation, the trail then curves north along the Sierra crest, where expansive eastern views unfold of Sand Canyon below and the desert beyond. Ahead on the crest a large pinyon protects a campsite from the usual ridgetop winds.

The trail cuts a nearly straight swath northwest, just below the ridgeline, taking you once again through pinyons, oaks and brush in sunny, dry country, then swings briefly east into a canyon where another small stand of Jeffrey pines and firs flourishes.

These few patches of pine and fir occur typically on north slopes where moisture lingers longer in this dry climate.

Now the trail traverses to a narrow saddle and then climbs a bit to a broader one (6900-3.3) with camping possibilities.

An extended descent on the PCT to Canebrake Road and Chimney Creek Campground begins. A short switchback leads you northwest to a half-mile-long leg along Lamont Point slopes.

A couple of solitary rust-brown, shreddy-barked, fragrant, scaly-needled western junipers thrive here and ahead in the most insecure places.

Rounding boulders, the path heads east before turning north onto another Sierra crest saddle (6260-1.4), this one with limited views.

Heading in a general northwest direction again, the PCT leaves the Sierra crest not to return until Gomez Meadow, 49.3 trail miles ahead. It slowly loses elevation, but occasionally rises briefly as it heads along lower slopes of the north side of the canyon between Lamont Point and Sawtooth Peak.

Gray pine debuts as you stroll along the path of decomposed granodiorite.

Accompanied by its water-loving willows, a seasonal creek crosses the path (5950-0.8); its water tumbles down from multicolored, sheer-sided rock canyons high above. Soon Lamont Meadow and a private inholding in this BLM-administered public land called Chimney Peak Recreation Area, come into view, then Canebrake Road. Finally you dip to cross year-round Chimney Creek. Faucets at the campground are often turned off—best to get your water here. Immediately, you are ushered by a corridor of late-summer-blooming rabbitbrush to unpaved, maintained Canebrake Road (5555-2.4). Canebrake Road heads south 10.7 miles to Hwy 178, or north 4.0 miles to Kennedy Meadows/Nine Mile Canyon Rd. Take that road east 10.8 miles to Hwy 395 or west 13.4 miles to Kennedy Meadows, which you reach via the PCT in 20.9 miles.

**See Map G4**

The campground, popular during hunting season, 0.3 mile up the road, provides 37 shaded sites with tables, grills, pit toilets and sometimes faucet water. The creek, however, flows year-round across the center of the linear camping area.

The PCT leaves Owens Peak Wilderness, crosses the unpaved road, and enters 13,700-acre Chimney Peak Wilderness. Your route leaves the rabbitbrush and sagebrush behind for a short while to climb above and parallel to the road and campground amid a flurry of spring blossoms featuring the yellow, daisylike coreopsis. The path, less sandy now, dips to cross a usually dry creek, and then by a small switchback it proceeds up the south-facing slopes of the creek's canyon.

Often you need to step carefully here lest you harm a "horney toad," blending so well with the rocks and sand. It is really a horned lizard, and with its spikes and bumps it is one of those contradictions: a creature so homely as to appear attractive.

Ahead you top out of this canyon and enter another one above a stream whose chortle echoes as the precipitous granodiorite walls of the canyon close in.

Beyond the canyon, to the left of the route, you find a scattering of debris where the multilevel ruins of a barite mill appear. The mineral barite, used in drilling muds, was mined here about until the early 1950s. Gold and tungsten were also mined in the area.

**Water access:** This clutter overlooks Fox Mill Spring, hidden in a sagebrush-and willow-choked meadow below. The BLM has upgraded this spring, placed a sign next to the trail, and improved its accessibility; it provides the last water, except for seasonal streams, until Rockhouse Basin, 10.2 miles ahead.

Immediately beyond the spring the trail crosses a dirt road (6580-2.2) descending from a flat area used for camping. The path winds along slopes and gains elevation while several sagebrush meadows and the dirt roads that snake through them appear to diminish below. Chimney Peak's double points seem just a stone's throw across the canyon to the east-northeast. Don't scan the peak for a chimney—the mountain was named for one still standing in Chimney Meadow.

Now out of Chimney Peak Wilderness, you cross another dirt road.

A few stately old juniper trees grace the path. Junipers can grow from partially digested seeds in bird droppings, far from parent trees. To the southeast Owens and Lamont peaks recede into the background and meld with other memories that hikers have who pass them heading north from Walker Pass.

Next, round a nose about ½ mile after the road, and then tramp through a pocket of sagebrush.

Suddenly, among pinyon pines, you reach the eastern border of the massive, human-caused, Manter Fire. In the summer of 2000 an estimated 816 acres of Chimney Peak Wilderness and an estimated 66,967 acres of Dome Land Wilderness ahead—around 75% of that wilderness—were consumed. From here to just beyond Pine Creek, around 14 miles, you will hike in the burned area. This was an especially hot fire that not

**See Maps G4, G5**

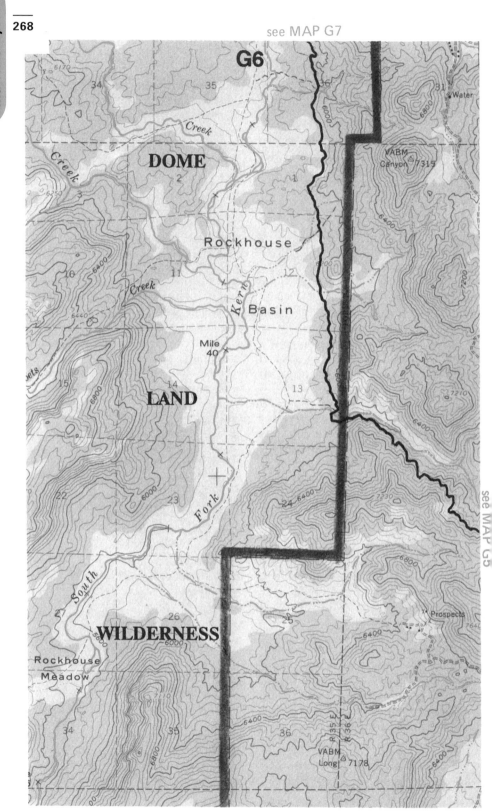

see MAP G7

G6

34

35

36

31 Water

Creek

DOME

2

1

VABM
Canyon 7315

Creek

3

Rockhouse

10

11

12

Kern

Creek

Basin

Mile
40

15

14

LAND

13

7210

22

23

South Fork

24 6400

7230

see MAP G5

27

26

25

Prospects

WILDERNESS

Rockhouse
Meadow

34

35

36

VABM
Long 7178

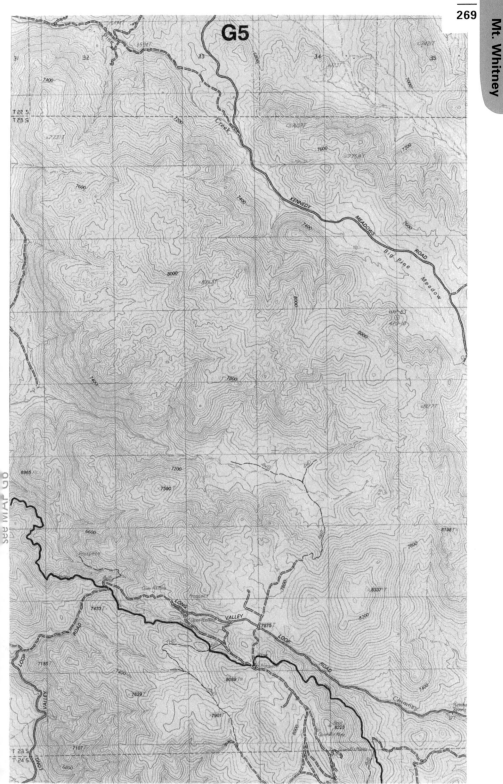

see MAP G4

only burned the vegetation in its path, but also scorched the rocks and baked the soil. Nothing seemed to have survived except a few unburned pine cones. But from these pines cones seeds scattered and some, which settled in crannies along the now barren slopes, will germinate. Future hikers will see the regeneration of the forest. The dynamics of nature continue.

You cross another dirt road and begin a northwestward trek traversing across the steep ridges and dry furrows of 8228-foot Bear Mountain, slowly ascending over metamorphic soils and chunks of rock among black skeletal trees. To the north Olancha Peak comes into view. At last you attain the trail summit of this segment (8020-3.6) atop a minor ridge. **Though it's suitable for camping, try to find open spaces away from weakened, burned trees, especially on windy days.**

You begin a descent now, bearing west and crossing a road (7980-0.2), and then immediately crossing another, both leading to large excavations sliced into the red-rock slopes to the left. Several more of these gouges attract attention as you progress down the trail.

Before the second excavation, an easy cross-country hike over the peak and up the next takes you to the locked facility housing a seismograph. This is one instrument in an important network of many placed by USGS Menlo Park Division to record earth tremors. If the building survived, the seismograph surely fried from the heat and had to be replaced.

Once the red-brown soil hereabout enhanced the gray-green pinyon forest, and an occasional juniper added to the pleasing weave. This will one day

return. Farther ahead the tapestry of Rockhouse Basin appears, with the stark granites of the domed lands weighing the basin's southwest border. The distant blues of Bald Mountain and other Kern Plateau peaks delineate the northwest curve of the basin, where the muted sage greens of Woodpecker Meadow are barely visible. The High Sierra silhouette stretches across the northern horizon, containing the Great Western Divide and the curved summit of Mount Langley.

The trail, curving northwest, crosses a road and then descends along a canyon where a sun-dappled seasonal creek glitters in the recesses. **At a bend in this canyon, the path arches over an artfully constructed culvert containing the seasonal stream, near some camping possibilities.** In about 100 yards the trail crosses unpaved, maintained Long Valley Loop Road (7220-1.9). Here it enters into a 1994 extension of Dome Land Wilderness.

This 7000-acre addition and the 32,000 acres earlier added in 1984 have considerably enlarged the original "rock" wilderness, which was a "charter member" of the National Wilderness Preservation System established by Congress in 1964.

Domes, spires and obelisks rise from this semiarid wilderness, now encompassing more than 100,000 acres. Rock climbers find it an excellent place to practice their skills on the granite. There are meadows and sizable fishing creeks along with the serpentine South Fork Kern River. The forests will return, but it will take 200 years to replace some of the old Jeffrey pines. A breeze usually moderates the heat of summer in this spacious land.

**See Maps G5, G6**

You next climb over a saddle and descend along the southwest side of a deeper canyon. In time a flat on a small northeast spur ridge (6600-2.7) offers one last place to camp before the broader lands of Rockhouse Basin.

There are better views now of Woodpecker Meadow, an area burned in the Woodpecker Fire of 1947. The trees there were unable to re-establish themselves, and were replaced by sagebrush and buckbrush. Stegosaurus Fin, Dome Land's resident dinosaur, which sits prominently in the wilderness interior, displays its fin and curved back. The South Fork Kern River, weaving through the basin below, remains hidden.

You continue to descend, sometimes clinking over loose, rocky slopes, then slowly plodding through sandy soils near the foot of the descent.

Now in Rockhouse Basin, you turn right and cross first a creek (5845-1.8) with exposed campsites on a sandy bank, then immediately a closed road that is returning to nature. (If water is needed and the creek is dry, follow its bed 1.1 mile to the river.) Once again in national forest, you head up-creek, passing a large campsite to the right and then switchbacking to head north, roughly following the South Fork, but, alas, the river is about a mile away for the next several miles. You now scuff along the sandy trail through a forest of pinyon pines. This sandy trail is subject to erosion, but if erosion has made it hard to see, just follow the corridor through the trees scarred by sawed-off branches.

You soon dip through the brushy wash of a waterless basin. After a burn the sagebrush root sprouts and returns rapidly. From here to Pine Creek, you will find sections of unburned forest. Later you pad across a northeast-southwest-trending closed road, which descends along a gully.

In a bit over a mile from the closed road you cross a willow-lined, seasonal creek (5870-3.2). **Open areas for camping are found here.**

In late spring you may see dainty funnellike white evening snow—flowers that fully open when the light wanes—cover these sandy grounds.

Contouring slightly northwest now, you approach a gateway of resistant metamorphic bedrock through which flows the South Fork Kern River (5760-1.0).

Beginning on the slopes of Trail Peak near Cottonwood Pass, a place you will visit as you travel north on the PCT, the South Fork Kern River flows south, wandering across the Kern Plateau, gathering much of the eastern plateau's drainage and eventually flowing into Isabella Lake, a reservoir. Most of the year it resembles a placid creek with good fishing holes and refreshing bathing pools, but during snowmelt the river becomes tumultuous, charging wildly through its banks. Then it is dangerous to cross. But during snowmelt this river is in its most unspoiled state and displays its scenic value, illustrating why in 1987 it was included with the North Fork Kern River in the protective custody of the prestigious National Wild and Scenic Rivers System.

Turning north again, the path threads between the willow and wild-rose tangles that edge the river and the boulders composing the cliffs. The trail climbs and dips, generally following the watercourse but not slavishly.

Sprinklings of flowers add an artists's touch to the captivating scenery, and the three-needled, vanilla-scented Jeffrey

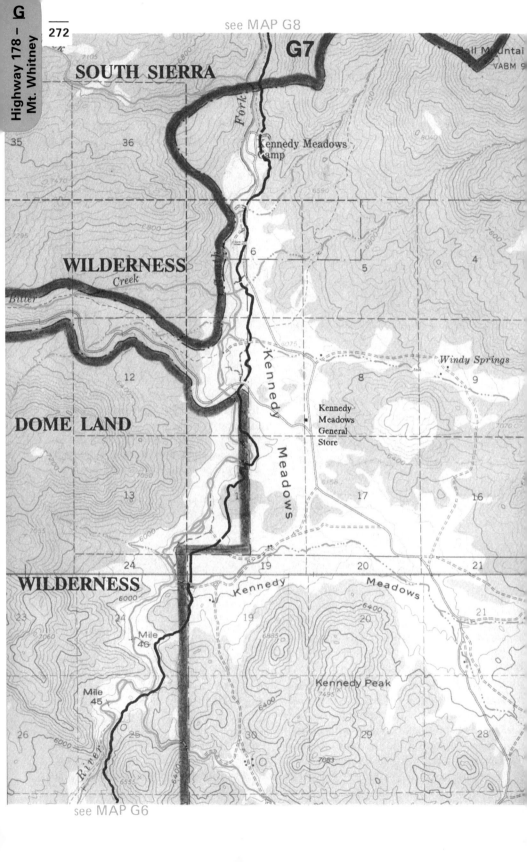

SOUTH SIERRA

WILDERNESS

*Creek*

*Bitter*

DOME LAND

WILDERNESS

Kennedy Meadows
Camp

Kennedy Meadows
General
Store

*Windy Springs*

K
e
n
n
e
d
y

M
e
a
d
o
w
s

Kennedy

*Meadows*

Kennedy Peak

Mile
46

Mile
45

*River*

see MAP G6

pines, which line the water's edge, though burned may recover.

Shortly you cross spring-fed Pine Creek, and then about ½ mile later you notice that the trail melds into a closed road, and that you are out of the burned area. In time, as you descend with views of a house below, you leave the road at a junction (5950-1.9) where it curves west toward the river, and continue on the path straight ahead (north) following the barbed-wire fence on the right. Soon you pass west of the house with its assorted vehicles and dogs, then wade through a stream garnished with sedges and watercress (5916-0.1) and cross a closed OHV road next to the stream. A vast outlying area of sagebrushy Kennedy Meadows stretches ahead, and you begin hiking through it.

Just ¼ mile later the PCT approaches a fence corner, then leaves the fence and angles off to the northeast, away from the river. In the middle of this meadow, the path crosses another closed OHV road (5980-0.6). Not far north of the meadow, the PCT climbs the lower west slope of a hill, where you catch your first sight of paved Sherman Pass Road and a few buildings along it. Pressing near the river again, the trail passes through three cattle gates (please close) and exits Dome Land Wilderness. Between the first two gates, it rounds west of outcrops where the path is often washed out by high water or covered with tall grass. Sections of this are privately owned land and trails or roads may lead away from the river, but you continue ahead. After the second gate, you ascend a couple of low hills, pass through the third gate and head for the paved road, just east of a bridge (6020-1.7).

**Resupply access:** At this point, if you need supplies, shower, washing machine, phone, refreshments, package pickup, or just wish to sign the PCT register and chat and maybe catch the Saturday night

movie, continue 0.7 mile, right, generally southeast, along the highway to tree-shaded Kennedy Meadows General Store.

This road with many names—Sherman Pass, Kennedy Meadows, Nine Mile Canyon, SNF Road 22S05, J41, M-152—reaches Highway 395 in 24.2 miles. Major supplies are available in Ridgecrest, 25 miles southeast of the junction, off Highway 178. The road reaches the Kern River to the west in 44.3 miles, and subsequently Kernville 19.5 miles farther, where there are ample supplies and accommodations.

When it is time to move along, you return to the trail where it crosses the road and amble north to Kennedy Meadows Campground. You would walk the same distance if you took the northbound road just beyond the store to reach the campground.

Across the Forest Service's paved road, you continue on sandy turf among early-season high-desert flora. Heading north, you dip through washes and cross dirt roads that lead west to riverside campsites, fishing pools, and swimming holes. Occasional junipers offer spots of shade as you pass fences, first on the right and then on the left. Then you go through one gate and soon through another. Enticing murmurs of the river increase as you reach and then hike above the musical South Fork. Slowly you leave the sagebrush meadow that is embraced by the gentle peaks of the semi-arid side of the Kern Plateau and head toward a distant fire-scarred mountain, seen up the river canyon to the north.

Soon the trail crosses the road to the campground (6080-1.8) and proceeds along higher ground. Here it winds for a short time around boulders among pinyon pines and brush. Then it crosses the road again (6120-0.4) and bisects Kennedy Meadows Campground (6150-0.2).

**See Map G7**

This year-round campground with 39 units and a small fee is especially popular with anglers who fish for the colorful golden trout in the river. The camp has the usual facilities but no trash pickup—a good place to overnight while you sort through your food packages from home.

The PCT leaves the north end of Kennedy Meadows Campground and joins the old Clover Meadow Trail. Pinyon and Jeffrey pines along with juniper trees offer shade as the trail immediately dips into a side canyon, then eases through a stock-fence gate, passes several lateral paths to the river, and enters South Sierra Wilderness.

This wilderness was one of many established by the comprehensive California Wilderness Act of 1984. Its 63,000 acres closed the gap between Dome Land and Golden Trout wildernesses, giving wildlife a wide, unperturbed area to roam and wildflowers room to spread.

The PCT soon approaches the river and winds to a forked junction (6240-1.1) where it leaves the Clover Meadow Trail, which continues to a river crossing—hazardous during snowmelt. (The old path west of the river is now used as a stock driveway.) Your route, the right fork, leads to a sturdy, yet scenic, steel-girdered wooden bridge built in 1984 (6300-0.8).

Beyond the bridge, the trail climbs north of a knoll, passes a medium-sized campsite perched to the right above the river, then continues over gravelly terrain. Soon your path gains the slopes of a craggy 7412-foot mountain whose soils nurture an occasional prickly-pear cactus.

The prominent yellow-orange blossoms of this spiny plant turn pink to rose as they mature.

Past the ascent, the path switchbacks down once to reach a saddle where it crosses the old trail, and then it makes a weaving traverse above the rumble of the South Fork Kern River, sometimes heard but not seen in its canyon to the east. The PCT intersects the old trail again, then dips to cross Crag Creek (6810-2.0). Yellow monkey flowers and cinquefoil luxuriate near the banks of the creek. There are campsites here and upstream along the old trail, all of which, however, are within 100 feet of the water—easily damaged areas the Forest Service wishes to protect.

After a short ascending hike beyond the ford, you again face the skeletal remains of trees.

These trees were burned in the 1980 Clover Meadow blaze. Started by a campfire along the former path of the PCT that was set too close to tree branches and improperly extinguished, the wind-whipped fire engulfed 5000 acres before it was contained. Buckbrush ceanothus, rabbitbrush and associated xerophytic plants have replaced the forest; the pines are slow to regenerate. The stark grays and blacks of the burn contrast sharply with the creek's riparian expanse and the plush greens of Clover Meadow below.

You pass campsites in an unburned pocket of trees and, 1.8 miles into the burn, again reach the welcome shade of forest.

Mountain mahogany is abundant here. This woody brush with small, wedge-shaped leaves clustered near

**See Map G8**

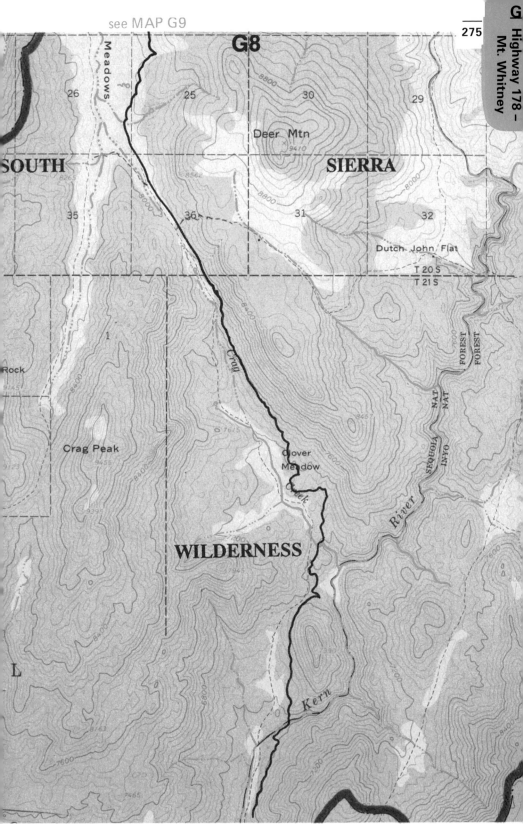

SOUTH

SIERRA

Deer Mtn

Dutch John Flat

T 20 S
T 21 S

Rock

Crag Peak

Clover
Meadow

WILDERNESS

Kern

branch tips turns silvery in the fall when clad in its corkscrew, feathered plumes.

The path meets the usually dry eastern branch of Crag Creek at a junction (7560-2.5) with the old Clover Meadow Trail (stock driveway) on your left, which you join. In 0.1 mile the PCT passes to the right of a campsite established in 1936, according to words on a concrete slab.

The old trail was probably built by the Civilian Conservation Corps, which was active from 1933 to 1942, during the Depression.

A spring appears in the creek's channel just before the path climbs up a narrowing, boulder-strewn slot, but a lush

growth of willows and wild roses laps up most of the water, leaving a timid flow. The grade abates amid yellow-flowered bitterbrush and ends at a saddle with campsites and a T-junction (8060-1.1) with Haiwee Trail 37E01, which follows an ancient Native American path east to the river and through Haiwee Pass to Owens Valley—a route that almost became the eastern leg of a trans-Sierra highway.

Beyond the saddle, the PCT drops gently to Beck Meadows, a sagebrush finger of Monache Meadows. Campsites can be found at the foot of the grade in the trees on either side of the trail.

A spacious view of Monache Meadows, the largest meadow in the Sierra, includes distant Mt. Whitney and

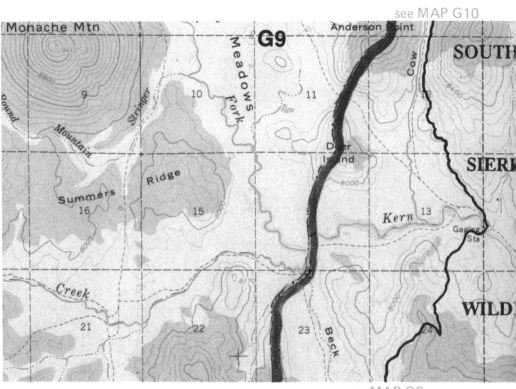

see MAP G10

see MAP G8

**See Maps G8, G9, G10**

its neighbors, peering over the plateau peaks. Among the seasonal flowers trailside, the yellow evening primrose with its heart-shaped petals makes a dramatic appearance.

The PCT veers north from northwest-leading Beck Meadows Trail 35E01 (7953-0.4), and from the all-but-gone grooves of an old jeep road that crossed the path.

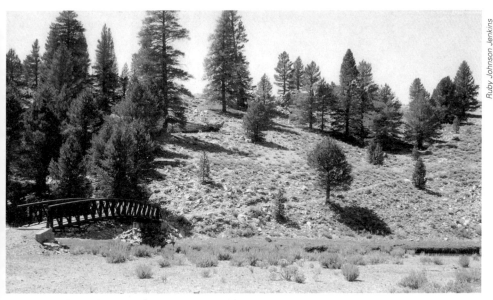

Jeeps first penetrated into Monache Meadows in 1949, but long before that horse-drawn buckboards left their parallel treads.

You focus your attention on direction now, for in 0.6 mile you leave a former section of the PCT, which is reverting to nature, and turn right (north-northeast) toward hulking Olancha Peak, to angle up the lower slopes of nearby Deer Mountain. After crossing a usually dry gulch, you climb through another gully from where you see a cow trough below at the edge of Beck Meadows. A usually dependable spring bubbles forth above the trough in the gully. You next pass through another stock-fence gate, and then Mt. Langley, framed by Brown and Olancha mountains, comes into view in the north. Its rounded backside resembles that of Mt. Whitney, with which it is often confused. After 0.7 mile from the gate, you top out on Deer Mountain's northern ridge (8390-2.2) near a dry campsite.

From there the path briefly heads southeast to a switchback, then north to drop out of the forest and cross a retired jeep road that bisects a low, broad ridge (7940-1.0). The PCT heads northeast along the ridge, turns right, and drops to an arched 1986 bridge over the South Fork Kern River (7820-0.4). Interestingly, the steel in this bridge was treated to resemble an old, rusted structure, rendering it less conspicuous. The bridge spans shallow water except during snowmelt, when most long-distance PCT hikers pass this way; then it is an important safety factor.

*Ruby Johnson Jenkins*

*Bridge over South Fork Kern River in Monache Meadow*

**See Maps G9, G10**

see MAP G11

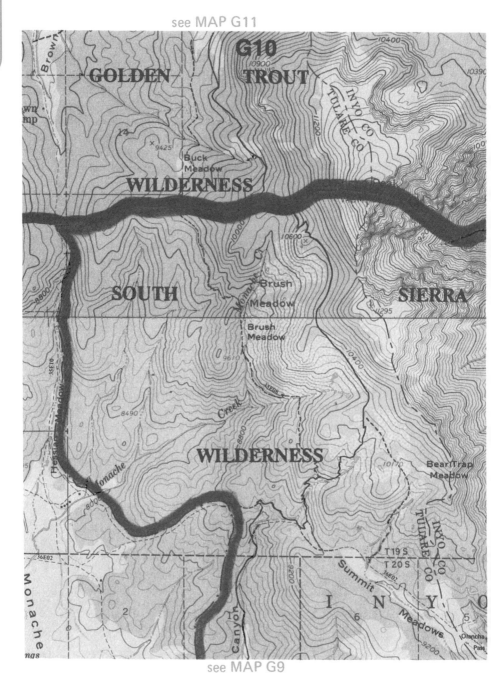

see MAP G9

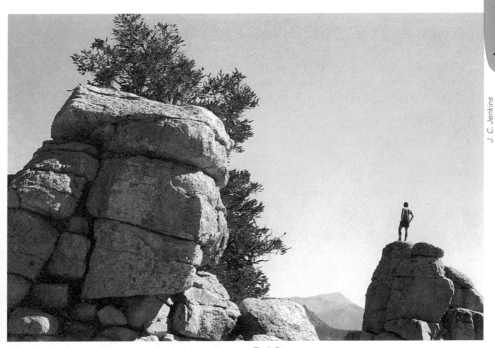

J. C. Jenkins

*Olancha Peak seen between trailside pinnacles near Trail Pass*

You will probably cause great commotion among the cliff swallows that return annually to raise their young in the braces under the bridge. Their mud nests are gourdlike, with a narrow, short tunnel entrance into which they dart to feed fat bugs to their families.

**An ideal campsite is sheltered by trees on the slope south of the bridge,** and exposed sites sprawl along the river's sandy north bank. Here you leave Sequoia National Forest and enter Inyo National Forest, but still remain in South Sierra Wilderness.

Resuming its route north of the bridge, here briefly overlapping an OHV road, the PCT passes a southeast-heading trail (7840-0.1) to Kennedy Meadows, a path that vibrated with motorcycles before the wilderness was established. Immediately your trail passes a once heavily used OHV road, which leads north into the canyon straight ahead. After paralleling the river a short way, the PCT turns right at a junction (7840-0.1) while the road/trail it was on continues to Monache Meadows.

Trail width now, the PCT climbs northwest above the meadow while jogging laterally around washes and ridgelets to stay within its required grade of 15% or less.

One can usually identify sections of PCT that overlay old trails: on old trails it plunges in and out of washes rather than curving around them.

The trail mounts a low ridge (8050-1.2) and heads north, leaving open slopes sparsely dotted with chartreuse-lichen-painted boulders. It enters forested Cow Canyon. Midway up this canyon the trail resumes on the former PCT path that it left in Beck Meadows, and immediately crosses

**See Map G10**

Cow Creek (8260-1.3), where you find the first of a spread of campsites along the creek.

The trail soon crosses the creek again, but quickly returns and ascends a canyon where Kern ceanothus debuts.

This ceanothus has hollylike leaves and blue-to-purple pompon flowers. It is a denizen of the plateau, occurring only in a few other places.

The trail merges briefly with paths of a stock driveway angling in from the left. (North-to-south hikers take note; an accidental turn onto a driveway path would take you to the head of Monache Meadows.)

You ford the creek once more and look for a PCT post marking the return ford. Again on the left side of the creek, you find your trail among the multiple twining cow paths paralleling it. Where the creek turns east, almost one mile after the last junction, you continue north and quickly reach a trickle from a spring just above. After a short, winding ascent you turn right to join the Olancha Pass Trail (8920-1.2). Vegetation coils about the sometimes slack spring immediately south of this junction.

Your route on the conjoined trail runs eastward, now on a gentle ascent around the head of Cow Canyon. Along the way it passes disturbed terrain on the canyonside created by stock drives, and then it crosses Cow Creek again just 250 yards before the next trail junction (9090-0.5), where the PCT departs north.

**Resupply access:** The Olancha Pass Trail continues east over the pass, then descends to Sage Flat Road, 6.9 miles. The paved, lightly traveled road heads east 5.8 miles to Highway 395. For emergency supplies, the town of Olancha, 5.0 miles north on the highway, has a BLM fire station, a restaurant, motels and a store with limited supplies.

The ascending PCT, left at the junction, switchbacks, arcs northeast up a rounded ridgelet, and then turns north where a lateral (9240-0.2) branches off to the trail you just left. Your trail runs across slopes of chinquapin and manzanita, fords Cow Creek and zigzags many times amid bush currant, a favorite berry of black bears. Now leaving the forest, the PCT continues to parallel the creek, which flows among groups of corn lilies, aptly named plants resembling cornstalks. The open tread is sandy and often very dusty, but it still supports the colorful scarlet gilia, a cluster of red flowers with tubular necks and pointed, starlike lobes. The gradient steepens, and the trail zigs sporadically as it climbs a side canyon. Then it fords a spring-fed brook and **switchbacks near a large campsite among boulders by a foxtail pine,** with an extensive view of Monache Meadows and the sandy flood plain of South Fork Kern River.

**Side trip:** Minutes beyond this campsite, a short path climbs from your trail to a broad, gently sloping ridge with a packer campsite and a corral. The verdant, watered meadow there sports corn lilies, buttercups and numerous mountain bluebells, another aptly named flower that resembles tiny, hanging bells whose styles extend like clappers. Mosquitoes may make lingering there in spring or early summer a bit unpleasant.

On the PCT, the grade diminishes as the trail leads into the shade of lodgepole and occasional foxtail pines—isolated specimens of the impressive foxtail-pine groves ahead.

The foxtail pine grows in gravelly soils just below tree line along with very few understory plants. Its short, five-clustered needles surround the branches; a bristly branch end with its tip up resembles

**See Map G10**

a fox's tail. Foxtail pines seem to survive nicely in the extreme weather of the high country where other trees cannot exist.

Atop a ridge, your trail proceeds past a junction signed cow trail, mostly obscured by a large fallen tree. (The path connects with the Olancha Pass Trail.) North of the fallen tree your path ascends gently to moderately, curves northwest, and crosses another open slope with seasonal stream-lets and seeps. The farther the trail climbs on this slope, the more remarkable are the Southern Sierra views; Dome Land is par-ticularly prominent. In almost one mile the trail crosses a flat, forested ridge with con-siderable camping potential.

Provocative vignettes ahead, east to west, of Olancha Peak, Mt. Langley, the Kaweah Peaks Ridge, and Kern Peak may be seen framed by the boughs of the for-est.

Continuing to climb, the path curves around a headwaters bowl of Monache Creek and then levels off on a saddle (10,540-3.4) of a ridge that juts out from the west-facing slope of Olancha Peak. This, the highest point of the trail on the side of Olancha Peak, is a good departure point for the nontechnical 1550-foot climb to the top of the most dominant peak on the Kern Plateau.

**Side trip:** To climb Olancha Peak, ascend northeast on a 0.6-mile cross-country route among foxtail pines to tree line, aiming for the slope north of the summit. There the rounded and gentler terrain makes for an easy final ascent, but only after you have pulled up and over scores of large boulders. Unexpectedly found among these boulders are vigorous plants of yellow columbine. Then you scale the 12,123-foot summit. At the top stands a tall stack of rocks, a cairn, pre-cariously perched on a slab that juts over the sheer eastern face. On the cairn is a box with a register in which you can record your ascent.

You might pause to reflect on the fate of the Native Americans for whom this summit was named. Olanche and Yau-lanchi were spoonerisms for Yaudanchi, a tribe of Yokuts Native Americans who probably traded with either the Paiutes north of Owens Lake or the Kosos south of it. The decimated Yaudanchi now reside on the Tule River Indian Reservation.

An alternative to climbing Olancha Peak for plateau views is Point 10,600, west of the saddle and the trail. From there you barely see the rounded back-side of Mt. Langley fronting the same part of Mt. Whitney, but you see the Kern Plateau wonderfully spread before you. **If you need a campsite you can find places on the saddle.**

From the saddle, the PCT drops to Gomez Meadow on a gentle-to-moderate grade. Along the way it switchbacks five times and then curves around another headwaters bowl of Monache Creek. The trail leads across a watershed divide, where it leaves South Sierra Wilderness and enters Golden Trout Wilderness.

As you saunter along this easy northern descent, you may contemplate some events that involved this area. Before the late 1940s the only way one could reach the gentle Kern Plateau was on foot, on animal, or on a breathtaking flight in a small aircraft. Then logging began in the southern part, and it slowly pushed north-ward. The loggers' roads opened the land to jeeps and their cousins, motorcycles. All these intrusions resulted in slope ero-sion, damaged meadows and silted streams. Environmentalists became alarmed and campaigned to protect the

**See Map G10**

remaining land. They were eventually successful. In 1978 President Carter signed into law 306,000-acre Golden Trout Wilderness, named for the colorful trout—California's state fish—that evolved in this area. The northern third of the Kern Plateau is part of this wilderness.

But, you may ask, if land is set aside in wildernesses to preserve its natural biota, why are cattle-grazing, hunting and fishing allowed? People interested in those activities would ask, "What about hiking?" The answer to the latter is that hikers seem neither to destroy nor disturb the flora and fauna as they walk along on their narrow paths and adhere to "no trace" camping.

As you ponder these thoughts and this recent history, you pass above a seasonal spring while hiking across exposed slopes with views of brownish, boulder-topped Kern Peak across the Kern Plateau. This 11,510-foot peak counterbalances Olancha Peak; the two are among the highest points on the plateau.

Now the PCT meanders northwest, dropping in and out of forests, passing seeps and springs that find their way to Brown Meadow and Long Stringer. The trail gradually curves northeast, then bends southeast to cross a year-round creek (9030-3.7) with **camping potential near its banks.** This is a better source of water than the stringer ahead. From the creek the PCT leads north and then east on a slightly rolling course. Then it bends sharply north and crosses a meadowside trail at a causeway abutment (9010-0.7) just west of very level Gomez Meadow.

The causeway's 35-yard length elevates the path above the sodden stringer beneath.

Shooting stars seem almost airborne across the meadow. The common name of this flower is well-chosen, because its swept-back crimson/purple petals suggest flight. A Basque carving of a man smoking a pipe appears on the snag at the beginning of the causeway. This was probably carved by a sheepherder around the late 1800s. You will also find two more carvings, these of crosses, on the trees along the meadow edges to the east.

The PCT resumes at the north abutment and immediately crosses another meadowside path. It then curves northeast into a dense forest of lodgepole pines, touching the inconspicuous Sierra crest, which it last crossed in Owens Peak Wilderness. The trail gradually turns northwest and soon skirts Big Dry Meadow.

Beyond this meadow you pass a creek-side campsite, then ford a step-across all-year creek (8940-1.7) at the mouth of Death Canyon. **To the left are several campsites;** to the right, up-canyon, a path takes PCT equestrians to another in a series of corrals and camping areas built for the PCT trail crews of Inyo National Forest. The corrals are infrequently maintained. **The trailside campsites are ideal places to overnight before the nearly 2000-foot steep climb out of Death Canyon.**

Next, amid a fine grove of fragrant, gnarled old mountain juniper trees, you labor up 22 broadly spaced switchbacks and numerous curves on the blocky, spired ridge west of the canyon. You may pause occasionally to view pointed Kern Peak and the broad expanse of Big Dry Meadow. You eventually cross the crest of this ridge for the last time at a slender slot between craggy outcrops. Foxtail pines now shade you and red mountain-pride penstemons decorate your path as you descend gently to a crestline saddle (10,390-3.7) from which the eastern slope drops precipitously to Owens Lake bed.

**See Maps G10, G11**

see MAP G12

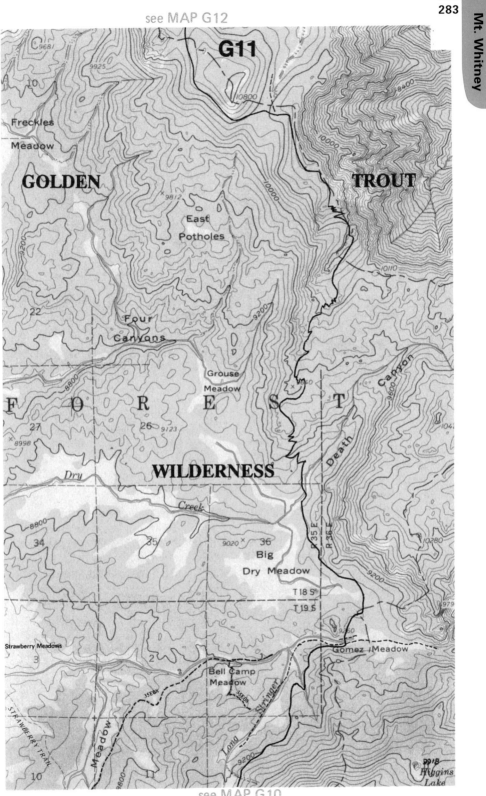

**G11**

Freckles
Meadow

**GOLDEN**

**TROUT**

East
Potholes

Four
Canyons

Grouse
Meadow

**F    O    R    E    S    T**

**WILDERNESS**

Dry

Creek

Big
Dry Meadow

Strawberry Meadows

Gomez Meadow

Bell Camp
Meadow

Death Canyon

Higgins
Lake

see MAP G10

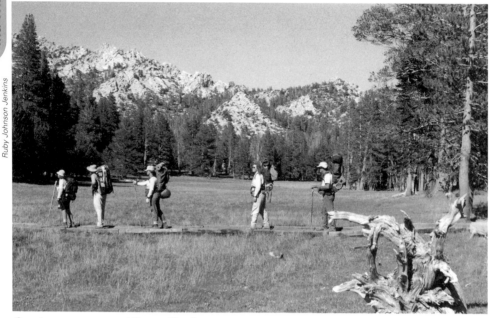

*Crossing on causeway at Gomez Meadow*

This alkali flat is usually dry because the Los Angeles Department of Water and Power diverted its inflow into their adqueduct. The pink coloration of the lake bed is due to algae and bacteria—some attribute it to brine shrimp.

Next you ascend on seven switchbacks to attain a crestline prominence, reaching an elevation of 10,700 feet.

Here you are rewarded again with grand views of Owens Lake bed and the Coso and Inyo mountains east of it. Olancha and Kern peaks dominate the southern half of the horizon.

At length you leave the ridgetop in a descending traverse of west-facing slopes, then curve west to a saddle where you meet a junction (10,425-1.5) with a faint, ½-mile-long lateral that descends north to a corral and campsites.

**Water access:** A spring waters a meadow polkadotted with buttercups in the crease of the canyon about 0.3 mile in on this lateral. This spring and the next off the PCT are good sources of water.

Beyond the faint junction, you ascend more or less northwest, crossing two more crestline saddles. Just east of the second saddle (10,260-1.6) is a path signed CORRAL to another corral and campsite.

**Water access:** A spring emerges 0.2 mile down-canyon on this path.

About ½ mile later you cross yet another saddle.

Here you leave one cattle allotment and enter another. In fact, the whole plateau is a patchwork of these parcels; wilderness classification here does not ban grazing. Most of the cattle

**See Maps G10, G11, G12**

people involved have been summering their animals in these allotments for several generations.

The PCT curves north where Sharknose Ridge juts off to the west, then skirts the west edge of wide Ash Meadow, traversing a nearly level stretch of Sierra crest. The trail leaves the crest to make a brief, easy descent of northwest-facing slopes, where it passes a nearly obscure path (10,000-1.8) to another corral down in a ravine above Mulkey Meadows.

As the dusty PCT descends, Mt. Langley, the southernmost 14,000-foot peak in the Sierra Nevada, sinks behind the shoulder of Trail Peak while views of Mulkey Meadows improve. Your path bends east around a spur ridge where you find a rather unusual juxtaposition of foxtail pine, sagebrush and mountain mahogany. For almost a mile now the path nearly levels and then regains the Sierra crest at a low saddle (9670-1.8).

**Side trip:** The PCT begins to ascend, but if you need a campsite, leave the trail on a use path east, to the right of Diaz Creek, to find some open space. A spring issues forth in a side canyon just under ½ mile in on this use path.

You now climb the crest on a gentle-to-moderate grade gradually heading northwest. After a mile you curve on the crest, then leave it for a short climb north to top a broad ridge south of Dutch Meadow. (North-to-south trekkers: be alert lest you wander onto a former trail, again in use, to Mulkey Meadows. Take the left fork.) You turn sharply left at a signed corral junction (9960-1.3), just below a switchback, but if you need water, a campsite, or a corral, turn right on the 0.2-mile lateral to Dutch Meadow.

Your trail ascends west with two sets of switchbacks to cross the Sierra crest again. It attains a spur ridge, bends from north to west around a canyon, and then contours over to cross Mulkey Stock Driveway at Mulkey Pass (10,380-1.5). Beyond the driveway, the PCT traverses around the south side of a crestline-straddling hill to reach Trail Pass and a junction (10,500-0.8) with the Trail Pass Trail.

**Resupply access:** If you have a package pickup in Lone Pine, need other supplies or need equipment repair, descend 2.1 miles north on Trail Pass Trail to Horseshoe Meadow Road and an overnight campground, then hitchhike 22.8 miles to Lone Pine. During most spring weekends after snowmelt and during summer, this place buzzes with activity, but on early-season weekdays finding a ride at this parking area or the adjacent Cottonwood Lakes parking area may not be easy. Nevertheless, this is a far better place to begin a detour to Lone Pine than the detour over Trail Crest to Whitney Portal, where cars are frequent—unless returning to the PCT up Mount Whitney's steep east face toting a heavy pack is of no concern to you.

Continuing beyond Trail Pass the PCT ascends gently northwest amid foxtail pines and talus, switchbacks twice, and then rounds the north-facing slopes of 11,605-foot Trail Peak.

Portals in the forest frame the last exhilarating views of Mt. Langley seen from the PCT and the nearer views of Poison Meadow below. There may still be a campsite and a corral at this location.

Now the PCT crosses refreshing Corpsman Creek and soon leaves the slopes of Trail Peak to intersect the crest at a saddle (10,740-1.9). It gently traverses southwest along a route that offers sweeping views of Mulky Meadows below. The path then curves northward, passing several small meadows.

**See Maps G12, G13**

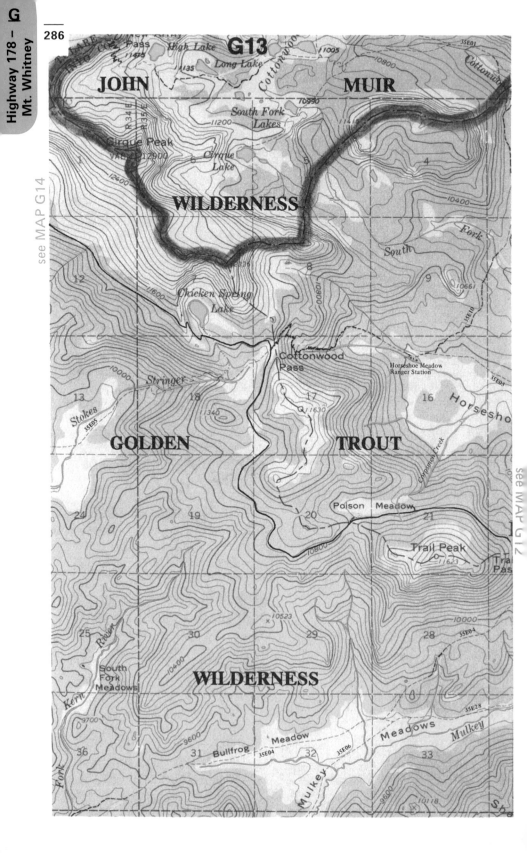

see MAP G12

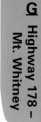
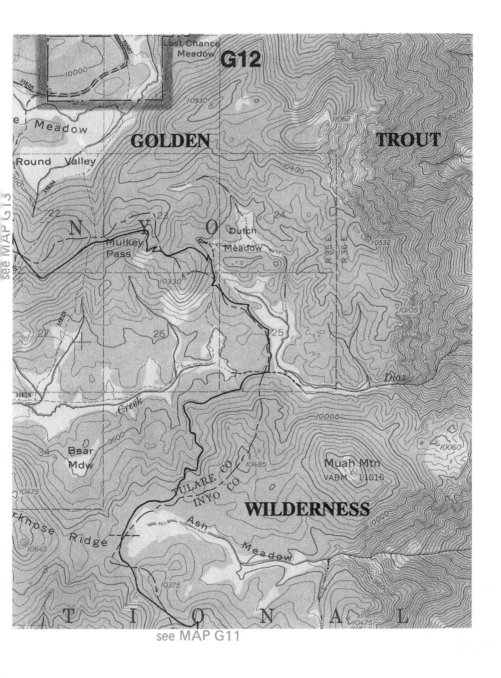

see MAP G13

see MAP G11

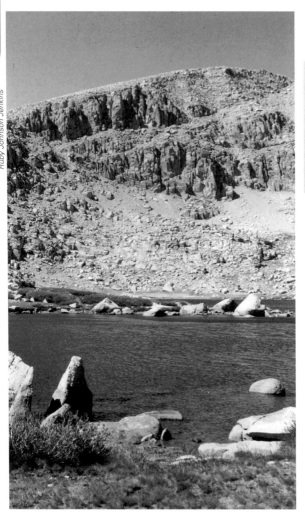

Ruby Johnson Jenkins

*Chicken Spring Lake*

watershed divide and pass through a west-facing, flower-flecked meadow.

 This meadow's drainage finds its way into Golden Trout Creek, where it travels west to tumble off Kern Plateau's basaltic rim into the narrow, steep trench of North Fork Kern River—the river's main branch.

After ascending to a spur-ridge saddle, you descend to meet the Cottonwood Pass Trail at Cottonwood Pass (11,160-2.9). This trail also reaches Horseshoe Meadow Road and the campground to the east.

North of the junction, you climb imperceptibly around the head of an alpine meadow, turn west upon entering forest, and soon reach the outlet stream of Chicken Spring Lake (11,235-0.6). To catch shoreline views of the lake in its granite cirque, leave the trail before the outlet and stroll northwest to the shore. **The lake is the last reliable water source before a tarn 2.7 miles onward or a brook that leads into Rock Creek,** 9.2 miles ahead. Campsites abound at the lake, and on weekends so do people using them. On any summer day, though, you will not be alone, since Clark's nutcrackers—crow-sized, black, white and gray birds—will hop to your pads and caw at you for handouts.

Back on the PCT, the trail crosses the lake's sometimes-dry outlet stream, climbs, and switchbacks above the lake to gain a spur ridge, then makes a seemingly endless tree-line traverse of the southwest-facing slopes below 12,900-foot Cirque Peak. Big Whitney Meadow appears intermittently

The meadows' seeps and springs combine to become the headwaters of South Fork Kern River, a stream that meanders through three wildernesses on the east side of the gentle plateau until it courses off the south end in a harsh area called The Roughs.

Foxtail pines shade you, parting occasionally to reveal views of the Great Western Divide. In time you round a

far below you through the forest of foxtail pines. Your trail is at times annoyingly sandy. The PCT intersects a seasonal creek (11,320-2.5), which often flows through summer; a NO STOCK GRAZING sign is posted on a pine to the left shortly before you get here.

**Water access:** There is no longer a lake in the little basin below the trail here; it is now a meadow where campsites may be found. Above the trail, however, a cross-country ascent of 200 feet, alongside the outlet creek, takes you to a fair-sized tarn snuggled within a cirque. This sparkling lake, its sandy, sloping beach, and a couple of campsites make this an attractive stopover, but not during a drought when the lake could be dry.

Climbing a little, the trail soon swings around a flat-topped ridge, then begins a descent that, except for some minor ups, does not end until it reaches the Rock Creek ford. The PCT passes an eye-catching "fang-toothed" rock formation, then enters Sequoia National Park (11,320-0.6), leaving Golden Trout Wilderness. Pets, firearms, grazing cattle and logging activities within the park are illegal.

On this descent, excellent views of the Great Western Divide appear across Siberian Outpost in the west.

Your downgrade first steepens somewhat, then becomes gentle as the path skirts the northeasternmost prong of Siberian Outpost.

Though named for its desolate aspect, the Outpost is surrounded by weathered foxtail-pine snags whose reddish-brown hues lend the place an impression of warmth and mellowness.

Now the PCT wanders westward, then crosses the Siberian Pass/upper Rock Creek Trail (11,139-0.9).

You next head toward the broad, gently rolling ridgetop separating the watershed of Rock Creek to the north from that of stagnant Siberian Pass Creek to the south. The dramatic sky-piercing crags of Rock Creek's headwaters basin are seen to the right, and Joe Devel Peak seems but a few steps away. After a 2-mile stroll from the last junction, you start an earnest downgrade. You descend and switchback, describing an S curve, then level to cross a sandy-grassy flat. Lodgepole pines, at first only scattered among foxtail pines, come to dominate the forest as you stroll northwest along a ridgetop, descend moderately via nine switchbacks northward, then hike down to a junction (9959-4.9) with the Rock Creek Trail.

Now your wanderings turn westward and zigzag several times more before crossing a brook (9840-0.3), the first reliable water since the tarn 6.5 miles back or Chicken Spring Lake, 9.2 miles. Pausing, you can easily identify the aromatic wild onions with their pinkish-purple blossoms gracing the banks upstream. Beyond, you follow the south edge of a meadow for a while, then cross it diagonally. Back in forest, you drop to a series of large campsites overlooking Rock Creek. You should bearproof your food if staying here or anywhere in the park. You can even be cited for noncompliance. A heavy metal retangular bearproof food locker has been placed at the creek crossing. You are asked to share the locker, keep it clean, close the door, and always secure the latch.

**Side trip:** The Rock Creek Ranger Station is 0.2 mile above (east of) the campsites. You reach it by first crossing the meadow while paralleling Rock Creek; then, finding the path among the trees, you follow it, hop across a stream, turn

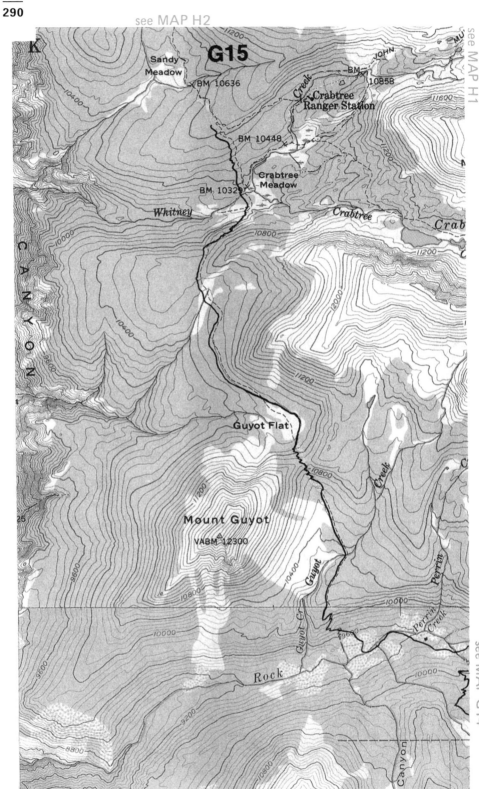

K

**G15**

Sandy
Meadow

X BM 10636

JOHN

BM
10858

Crabtree
Ranger Station

BM 10448

Crabtree
Meadow

BM 10329 X

Whitney

Crabtree

Crab

Guyot Flat

**Mount Guyot**

VABM 12300

Guyot

Perrin

Perrin Creek

C A N Y O N

Rock

Guyot Cr

Canyon

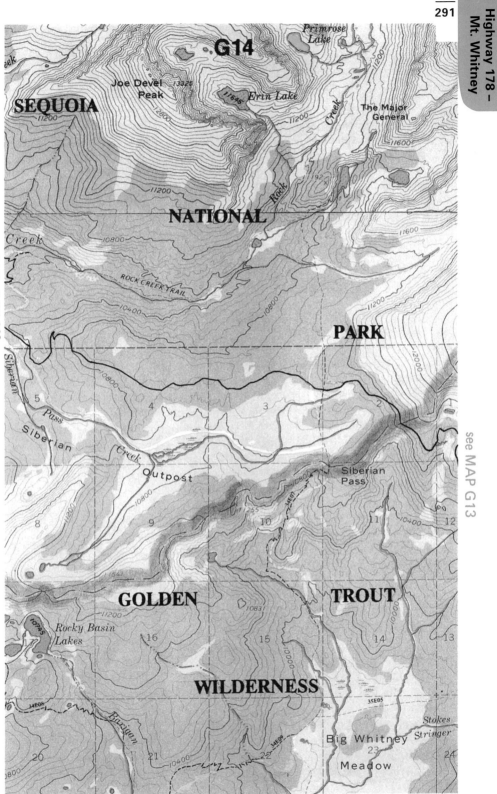

see MAP G15

see MAP G13

G14

SEQUOIA

NATIONAL

PARK

GOLDEN

TROUT

WILDERNESS

Joe Devel
Peak

Erin Lake

Primrose
Lake

The Major
General

Creek

ROCK CREEK TRAIL

Siberian

Pass

Siberian

Creek

Outpost

Siberian
Pass

Rocky Basin
Lakes

Big Whitney
Meadow

Stokes
Stringer

right immediately after, and then curve left. There it is—an ideal hideaway.

On the westbound PCT, the trail approaches Rock Creek, fords a rivulet while swerving away from the creek a bit, and finally crosses the creek on stepping-stones (9550-0.9). Just downstream is a log for high-water crossings.

Your path ahead switchbacks, first north and then west-northwest, as it begins to climb a moderate-to-steep—sometimes steep—grade through stands of lodgepole pine and juniper trees. After passing cold, plant-caressed brooks just below their springs, the PCT climbs a rack of 10 switchbacks, and then its grade eases. **Camping areas are found here before the trail crosses Guyot Creek (10,320-1.5), the last source of water until Whitney Creek, 4.5 miles ahead.**

After some easy hiking over gravelly terrain, you pass through a wreckage of mature trees on the slopes east of Mt. Guyot that were uprooted and broken by a 1986 snow avalanche. Young resilient trees survived. Beyond, you labor up and over a pass (10,920-1.0) northeast of 12,300-foot Mt. Guyot. As you descend and cross above grit-filled Guyot Flat, you have magnificent views across Kern Canyon of Red Spur and the Kaweah Peaks Ridge, then west-southwest beyond the gap of the Big Arroyo, of the Great Western Divide peaks—notably the pointed summit of Mineral King's monarch mountain, Sawtooth Peak. Shaded by foxtail pines, you hike along the sandy trail, gradually veering north and passing another gritty flat. Next you ascend a broad, flat-topped ridge, then proceed northeast, dropping abruptly through a series of switchbacks.

Ahead of you, while descending the switchbacks, looms Mt. Young. East of it you receive your first near view of 14,491-foot Mt. Whitney, the highest mountain in the contiguous United States.

PCT thru-hikers have glimpsed Mt. Whitney's peak from great distances as far back as Sweet Ridge north of Highway 58. From here its furrowed backside and rounded top are partly hidden by Mt. Hitchcock. The grand mountain's most spectacular side, however, is its precipitous east face. The mountain, surrounded by other 14,000-foot peaks, lies on the granitic Sierra crest, thrust up by many grinding earthquakes.

At the foot of the descent, the PCT travels through a wooden-gated fence, levels out, and passes a use path that plummets west next to Whitney Creek and ends at the Kern River. Your path proceeds north passing to your left a cluster of campsites and a food locker. Then it fords Whitney Creek and arrives at Crabtree Meadow, where it meets a lateral (10,329-3.5) to Mt. Whitney.

If you do not plan to climb up Mt. Whitney, proceed along the winding path north-northwest to a signed junction (10,870-0.8) with the John Muir Trail, the start of Section H.

**Resupply access:** To reach Lone Pine, hike east 6.8 miles on the trail to Mt. Whitney. At Trail Crest junction, descend 8.7 miles to Whitney Portal. There, the busy Whitney Portal Road winds down 13.0 miles to Lone Pine, a sizable town.

**Side trip:** Few can resist the opportunity to climb such a famous peak, so you turn northeast, with your previously obtained Mt. Whitney permit, to ramble along the lateral, favored along the way with full views of Mt. Whitney's west side. On this path you skirt lush, well-watered Crabtree Meadow, ascend a little canyon beside Whitney Creek, cross the creek,

**See Map G15**

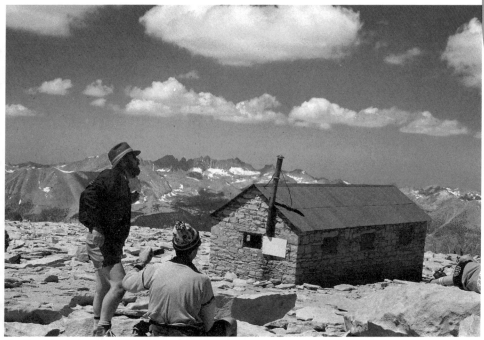

Ruby Johnson Jenkins

*Smithsonian hut atop Mt. Whitney*

and then recross it to its north side to meet the John Muir Trail (10,640-1.2).

You do not recross the creek, however, if you are seeking campsites with a food locker or the Crabtree Ranger Station. The campsites are scattered among the trees on the southeast side of Whitney Creek, and the station is 0.1 mile northeast along a replaced section of the John Muir Trail. A ranger is available, if not on patrol, from mid-June to mid-October to help with emergencies and to answer questions, but this popular station is not a place to dump off trash.

The 1982 building near the station houses equipment for the snow pillow, which collects data on the winter snowpack and automatically sends the information via satellite to the California Department of Water Resources. This is important information, since most of California depends on water from the Sierra snowpack.

With knowledge that the summit can be bitterly cold, and assessing the time and the weather so as not to be caught on the summit or open slopes in an afternoon lightning storm, you proceed northeast on the John Muir Trail north of the creek. After climbing over granite slabs, you amble near the north shore of placid Timberline Lake.

Once heavily used as a base camp for climbing Whitney, these shores have been closed to all camping and stock grazing since before 1970.

Above the lake your trail passes the last of the forest on a moderate-to-steep grade away from Whitney Creek. Glacial polish is much in evidence on the granite along this ice-carved canyon of spectacu-

**See Map G15**

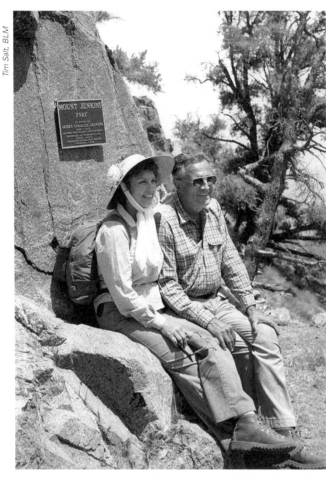

Tim Salt, BLM

*Co-author Ruby Johnson Jenkins with husband Bill on Mt. Jenkins dedication hike, 1985*

lar beauty. The path takes on a pattern of climbing slab staircases up granite benches, then traversing around hollows sometimes holding a tarn or a good-sized lake. After topping a broad, rounded ridge the path approaches Guitar Lake (11,480-2.7), where many hikers camp among the rocks away from the meadow grasses. **Above Guitar Lake, the two tarns at 11,600 feet offer an ideal camp setting as well, and are the last reliable sources of water on this summit quest.**

Here the trail levels briefly, allowing you to pause and catch your breath preparing for the high-altitude climb ahead.

When the ascent resumes, the Hitchcock Lakes come into view; they were hidden until now in a deep cirque at the foot of 13,184-foot Mt. Hitchcock.

The rugged appearance of many glacier-carved peaks contrasted with pockets of delicate deep-pink rockfringe flowers instills in some a sense of awe and wonder.

A few short switchbacks now signal the onset of nine long-legged switchbacks that wind up the rocky slopes on the

**See Maps G15, H1**

highest section of the Sierra crest, to a junction (13,560-2.9) with the eastbound Mt. Whitney Trail, which in 8.7 miles meets a road at Whitney Portal. Lines of stashed backpacks at this junction make a colorful collage as they lean against the rocky crags.

**Resupply access:** From the junction, the Mt. Whitney Trail descends east 8.7 miles to Whitney Portal. There, the busy Whitney Portal Road winds down 13.0 miles to the town of Lone Pine, a major resupply center.

You turn left, climb north up a pair of switchbacks, pass Mt. Muir, and labor breathlessly on a long traverse beside a row of gendarmes.

Between gendarmes, you can look through crestline notches, sometimes called windows, to indigo lakes nestled in polished cirques almost straight down, far below and yet well above the pale Owens Valley. More reassuring are the brilliant blue clusters of fragrant sky pilot that grow in nooks along the path, evoking admiration for these hardy flowers that flourish in such harsh elements.

Your path makes a final few switchbacks up Mt. Whitney's back, then approaches a stone cabin with its register, and at last attains the summit (14,491-1.8-8.6).

This mountain was named by members of the Whitney Survey team for Josiah Dwight Whitney (1819-1896), the highly respected chief of the California State Geological Survey.

Strictly enforced quotas on the number of hikers allowed to leave Whitney Portal per day have reduced the population problem here, but it is still possible to find a crowd when you arrive—and a line at the outhouse. It is not only the highest toilet in elevation in the country, but it must be the most expensive toilet to maintain, as the "honey pot" has to be flown out regularly by helicopter. Nevertheless, it is a prime necessity.

The stone cabin was built in 1909 by the Smithsonian Institute to be used as an observatory. It was added to the National Register of Historic Places in 1978. In 1990 a fatality occurred when a group of hikers thought the hut a safe refuge during a lightning storm—it was not. It still is not, even though fitted with lightning rods.

On a clear day you can see almost any of your favorite mountains in the Sierra. Through PCT hikers can note dim, pointed Owens Peak and rounded Mt. Jenkins' tandem silhouette in the southeast, showing the distance they have hiked since Walker Pass. They may be able to see the San Bernardino Mountains as well.

From the summit you backtrack to the junction (10,640-7.4) across the creek from the ranger station. From there you continue on the John Muir Trail, progressing across a sandy flat from lodgepole pines to foxtail pines. A few zigzags and a long westward traverse with lingering views of Whitney lead to a signed junction (10,870-0.9-16.9) where you turn north on the Pacific Crest Trail, which joins the John Muir Trail to begin Section H.

**See Map H1**

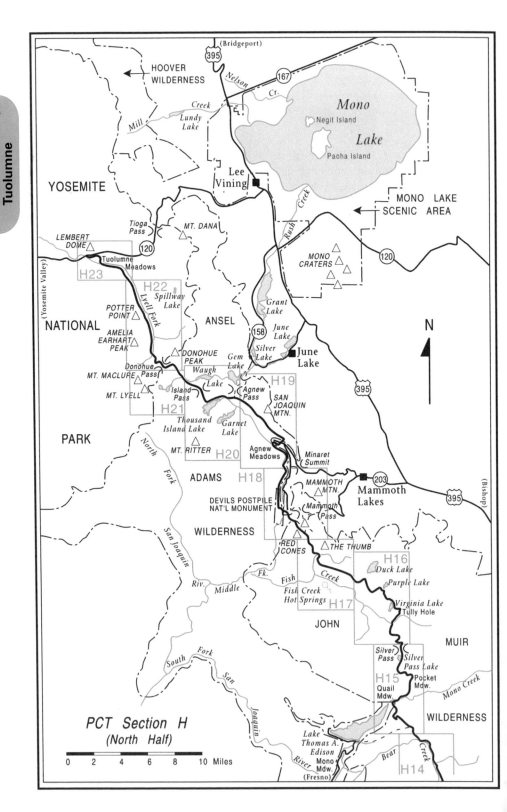

**Mt. Whitney – Tuolumne**

PCT Section H
(North Half)

0   2   4   6   8   10 Miles

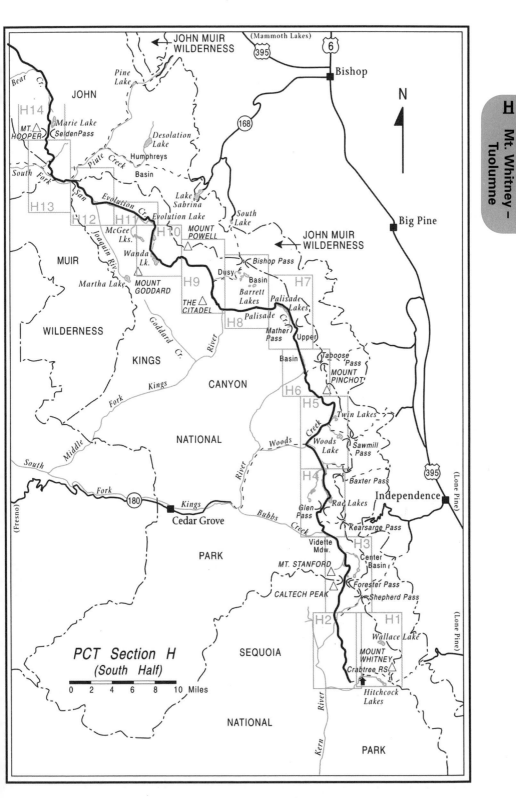

PCT Section H
(South Half)

0  2  4  6  8  10 Miles

*Section H:*

# Mt. Whitney to Tuolumne Meadows

The Pacific Crest Trail from the Mt. Whitney Trail junction to Tuolumne Meadows passes through what many backpackers agree is the finest mountain scenery in the United States. Some hikers may give first prize to some other place, but none will deny the great attractiveness of the High Sierra.

This is a land of 13,000-foot and 14,000-foot peaks, of soaring granite cliffs, of lakes literally by the thousands, of canyons 5000 feet deep. It is a land where man's trails touch only a tiny part of the total area, so that by leaving the trail you can find utter solitude. It is land uncrossed by road for 150 airline miles from just north of Walker Pass to Tuolumne Meadows. And perhaps best of all, it is a land blessed with the mildest, sunniest climate of any major mountain range in the world. Though rain does fall in the summer—and much snow in the winter—the rain seldom lasts more than an hour or two, and the sun is out and shining most of the hours that it is above the horizon.

Given these attractions, you might expect that quite a few people would want to enjoy them. And it is true that some hikers joke about traffic signs being needed on the John Muir Trail—which the PCT follows for most of this section. But the land is so vast that if you do want to camp by yourself, you can. While following the trail in the summer, you can't avoid passing quite a few people, but you can stop to talk or not, as you choose.

# Maps

Mount Whitney
Mount Kaweah
Mount Brewer
Mount Williamson
Mount Clarence King
Mount Pinchot
Split Mountain
North Palisade
Mount Goddard
Mount Darwin
Mount Henry

Mount Hilgard
Florence Lake
Graveyard Peak
Bloody Mountain
Crystal Crag
Mammoth Mountain
Mount Ritter
Koip Peak
Vogelsang Peak
Tioga Pass

**H**

Mt. Whitney –
Tuolumne

# Declination
14+°E

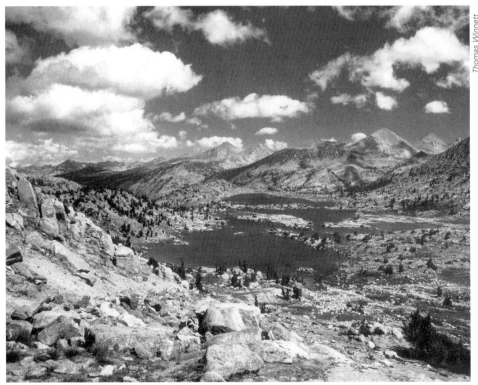

Thomas Winnett

*Marie Lake from Selden Pass*

**H** **Mt. Whitney – Tuolumne**

| Points on Route | S→N | Mi. Btwn. Pts. | N→S |
|---|---|---|---|
| John Muir Trail above Crabtree Meadows | 0.0 | | 175.8 |
| | | 3.3 | |
| Wallace Creek | 3.3 | | 172.5 |
| | | 5.3 | |
| Lake South America Trail | 8.6 | | 167.2 |
| | | 4.3 | |
| Forester Pass | 12.9 | | 162.9 |
| | | 8.0 | |
| Bubbs Creek Trail | 20.9 | | 154.9 |
| | | 2.2 | |
| Kearsarge Pass Trail | 23.1 | | 152.7 |
| | | 2.3 | |
| Glen Pass | 25.4 | | 150.4 |
| | | 8.3 | |
| Woods Creek | 33.7 | | 142.1 |
| | | 7.1 | |
| Pinchot Pass | 40.8 | | 135.0 |
| | | 4.3 | |
| South Fork Kings River | 45.1 | | 130.7 |
| | | 5.2 | |
| Mather Pass | 50.3 | | 125.5 |
| | | 10.2 | |
| Middle Fork Kings River | 60.5 | | 115.3 |
| | | 3.3 | |
| Bishop Pass Trail | 63.8 | | 112.0 |
| | | 7.0 | |
| Muir Pass | 70.8 | | 105.0 |
| | | 4.6 | |
| Evolution Lake Inlet | 75.4 | | 100.4 |
| | | 7.4 | |
| Evolution Creek in Evolution Meadow | 82.8 | | 93.0 |
| | | 4.8 | |
| Piute Pass Trail | 87.6 | | 88.2 |
| | | 1.8 | |
| Florence Lake Trail | 89.4 | | 86.4 |
| | | 7.6 | |
| Selden Pass | 97.0 | | 78.8 |
| | | 13.3 | |
| Mono Creek | 110.3 | | 65.5 |
| | | 7.0 | |
| Silver Pass | 117.3 | | 58.5 |
| | | 4.8 | |
| Tully Hole | 122.1 | | 53.7 |
| | | 6.3 | |
| Duck Lake outlet | 128.4 | | 47.4 |
| | | 11.5 | |
| Reds Meadow | 139.9 | | 35.9 |
| | | 7.8 | |
| Agnew Meadows Trailhead | 147.7 | | 28.1 |
| | | 7.8 | |
| Thousand Island Lake outlet | 155.5 | | 20.3 |
| | | 3.2 | |
| Rush Creek Forks | 158.7 | | 17.1 |
| | | 3.4 | |
| Donohue Pass | 162.1 | | 13.7 |
| | | 4.0 | |
| Lyell Base Camp | 166.1 | | 9.7 |
| | | 9.7 | |
| Highway 120 in Tuolumne Meadows | 175.8 | | 0.0 |

## Weather To Go

High Sierra weather is mostly dry from June to September—especially in September—but afternoon showers are fairly common, and it may even rain at night. A tent and good raingear are mandatory.

## Supplies

This section does not allow easy resupply. To reach any kind of civilization you must—except at Reds Meadow—walk at least 18 miles round trip. Even then, if you have major needs, you will have to hitchhike many miles farther. At the beginning of this section, you can take the Mt. Whitney Trail 15½ miles to Whitney Portal, where there is a very small store, or hitchhike from the portal 13 miles to Lone Pine, which has almost everything you might want. Twenty-one miles into Section H, at the Bubbs Creek Trail, you can hike 14 miles west to Cedar Grove, with another very small store and a modest cafe plus post office. To hitchhike from there to Fresno would be a major project. About 2 miles farther, at the Kearsarge Pass Trail, you can hike 9 miles east to Onion Valley, and hitchhike from there 15 miles out of the mountains to Independence, which has just one store, albeit a rather large one for such a small town. About 41 miles farther, at the Bishop Pass Trail, you can hike northeast 12 miles to South Lake, which has nothing, and hitchhike 19 miles to Bishop, which has everything. Then, 24 miles farther, at the Piute Pass Trail, you can hike northeast 18 miles to North Lake, which has nothing, and hitchhike 18 miles to Bishop. About 2 miles farther, you can hike north 11 miles along the Florence Lake Trail to the roadend, where there is a tiny store. Then 22 miles farther, from where you bridge Mono Creek, you can walk 6 miles west, mostly beside Lake Edison, to Vermilion Resort, again with a small store

plus meals, showers, and a package-holding service. (Write ahead to confirm this service; the address is in Chapter 2, under "Post Offices Along or Near the Route." Enclose an SASE.) Seven miles west by road from there is Mono Hot Springs, with meals, supplies and a post office.

About 29 miles farther, you are at Reds Meadow, with a somewhat-more-than-minimal store and a cafe. Just down the paved road is Reds Meadow Campground, which has a nearby, free public bathhouse fed by a hot spring. If you need more than a few supplies, go to Mammoth Lakes, a recreation-oriented town. From a choice of stops along the Reds Meadow-Agnew Meadow stretch of road, you can take a shuttle bus up over Minaret Summit and down one mile to expansive Mammoth Mountain Inn, opposite the ski area. In 2001 the round-trip fare was $10, but the fare goes up every year or two, so expect continued increases. For about the same amount you can take a taxi from the inn to central Mammoth Lakes, another 4½ miles farther. The shuttle bus operates from about the weekend before the Fourth of July through the weekend after Labor Day. Note that the charge is for one way only—from the Inn over to the Reds Meadow-Agnew Meadow area. Going the opposite way is a free ride. Out of season, the shortest walk to downtown Mammoth Lakes is an 8-mile route starting from Upper Crater Meadow (bottom of Map H18), and this is described in the trail text. On the other hand, you may be able to hitch a ride in the Reds Meadow-Agnew Meadow area if its road is still in use.

Finally, in the Tuolumne Meadows area, at the end of this section, you can get hot meals and showers at Tuolumne Meadows Lodge, a mile east of the principal meadow, or you can stop at a good store, with a cafe and post office, just southwest of the entrance to Tuolumne Meadows Campground.

Be aware that the facilities at Whitney Portal, Florence Lake, Lake Edison, Mono Hot Springs, Reds Meadow, and Tuolumne Meadows may close by early or mid-September.

## Water

The only possible water problem in this section is that you might have to melt some snow if you hike here early in the season.

## Permits

If you are northbound, you can get a permit for this entire section by writing to Sequoia and Kings Canyon National Parks. If you are southbound, write Yosemite National Park. If you are southbound (or northbound) and are starting in the Mammoth Lakes-Devils Postpile area, write Mammoth Ranger District. (Refer to Chapter 2's "Federal Government Agencies" for addresses.) Be aware that during the summer season (about late June through mid-September) user quotas are in effect for the three national parks and the wildernesses between them. Popular trailheads do reach their quotas, especially on weekends, so plan accordingly.

## Special Problems

### Snow

For hikers trying to do the whole PCT in one year, the biggest problem in the High Sierra is snow. If you leave Mexico in early April, you will reach the Sierra before the end of May. In most years there will be a lot of snow in the High Sierra in May and June. A few people use snowshoes or skis to travel over the snow, but as the sun cups get deeper, these devices become useless. What you will need for the snowy sections is crampons and an ice ax, and the knowledge of how to use them.

You need a tent. You need plenty of warm clothing, including mitts. And you need a basic understanding of avalanches—where they tend to occur, why they tend to occur, what to do if caught in one. *The ABC of Avalanche Safety*, published by The Mountaineers, is a good primer. Finally, where the trail is hidden by snow, you need some skills with map and compass to follow the route. You also need a lot of perseverance.

### Cold

Even in midsummer it may freeze on any given night, so you need appropriate warmth.

### Fords

In late spring and early summer, when runoff is at a maximum, a few stream fords can be potentially lethal for careless or inexperienced hikers. If a stream crossing looks too deep or swift, take the time to find a safe place to cross. This may entail going 100+ yards up- or downstream. Maybe you'll find a fallen log or some safe boulders to cross. If you must ford, doing so in chest-deep slow water is preferable to waist-deep fast water. Never ford just upstream from dangerous fast water, especially rapids or cascades. Trekking poles or a suitable nearby branch may help you balance but Schaffer has never used either, despite crossing Sierran streams more than 5 feet deep while carrying a backpack over his head. (You cannot do this and simultaneously balance with trekking poles!) Because there is always a chance that you might slip—even when the water is only waist deep—be sure that at least your sleeping bag is wrapped in waterproof material, such as a plastic trash bag. Some experts recommend that you unlatch the buckle on your backpack's waist belt, so that if you have to abandon your pack in a hurry (to save your skin), you can do so. However, consider the converse: that with your waist belt unbuckled you are more likely to fall. Your pack will sway more—especially a modern pack with a high-center-of-gravity when loaded—so an unexpected move in one direction can really throw you off. Perhaps the best advice is to make sure that the pack you use has a quick-release buckle, so you can cross buckled up but unbuckle quickly if necessary. Do not tie in with a rope. A rope is useful in crossing swift streams, but hang on rather than tie into it. Hikers have drowned before they could untie the rope after they slipped, because their taut rope forced them underwater. Also, no one wants to get wet boots and socks. Even if you remove your socks, you still have wet boots, which invite blisters. So carry lightweight shoes for both camp use and stream fords. Going barefoot invites a smashed toe or other injury, and in response to a sharp pain, you may lose your balance and fall in. Finally, you might plan your hike to cross the major streams early in the day, when their discharge is less than it becomes by midafternoon through early evening.

### Bears

Black bears are very intelligent (one dare say more so than some humans), and evidence for this may be in how adept they are at outwitting us to steal our food. Bears know that where there are backpackers there is food, and the High Sierra seems to have an endless supply of backpackers from about June through September. So, just as we head to the highlands during the summer season, so do the bears. Black bears were discussed in some detail in Chapter 2's section, "Animal and Plant Problems on the PCT," as well as various strategies to safeguard your food from bears. What follows here are special issues for those hiking especially in Section H.

Beginning in 2000, the Sequoia/Kings Canyon National Park Wilderness Office requires you to use bear-proof canisters or food-storage boxes along the 12½-mile stretch of trail between Forester Pass and Glen Pass. (For more information, call the office at (559) 565-3766.) To hike from Kennedy Meadows in Section G to your next near-route resupply point—probably Vermilion Valley Resort at a distance of roughly 180 miles—you'd have to carry two or three of these heavy bear-proof canisters, something most people would find unacceptable. Your best solution is to not camp along the 12½-mile stretch but rather at sites south of Forester Pass and north of Glen Pass. In Sequoia, Kings Canyon, and Yosemite national parks you'll find metal food-storage boxes at many popular camping areas, starting with one at the ford of Lower Rock Creek, about 7 miles before the end of Section G. (Bears may be waiting for you.) Hopefully, the Forest Service also will place many metal food-storage boxes in the lands between Kings Canyon and Yosemite national parks.

### Lack of signs

Some hikers are glad to see signs disappear. Others are glad to have signs confirm their notion of where they are. In Sequoia and Kings Canyon National Parks virtually all place signs have been removed, and there appears to be a trend toward removing or at least not replacing signs at trail junctions too.

To help you cope with some of the difficulties mentioned above, a number of summer rangers are stationed along or near the trail in Sequoia and Kings Canyon National Parks from about July 4th to Labor Day. The trail description below tells where they are. Two points deserve special mention. First, if you go to a summer ranger station to report a friend in trouble and find the ranger out, please realize he might be gone for several days, and so leave a note for him and walk out for help yourself. Second, remember that the ranger has to buy his own food and camping gear, so he, not the government, is the loser if it is taken.

*Thomas Winnett*

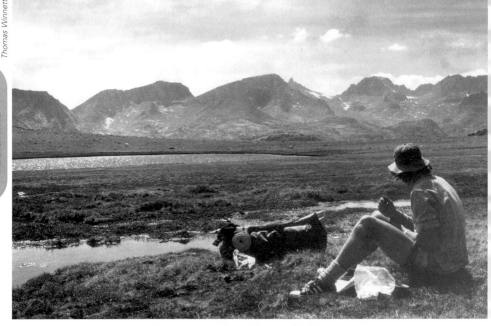

*A hiker gazes beyond Bighorn Plateau at the Great Western Divide*

# THE ROUTE

In this trail section you will be on the John Muir Trail almost all the way to Tuolumne Meadows, 176 miles ahead. Northbound on the combined PCT/John Muir Trail, you skirt what the map calls Sandy Meadow and ascend to a high saddle (10,964–1.7). Beyond it the trail winds among the huge boulders of a glacial moraine on the west shoulder of Mt. Young and brings you to excellent viewpoints for scanning the main peaks of the Kings–Kern Divide and of the Sierra crest from Mt. Barnard (13,990') north to Junction Peak (13,888'). Soon you descend moderately, making several easy fords, and then switchback down to Wallace Creek and a junction (10,390–1.6) where the High Sierra Trail goes west toward a roadend near Giant Forest and a lateral trail goes east to Wallace Lake. The Wallace Creek ford, just north of the popular campsites, is difficult in early season.

Now your sandy trail climbs up to a forested flat, crosses it, and reaches the good campsite at the ford of Wright Creek (10,790–1.1), also difficult in early season. You then trace a bouldery path across the ground moraines left by the Wright Creek glacier and rise in several stages to Bighorn Plateau. Views from here are indeed panoramic. An unnamed, grass-fringed lake atop the gravelly, lupine-streaked plateau makes for great morning photographs westward over it. Now the PCT descends the talus-clad west slope of Tawny Point past many extraordinarily dramatic foxtail pines. At Tyndall Frog Ponds, tiny lakes beside the trail, there are fair campsites, warmish swimming, and a bear box. At the foot of this rocky slope a trail departs southwest for the Kern River, and 200 yards past the junction you come to the Shepherd Pass Trail (10,930–3.5) going northeast. Not far

**See Map H2**

beyond is a formidable ford of Tyndall Creek, on the other side of which are many highly used campsites and a bear box; campfires are prohibited within 1200 feet of the crossing.

From these gathering places your trail makes a short climb to the junction with the Lake South America Trail (11,160–0.7), passes some fair campsites, and rises above tree line. As you tackle the ascent to the highest point on the PCT, you wind among the barren basins of high, rockbound—but fishy—lakes to the foot of a great granite wall, then labor up numerous switchbacks, some of which are literally cut into the rock wall, to Forester Pass (13,180–4.3), the highest spot on the entire PCT, and on the border between Sequoia and Kings Canyon National Parks. Forester Pass' south side can be dangerous when snow-covered.

Wearing your wind garment, you will enjoy the well-earned, sweeping views from this pass before you start the (net) descent of 9000 feet to Canada. Down the switchbacks you go, unless they are buried under snow, and then stroll high above the west shore of Lake 12248. The trail soon doubles back to cross the lake's outlet and then descends past one or two spartan campsites fit only for those unafraid of rockfall. You ford splashing Bubbs Creek just below that lake, then ford it twice more within a mile. Soon you reach tree cover and notice campsites clinging to the canyon wall below the trail at 11,250 feet. You soon pass a campsite at 10,950 feet, just west of the trail before a pair of seasonal streamlets.

Now you ford Center Basin Creek (high in early season), pass several overused campsites (bear box) below the trail, and then pass the unsigned junction with the Center Basin Trail (10,500–4.5). You stay on the PCT and ford more tributaries of Bubbs Creek.

Many good campsites are located near some of these fords and along the main creek. Wood is scarce, and wood fires are *not permitted* above 10,800 feet!

Continuing down the east side of dashing Bubbs Creek, you pass **Upper Vidette Meadow (9000'), where there are a bear box and good if well-used campsites.** At Vidette Meadow (9600–2.8), long a favorite camping spot in these headwaters of South Fork Kings River, you find two bear boxes. High use has made the place less attractive, but its intrinsic beauty has not been lost, and the mighty Kearsarge Pinnacles to the northeast have lost only a few inches of height, if that, since Sierra Club founders like Joseph Le Conte camped here at the turn of the twentieth century. Camping is limited to one night in one place from here to Woods Creek. A summer ranger may be in Vidette Meadow east of the trail to assist traffic flow. Beyond the meadow, a trail goes west to Cedar Grove. The PCT turns north (9550–0.7) to fiercely attack the wall of Bubbs Creek canyon. You come to the junction with the trail to Bullfrog and Kearsarge Lakes (10,530–1.5), an alternate and scenic route to Kearsarge Pass for northbound hikers, then finish off the climb at a broad, sandy saddle that contains the junction of the Charlotte Lake and Kearsarge Pass trails (10,710–0.7). Charlotte Lake offers good camping, bear boxes, and a summer ranger station on its north shore. In ¼ mile you pass a shortcut (for southbound hikers) to the Kearsarge Pass Trail which heads east 9 miles to its Onion Valley trailhead, and then you traverse high above emerald Charlotte Lake. As the route veers eastward, it passes another trail to Charlotte Lake, then climbs past a talus-choked pothole and ascends gently to the foot of the wall that is notched by Glen Pass.

It is hard to see where a trail could go up that precipitous blank wall, but one does, and after very steep switchbacks you are suddenly at Glen Pass (11,978–2.3). The view north presents a barren, rocky, brown world with precious little green of

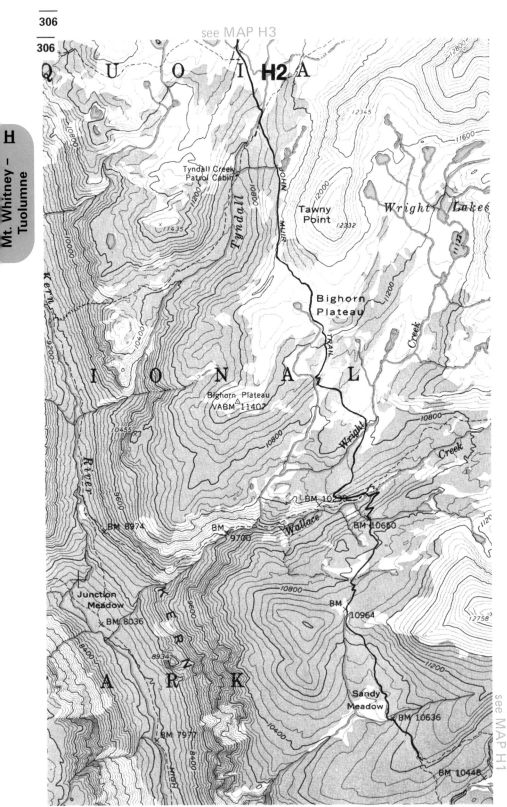

see MAP H3

Q U O I **H2** A

Tyndall Creek
Patrol Cabin

Tawny
Point

*Wright Lakes*

Bighorn
Plateau

*Tyndall*

JOHN MUIR TRAIL

I O N A L

Bighorn Plateau
VABM 11407

*Wright*

*Creek*

*Kern*

*River*

BM 8974

BM
9700

*Wallace*

BM 10735

BM 10650

Junction
Meadow

BM 8036

BM
10964

A R K

Sandy
Meadow

BM 10636

BM 7977

BM 10448

see MAP H1

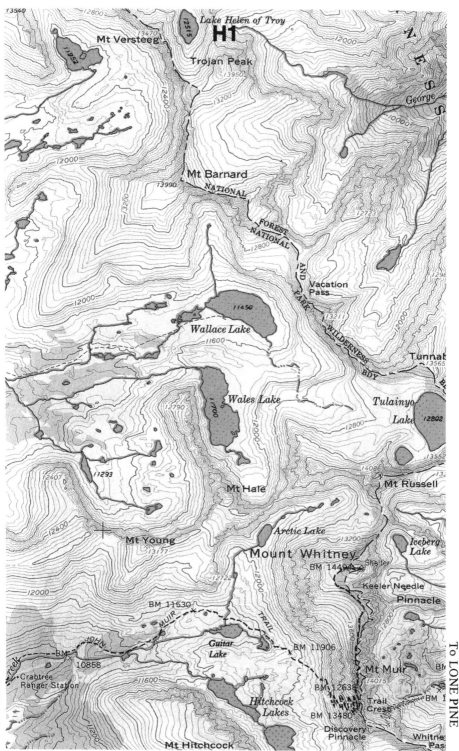

13540

12800

Lake Helen of Troy

**H1**

13470

12515

Mt Versteeg

Trojan Peak

11952

13950

12000

N
E
S

13200

12400

George

10000

Mt Barnard

13990

NATIONAL

12000

FOREST
NATIONAL

12723

12800

AND

Vacation
Pass

12000

13211

PARK

12000

11450

WILDERNESS

Wallace Lake

11600

Tunnab

13565

BDY

B

12000

Wales Lake

11700

Tulainyo

12790

Lake

12802

12000

12800

13552

12407

14086

11293

Mt Hale

13

Mt Russell

12400

Arctic Lake

13200

Mt Young

Mount Whitney

Iceberg
Lake

13177

BM 14494

Shelter

12000

12722

Keeler Needle

Pinnacle

JOHN

BM 11530

MUIR

TRAIL

BM

Guitar
Lake

BM 11906

3600

12800

10858

Mt Muir

BM

To LONE PINE

Crabtree
Ranger Station

11600

14015

BM 12636

Trail
Crest

BM 1

11200

Hitchcock
Lakes

BM 13480

Discovery
Pinnacle

Mt Hitchcock

Whitney
Pas

see MAP H2

see MAP G18

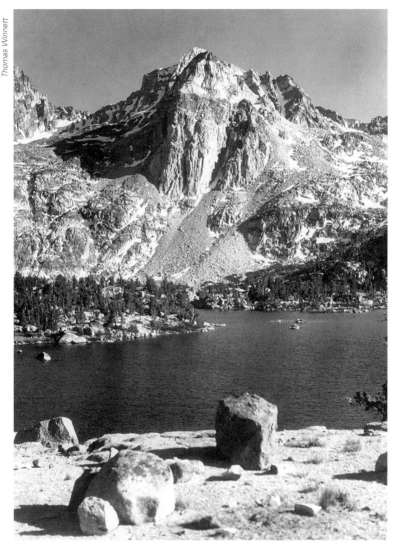

*Thomas Winnett*

*Painted Lady above Rae Lake*

tree or meadow visible. Yet you know by now that not far down the trail ahead there will be plenty of willows, sedges, wildflowers and, eventually, groves of whitebark, lodgepole and foxtail pines. To be sure you get there, take special care on your descent from Glen Pass as you switchback down to a small lake basin, ford the lakes' outlet and switchback down again.

When you are about 400 vertical feet above Rae Lakes, you will see why Dragon Peak (12,995'), in the southeast, has that name. Where the unsigned Sixty Lake Basin Trail turns off to the west (10,550–2.0), the Rae Lakes summer ranger posts the current camping regulations in the Rae Lakes Basin; please study them. **The middle and lower Rae Lakes have bear boxes. Hanging your food is utterly useless for protection against bears in the Rae Lakes Basin! Either use the bear boxes or carry and use canisters. (It's hoped that increasing use**

**See Map H4**

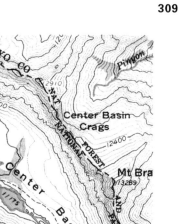
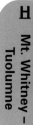

TULARE CO

H3

INYO CO.

East Vidette
*12350*

Pinyon

Center Basin
Crags
*12400*

Mt Bra
*13289*

Y O N

East Spur

*12735*

Golden Bear
Lake
*11175*

Center Basin

Center
Peak
*12760*

*11600*

*12000*

*12889*

P A R K

*13414*

*12795*

*11776*

orn

Mt Stanford
*13963*
Gregorys
Monument

Harrison
Pass

D I V I D

*12248*

*12021*

VABM Mt Keith
*13977*

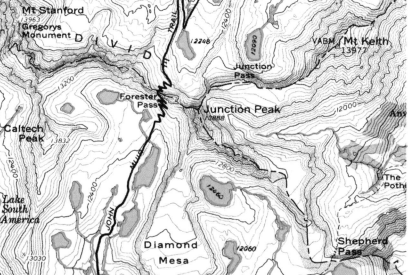

Junction
Pass

Forester
Pass

Junction Peak
*13888*

Caltech
Peak
*13832*

Anx

The
Poth

To INDEPENDENCE

Lake
South
America
*11941*

*12800*

*12460*

JOHN MUIR

*13030*

Diamond
Mesa

*12060*

Shepherd
Pass

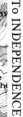

*12002*

*12000*

Creek

*11600*

Mt Tyn
*14018*

see MAP H5

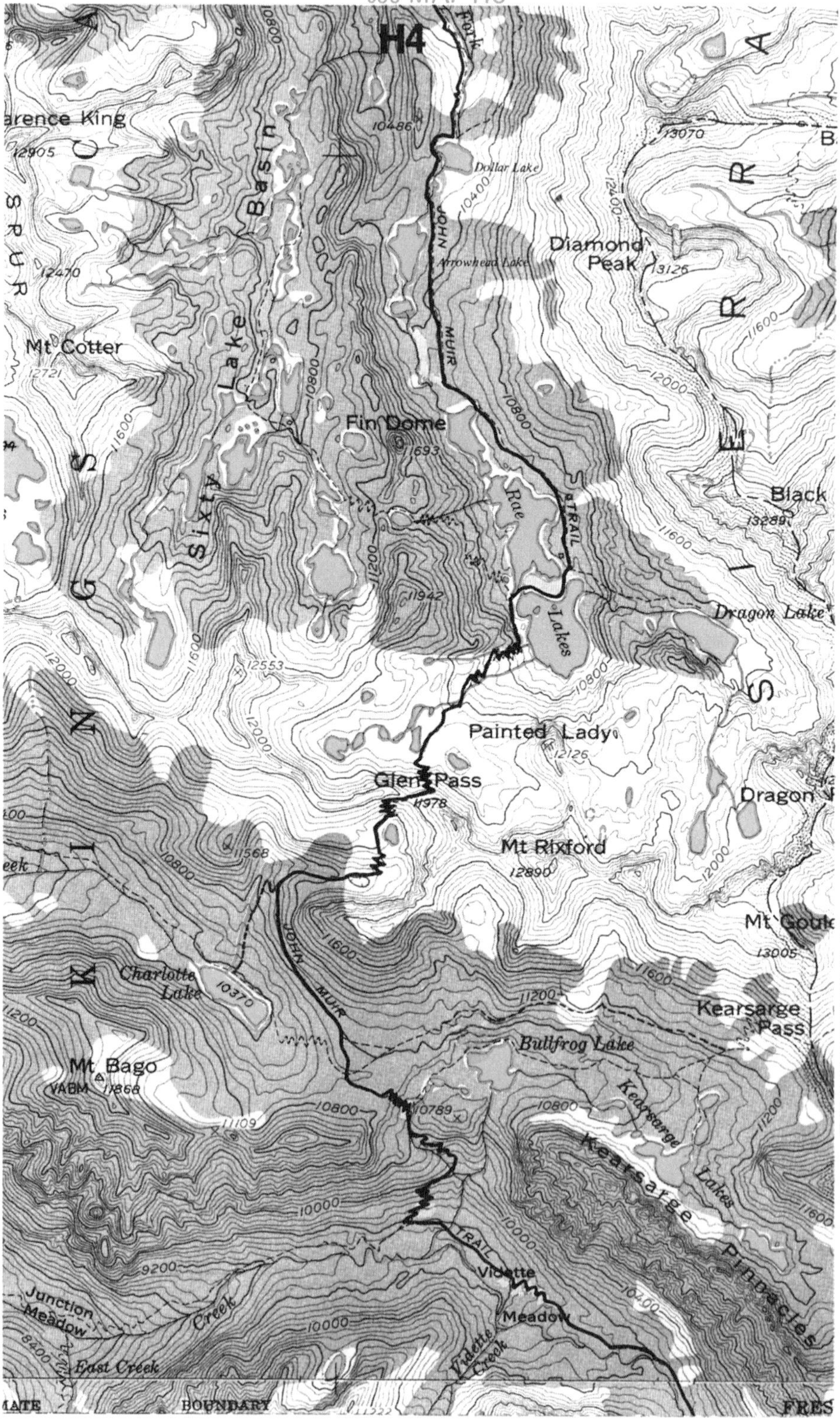


see MAP H3

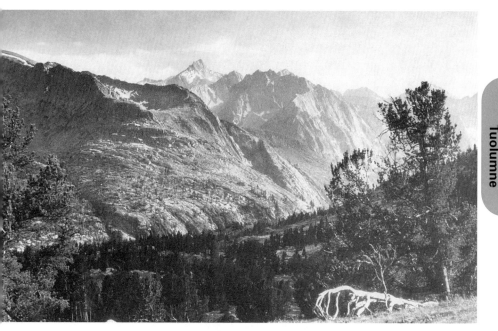

*Mt. Clarence King from Woods Creek Headwaters*

of the bear-resistant canisters will permit campers to disperse more widely, away from the heavily used bear-box sites.)

The PCT turns east, crosses the "isthmus" between the upper and middle Rae Lakes, fording the connecting stream en route (difficult in early season), passes the unsigned Dragon Lake Trail, and winds above the east shore of the middle lake, passing a signed trail (10,597–2.8) to the summer ranger station. Wood fires are not allowed between Glen Pass and 10,000 feet, well below Dollar Lake.

Beyond Rae Lakes your gently descending trail passes above an unnamed lake and drops to the northeast corner of aptly named Arrowhead Lake, where there are good campsites and a bear box. Then it fords gurgling South Fork Woods Creek and reaches scenic Dollar Lake, where there is no bear box and camping is severely restricted to protect its fragile environment. Just north of Dollar Lake, the unsigned

Baxter Pass Trail heads northeast across the lake's outlet (10,230–2.6).

The lower slopes just east of Dollar Lake are composed of Paleozoic sediments that were later metamorphosed to biotite schist. Granitic rock separates these metasediments from a higher, north-south band of Triassic-Jurassic lava flows that have been changed into metavolcanic rocks. The metamorphism of all these rock types probably occurred during the Cretaceous period, when bodies of molten granite rising up into them deformed and altered them. As we progress north to Yosemite, we'll see many more examples of similar metamorphosed rocks.

From the Baxter Pass Trail junction you descend gently down open, lightly forested slopes, crossing several good-sized though unnamed streams, including the

**See Maps H4, H5**

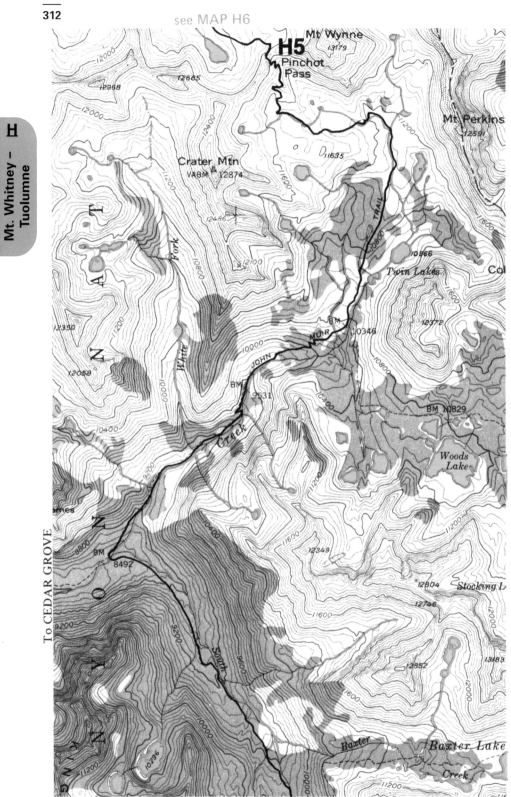

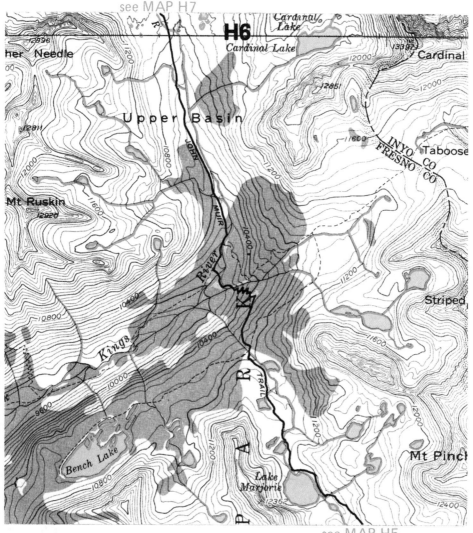

see MAP H7

see MAP H5

creek from Lake 10296 (Lake 3144 on the metric topo—creek may be difficult in early season). The reward for all this descent is a chance to start climbing again at Woods Creek (8492–3.7), crossed on a wood bridge, where the campsites are good but much used and have bear boxes. Immediately beyond the bridge a trail to Cedar Grove goes south down the creek. As you perspire north from the crossing up the valley of Woods Creek, **there is no drinking-water**

**problem, what with the main stream near at hand and many tributaries,** some of good size, to ford, jump or boulderhop. After the junction of the Sawmill Pass Trail (10,370–3.4), the grade abates, you soon pass a use trail northeast to Twin Lakes, and you reach the alpine vale where this branch of the Kings River has its headwaters, bounded by glorious peaks on 3½ sides. With one last, long spurt you finally top Pinchot Pass (12,130–3.7), one of those "passes" that are regrettably not at the low point of the divide.

From this pass the PCT swoops down into the lake-laden valley below, runs along the east shore of at-tree-line Lake Marjorie, touches its outlet (11,160–1.7), and then passes four laklets, fording several small streams along the way. A summer ranger station is sometimes located beyond the fourth laklet, just south of the Bench Lake Trail junction. **Bench Lake, on a true bench high above South Fork Kings River's canyon, has good campsites that are off the beaten track.** Just beyond this junction you ford the outlet of Lake Marjorie and in 200 yards meet the Taboose Pass Trail (10,750– 1.3) at the upper edge of a lodgepole forest. Another downhill segment of forested switchbacks brings you to the South Fork, which is best crossed a few yards downstream from the trail. On the far bank the South Fork Trail (10,050–1.3) leads downstream and you turn northeast upstream, passing another trail to Taboose Pass in ⅓ mile.

Climbing steadily, you cross several unnamed tributaries that can slow you down at the height of the melt, and then ford the infant South Fork (10,840–2.2) near some good campsites.

East of the trail, on the Sierra crest, looming Cardinal Mountain (13,397′) is named for red but is in fact half white and half dark, in a strange mixture of metamorphosed Paleozoic rocks.

West of this peak you cross grassy flats and hop over numerous branches of the headwaters of South Fork Kings River. Every camper can have his own lake and laklet in this high basin—though the campsites are austere.

This ascent finally steepens and zigzags up to rockbound Mather Pass (12,100–3.0), named for Stephen Mather, first head of the National Park Service. The view ahead

is dominated by the 14,000-foot peaks of the Palisades group, knifing sharply into the sky. Your trail now makes a knee-shocking descent to the poor campsites ¼ mile southeast of long, blue upper Palisade Lake. The route then contours above the lakes, fording the stream draining a high basin to the east-northeast (may be difficult). **Viewful, spartan campsites dot the bench south of this ford and above the trail (10,880′).** Beyond the ford, the PCT drops to the north shore of the lower lake (10,613–3.5), with its poor-to-fair campsites. Knees rested, you descend again, down the "Golden Staircase," built on the cliffs of the gorge of Palisade Creek. This section was the last part of the John Muir Trail to be constructed, and it is easy to see why. In ½ mile from the bottom of the "staircase" you cross multibranched Glacier Creek and immediately arrive at Deer Meadow (8860–3.0), which is more lodgepole forest than meadow, but pleasant enough anyway.

Beyond the campsites here, the downhill grade continues, less steeply, across the stream draining Palisade Basin and several smaller streams to reach the confluence of Palisade Creek and Middle Fork Kings River (8020–3.7), where a trail takes off downstream for Simpson Meadow. Campsites are few in this lower canyon of Palisade Creek and in the lower part of the next canyon, along Middle Fork Kings River, because of overgrowth and erosion. Look for sites near the confluence, where there is a large, Jeffrey-pine-shaded flat.

The PCT turns north up Le Conte Canyon, staying well above the Middle Fork, and passes more campsites a couple of switchbacks north of the confluence as well as on a flat uphill from the trail and just north of a dashing double cascade. The ascent continues past a series of falls and chutes to **Grouse Meadow**, a serene expanse of grassland with **good campsites in the forest along the east side.** Up the canyon from these meadows, you can see repeated

**See Maps H6, H7, H8, H9**

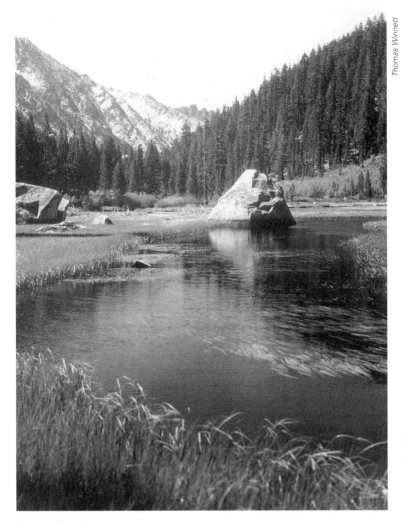

*Thomas Winnett*

*Grouse Meadows*

evidence of great avalanches that crashed down the immense canyon walls and wiped out stands of trees. The trail climbs gently to turbulent Dusy Branch, crossed on a steel bridge, and immediately encounters the Bishop Pass Trail (8710–3.3) to South Lake. Near this junction is a ranger station occupied in summer.

Our route up-canyon from this junction ascends between highly polished granite walls past lavish displays of a great variety of wildflowers. The trail passes through sagebrushy **Little Pete and Big Pete meadows (campsites at both; the former is bigger),** and swings west to assault the Goddard Divide and search out its breach, Muir Pass. Up and up the rocky trail winds, passing the last tree long before you reach desolate Helen Lake (11,595-5.7)—named, along with Wanda Lake to the west, for John Muir's daughters. This east side of the pass is under snow throughout the summer in some years. Finally, after five fords of the diminishing stream, you haul up at Muir

**See Maps H9, H10**

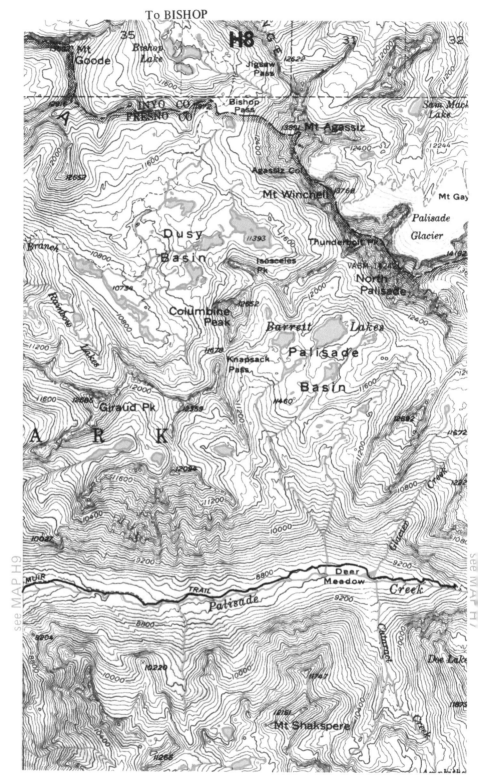

see MAP H9

see MAP H7

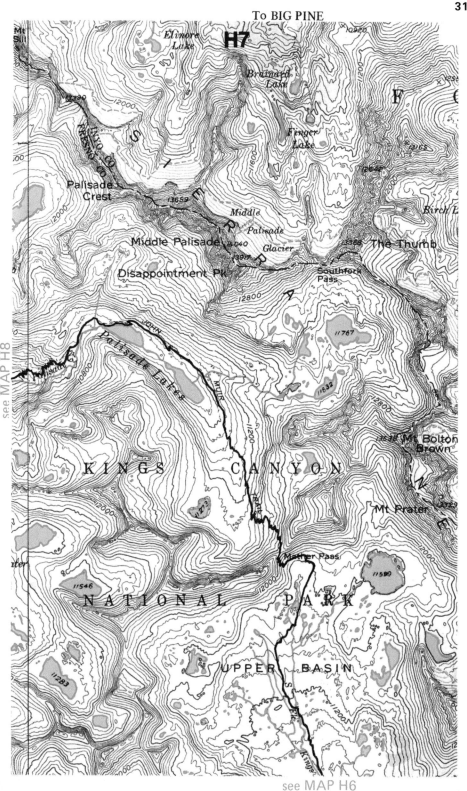

Elinore
Lake

Brainard
Lake

Finger
Lake

Palisade
Crest

Middle
Palisade
Glacier

Middle Palisade

The Thumb

Disappointment Pk

Southfork
Pass

Birch L

Mt Bolton
Brown

Palisade Lakes

KINGS    CANYON

Mt Prater

Mather Pass

NATIONAL    PARK

UPPER    BASIN

see MAP H8

see MAP H6

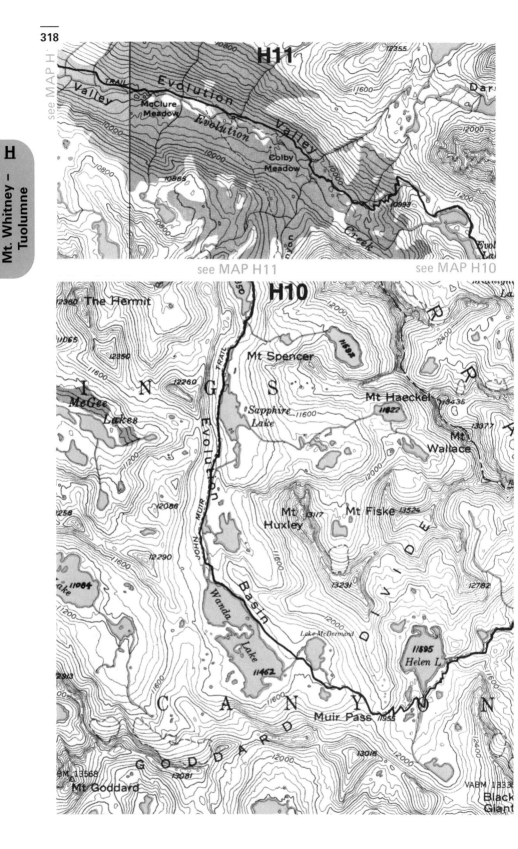

see MAP H11

see MAP H10

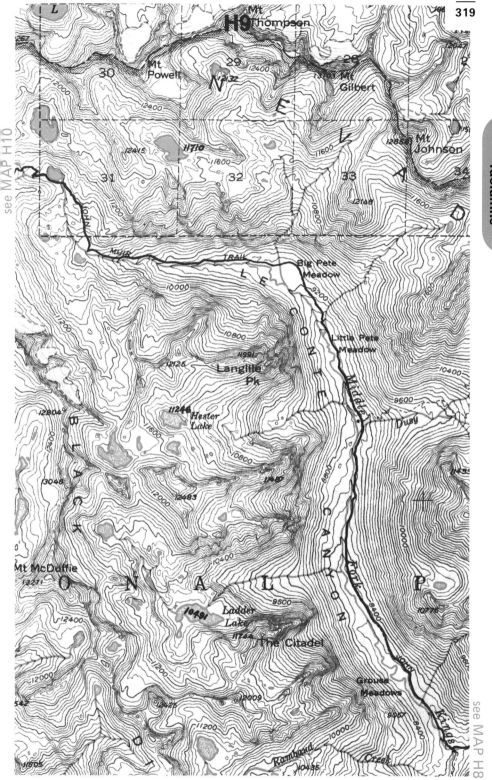

see MAP H10

see MAP H8

L

Mt
Thompson

H9

Mt
Powell

30

29

Mt
Gilbert

Mt
Johnson

12858

N

E

V

A

D

31

32

33

34

H710

12415

11600

11600

12148

10800

MUIR

TRAIL

Big Pete
Meadow

L

E

C

O

N

T

E

10000

Little Pete
Meadow

9600

Langille
Pk

11991

12125

10800

10400

Middle

Dusy

11246

Hester
Lake

11600

10800

12804

9600

B

L

A

C

K

12000

11467

13048

12483

8800

C

A

N

Y

O

N

10000

Mt McDuffie

13271

O

N

A

L

L

P

10776

9500

10400

12400

Ladder
Lake

10491

11744

The Citadel

10009

Fork

Kings

Grouse
Meadows

8400

9057

8400

12000

11200

10009

8400

10000

Rambaud

Creek

10435

11505

Pass (11,955–1.3), where a stone hut honoring Muir would shelter you fairly well in a storm, though the roof leaks. Otherwise, camping is prohibited in the hut's vicinity due to human-waste problems.

The views from here of the solitary peaks and the lonely lake basins are painted in the many hues of the mostly Jurassic-age metamorphic rocks that make up the Goddard Divide.

From the hut your trail descends gently past Lake McDermand and Wanda Lake. (Wood fires are banned from Muir Pass to beyond Evolution Lake.) You then ford Evolution Creek (11,400–2.2) and descend into the Sapphire Lake basin, where there are almost no campsites. There is simply not enough ground that is dry, flat, large enough, and stone-free enough to lie down on between Wanda and Evolution lakes!

The land here is nearly as scoured as when the ice left it over 10,000 years ago, and the aspect all around is one of newborn nakedness. To the east is a series of tremendous peaks named for Charles Darwin and other major thinkers about evolution, and the next lake and the valley below it also bear the name "Evolution."

The trail fords the stream at the inlet of Evolution Lake (10,850–2.4), skirts the lake, which has some campsites in clumps of stunted whitebark pines, and then drops sharply into Evolution Valley.

The marvelous meadows here are the reason for rerouting the trail through the forest, so the fragile grassland can recover from overtromping by the feet of earlier backpackers and horsepackers.

After crossing the multibranched stream that drains Darwin Canyon, you pass Colby Meadow, with many good campsites. Farther along, at McClure Meadow (9650–4.9) you will find a summer ranger midway along the meadow and more campsites. After further descent and several boulder fords of tributaries, you meet the head of Evolution Meadow and begin looking for a good spot to ford the wide, placid waters (may be difficult in early season). The old ford below Evolution Meadow has washed out. **A use trail on the south side leads out of the meadow, past fair campsites, and rejoins the PCT just below the old ford.** After passing overlooks of some beautiful falls and cascades on the creek, the trail switchbacks steeply down to the South Fork San Joaquin River's canyon floor and detours upstream to pass campsites and cross a footbridge (8470–3.5) over the South Fork San Joaquin River to reach the junction with the Goddard Canyon/Hell for Sure Pass Trail. Staying on the PCT northwest-bound along the west bank of the river, heading downstream, you pass numerous campsites, pass through a stout drift fence, recross the river on another bridge, and stroll past Aspen Meadow. From this hospitable riverside slope, you roll on down and out of Kings Canyon National Park at the steel-bridge crossing of Piute Creek. Here, where you enter John Muir Wilderness, the Piute Pass Trail (8050–3.5) starts north toward North Lake.

**Resupply access:** The Florence Lake roadend is 11 miles west down this trail; the Muir Trail Ranch is 1½ miles down it. (The latter is a possible package drop; inquire of the owner by writing Box 176, Lakeshore, CA 93634.)

**Side route:** Shortly before the ranch, and about 200 yards west of signs that indicate the John Muir Trail is 1½ miles away, both to the east and to the north,

**See Maps H10, H11, H12, H13**

an unsigned trail goes south ¼ mile down to riverside campsites. From the campsites on the south side of the river a faint trail goes 150 yards southwest to a natural hot spring—great for soaking off the grime—and a warmish small lake.

From the Florence Lake Trail junction, the PCT-John Muir Trail veers right to climb the canyon wall. It rises past a lateral trail down to the Florence Lake Trail (8400– 1.7), crosses little Senger Creek (9740– 2.2), and levels off below **Sally Keyes Lakes. Then your route passes the fair campsites at these lakes,** crossing the short stream that joins the two. Leaving the forest below, the trail skirts small Heart Lake and presently reaches barren Selden Pass (10,900– 2.1). At this pass, many-islanded Marie Lake is the central feature of the view northward, and soon you boulderhop its clear outlet (10,570-0.9), then descend moderately to the green expanses of Rosemarie Meadow (10,010–1.6). From this grassland a trail forks left, soon climbing southwest to **Rose Lake,** and about ¼ mile beyond another trail departs east for **Lou Beverly Lake. Both these lakes provide good, secluded camping.** About 200 yards past the last junction you bridge West Fork Bear Creek (avoid a use trail westward on this ford's north side), and then you make a 1-mile descent in lodgepole forest to a boulder ford of Bear Creek (very difficult in early season).

On the creek's far bank you meet a trail (9530–1.4) that goes up East Fork Bear Creek, but you turn down-canyon and descend gently to the log ford of refreshing Hilgard Creek. Immediately beyond, the Lake Italy Trail (9300–1.2) climbs east, and your trail continues down through the mixed forest cover, always staying near rollicking Bear Creek. **You pass campsites near the trail, but for more wood and more solitude it is better to find a place to camp across the creek.**

**Side route:** Below Hilgard Creek (9040–2.0), you pass a junction with the trail to Bear Diversion Dam. (Those wishing to go to Mono Hot Springs can take this trail west to an OHV route that leads to a paved road; the short spur road to Mono Hot Springs lies about one mile south on the paved road.)

The trail gradually veers west as it follows the contour line, fords a difficult tributary, then turns north at the foot of a tough series of switchbacks. The south-facing hillside gets plenty of sun, but is surprisingly wet even in late season. You can pleasure your eyes with flowers in bloom as your route levels off. At the crest of Bear Ridge passes a trail (9980–1.6) that descends to Mono Hot Springs. The north side of Bear Ridge is incised with 53 dusty switchbacks.

Here you begin in a pure lodgepole forest but successively penetrate the realms of mountain hemlock, western white pine, red fir, Jeffrey pine, aspen, white fir and, finally, cottonwoods at Mono Creek (7850–4.6).

**Resupply access:** After you cross the footbridge over Mono Creek, you reach a junction with the trail that goes west to Lake Edison and Vermilion Valley Resort, 1 mile and 5½ miles away, respectively– though seasonal ferry service (fee) at Lake Edison's head, reached by a signed spur trail, can cut 4½ miles off your hike to the resort. Campsites lie several hundred yards west down this trail to the resort.

Beyond the bridge, the PCT turns right, soon crosses North Fork Mono Creek (difficult in early season), and climbs to a junction with the Mono Pass Trail (8270– 1.6). Your steep trail levels briefly at lush

**See Maps H13, H14, H15**

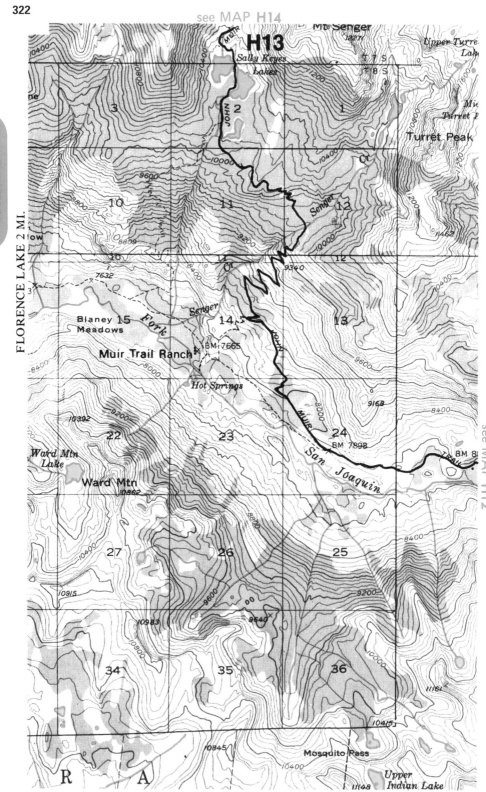

H13

Mt. Senger

Sally Keyes
Lakes

Upper Turret
Lake

Turret Peak

Senger

Blaney 15
Meadows

Fork

Senger

Muir Trail Ranch

BM 7665

Hot Springs

Ward Mtn
Lake

Ward Mtn

San Joaquin

BM 7898

Mosquito Pass

Upper
Indian Lake

R        A

Pocket Meadow (good campsites), passes a junction with a trail to Mott Lake, and again fords North Fork Mono Creek (8940–1.4; very diffcult in early season due to swift, deep, icy water and a rocky stream-bed—one of the JMT's more-dangerous fords, where a fall could be fatal). Then you resume climbing steeply on a narrow, rocky, exposed track up the west wall of Mono Creek's canyon.

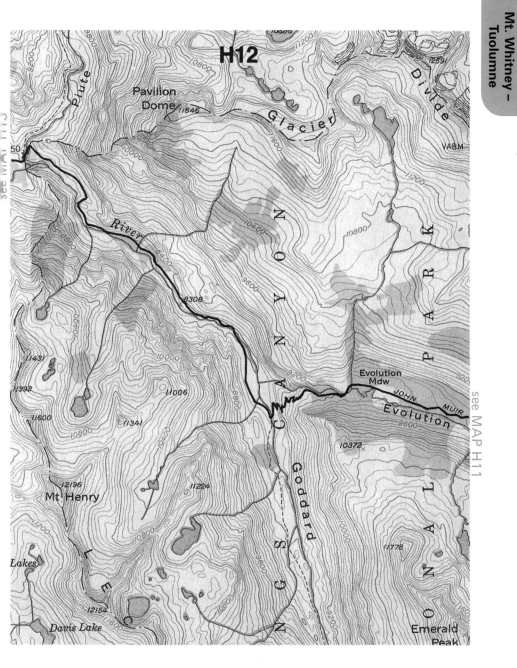

**See Map H15**

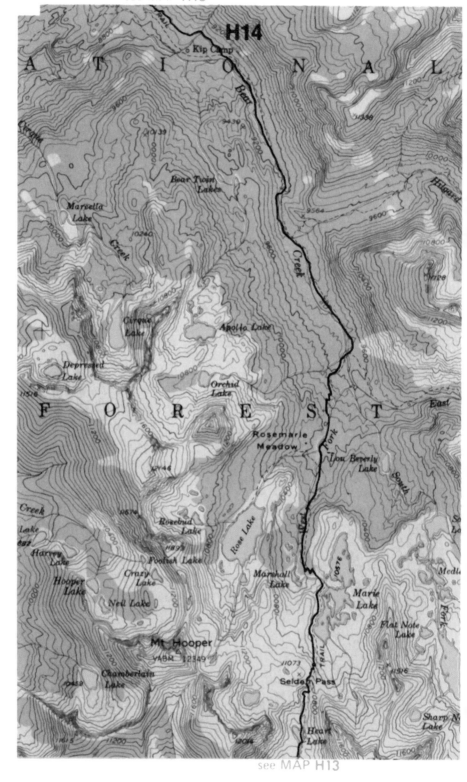

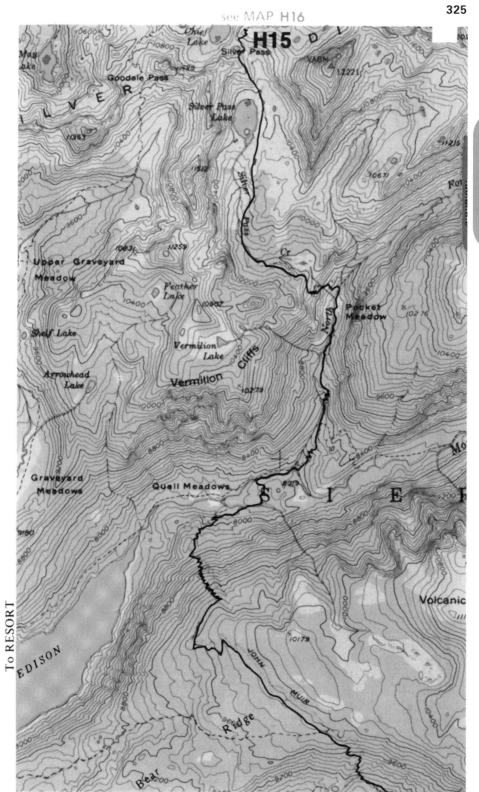

H15

Chief
Lake

Silver Pass

YABM
11221

Goodale Pass

Silver Pass
Lake

11215

10671

(1353)

Silver Pass

10836

11259

Upper Graveyard
Meadow

Feather
Lake

10907

Cr

Shelf Lake

Vermilion
Lake

North

Pocket
Meadow

10276

Vermilion
Cliffs

Arrowhead
Lake

Vermilion

10279

Graveyard
Meadows

Quail Meadows

8010

S   I   E   R

9180

To RESORT

EDISON

Volcanic

10179

JOHN   MUIR

Ridge

Bear

The first ford of Silver Pass Creek is very difficult in early season; the combination of slippery boulders and icy cascades make this another of the more-dangerous fords on the present JMT route, and a slip here could be fatal. Above a large meadow you reford the creek (9640–1.2) and then rise above treeline. The trail bypasses Silver Pass Lake and then ascends past the actual pass (low point) to the sign SILVER PASS (10,900–2.8) at a glorious viewpoint. The descent northward passes Chief Lake and then the Goodale Pass Trail (10,550–1.2), switchbacks northeast down to ford the outlet of Squaw Lake (Spartan campsites), passes a small meadow whose outlet it crosses on a footbridge, shortly fords the outlet, and then makes a long, hemlock-lined descent to the beautiful valley of **Fish Creek, where there are good campsites near the sometimes hard-to-spot junction with the Cascade Valley Trail (9130–2.5).**

**Alternate route:** Via the PCT, you are now 19.0 miles from the Rainbow Falls trailhead parking lot near Reds Meadow. Via the Cascade Valley–Fish Creek–Rainbow Falls trail, you are 19.4 miles from it. Some backpackers who aren't committed to following the PCT every step of the way prefer this lower, easier, mostly downhill, less-crowded route. **Camping opportunities are greater and, if you're experiencing bad weather, you'll find this lower, well-forested route far more hospitable.**

If you stay on the PCT, turn right from the Cascade Valley Trail junction and ascend northeast, soon crossing Fish Creek on a steel bridge. Staying above this good-sized creek, the route ascends gently to the campsites at Tully Hole (9520–1.1), a well-flowered grassland where the McGee Pass Trail departs eastward. Now the PCT climbs steeply north up a band of Mesozoic metavolcanics which sweep east and grade into the Paleozoic metasediments of dominating Red Slate Mountain (13,163'). Beyond the crest of this ascent you reach deep-blue Lake Virginia (10,314–1.9), with several somewhat exposed campsites. In early season you will have to wade across the head of the lake or detour rather far north. From this boggy crossing your trail climbs to a saddle below the nearly vertical northeast face of Peak 11147 and then switchbacks down to heavily used Purple Lake (9900–2.1), just beyond whose outlet (can be difficult) a trail begins its descent into deep Cascade Valley. **Camping is prohibited within 100 yards of the outlet.** If you want to camp in this vicinity, use the sites by the lake's northwest shore. In late summer and in dry years, you may not have any trailside water until Deer Creek, 7.8 miles ahead, so plan accordingly.

From Purple Lake the rocky trail climbs west and then bends north as it levels out high on the wall of glaciated Cascade Valley. Soon you reach a trail (10,150–2.3) to Duck Lake and beyond, which could be used to escape bad weather or to resupply at Mammoth Lakes.

Just beyond the Duck Lake Trail, you ford Duck Creek near several undistinguished campsites before traversing first southwest and then northwest.

If you sharpen your gaze, you will see both red firs and Jeffrey pines above 10,000 feet on this north wall of Cascade Valley, well above their normal range. You also have views of the Silver Divide in the south as you slant northwest and descend gradually through mixed conifers.

From your last set of excellent views, which are along the south slopes of Peak 10519, the trail begins a westward descent, crossing about a mile of lava-flow rubble before turning north for a rambling drop to **Deer Creek (9090–5.5). Here you'll find fair, lodgepole-shaded campsites.**

In the next ⅔ mile the trail starts west, climbs briefly over a granitic ridge, and

**See Maps H15, H16, H17**

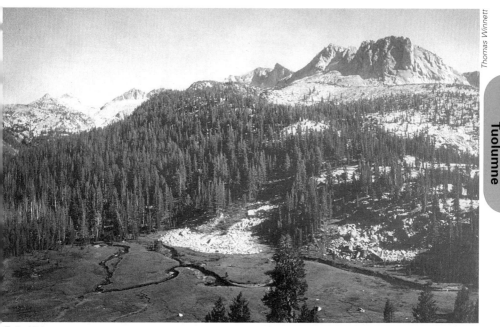

*Thomas Winnett*

*Tully Hole*

then descends north to a creek crossing in a long, slender meadow. Heading north through it you have views of The Thumb (10,286′), then leave this county-line meadow as you cross a seasonal creeklet. This freshet you parallel for about a mile as you descend a bit to Upper Crater Meadow (8920–2.0).

**Resupply access:** From this junction and one 100 yards later, trails head over to very popular Horseshoe Lake. From it the Lake Mary Road starts a 4.9-mile descent to a junction with Minaret Summit Road in bustling, recreation-oriented Mammoth Lakes. See Supplies at the start of this section for the seasonal shuttle-bus route to the town. If you would rather hike to it and back, then take the following 7¼-mile route, of which the first 5 miles are on trails and lightly used roads.

You can start from either of the two junctions in Upper Crater meadow. Both trails go about 1½ miles before a uniting, from where one tread goes about 1 mile northeast to broad Mammoth Pass. Just east beyond it you reach the north shore of McCloud Lake, and beyond it continue ahead (off the map) about ½ mile down to a road on the northwest shore of Horseshoe Lake. Walk over to the north end of the lake, from where you could take the aforementioned Lake Mary Road to town.

A shorter, quieter way, however, is to go but ¼ mile east on the road, take a spur road ¼ mile north past houses to its end and, on a trail, head east, dropping about 300 feet to the west end of Twin Lakes Campground. Continue east through the campground to a road that parallels the east shores of the Twin Lakes. This road you take about ½ mile north to the Lake Mary Road, on which you walk 2¼ miles to town.

**See Map H18**

see MAP H18

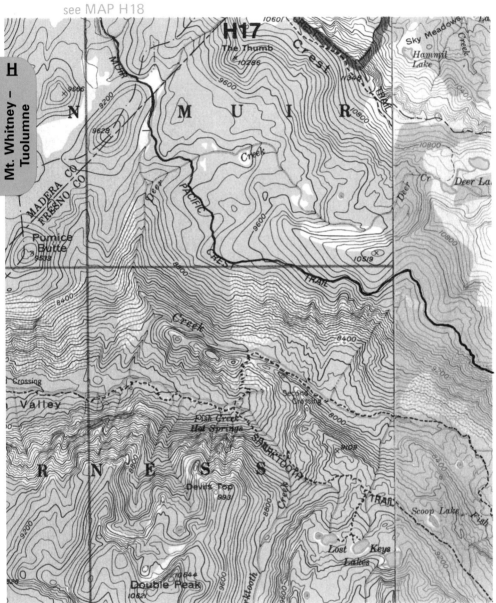

**H17**

**H**

**Mt. Whitney – Tuolumne**

see MAP H16

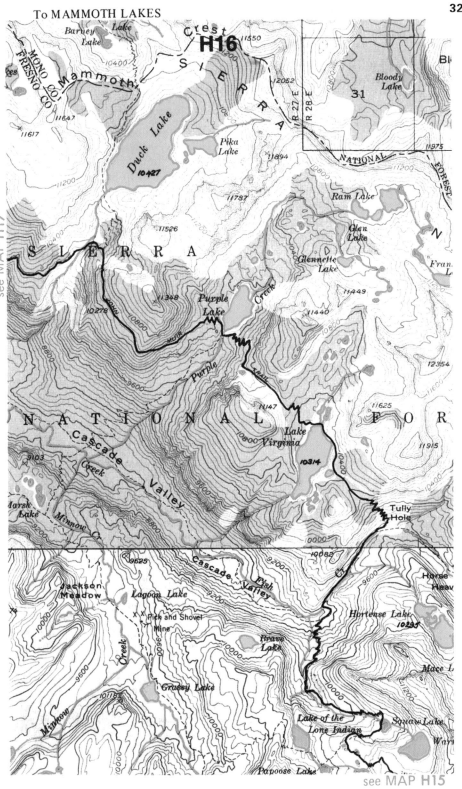

**H16**

see MAP H17

see MAP H15

In about 100 yards, by the north edge of Upper Crater Meadow, you meet the second of the two trails that lead to Mammoth Pass. It also provides an alternate (not recommended) route—the old JMT/PCT—down to the Reds Meadow area. With that goal in mind, you take the newer route down along the creek you've been following, cross it in ½ mile, and **then descend to a recrossing with a good campsite** (8660-0.8), the last one before Reds Meadow. Here you leave John Muir Wilderness for good and enter Ansel Adams Wilderness for a short spell.

This creekside campsite lies between the two Red Cones, products of very recent volcanic eruptions. The northern one is easy to climb and offers a fine view of the Ritter Range and Middle Fork San Joaquin River's deep canyon. You'll also see Mammoth Mountain (11,053') in the north-northeast, on whose north slopes as many as 20,000 skiers, most of them from Southern California, may be found on a busy day. This mountain is a volcano which began to grow about 400,000 years ago. The area around it, including the upper canyon of Middle Fork San Joaquin River, has been volcanically active for over 3 million years, and the last eruption here occurred less than 1000 years ago. It is the Sierra's "hot spot"—ironically, considering that it is also a mecca for skiers due to its large, late-melting snowpack.

Beyond the creekside campsite between the Red Cones the PCT makes lazy switchbacks down to Boundary Creek (7910–2.3). Roughly midway between it and the next junction, you cross a smaller creek, where you exit from an east lobe of Ansel Adams Wilderness. Through a fir forest your well-graded route descends to an abandoned stagecoach road (7700–0.7).

**Resupply access:** Now on a broad path, you can walk about 300 yards north on it to Reds Meadow Pack Station. Another 230 yards north along a paved road takes you to Reds Meadow Resort, with a store and cafe, at road's end. The food selection is aimed at campers with ice chests, not at hikers with backpacks. From here and from a number of roadside stops as far north as Agnew Meadows, you can take a shuttle bus to the Mammoth Lakes area (see Supplies at the start of this chapter).

Past the abandoned stagecoach road you immediately cross a horse trail that climbs briefly north to the pack station, reaching it at a switchback in the paved road. Just past this horse trail the PCT descends to a crossing of the Rainbow Falls-Fish Valley-Cascade Valley Trail (7600– 0.2), on which you'd be ascending if you took the alternate route to here mentioned earlier.

**Side route:** This popular trail starts from the Rainbow Falls trailhead parking lot about 250 yards north of the PCT. If you've got the time, hike 1.0 mile south on this trail for a view of Rainbow Falls. Afternoon is the best time to see and photograph this waterfall, as well as the columns of Devils Postpile just ahead.

Beyond the Rainbow Falls trail, you curve southwest over to a low, nearby crest from which an old trail, essentially abandoned, heads north, and then you meander northwest down to a trail junction (7430–0.5) by the east boundary of Devils Postpile National Monument.

**Alternate route:** Here we recommend you leave the PCT and head ½ mile north to a junction, crossing a creek from Sotcher Lake just before you reach it. From this junction, at the base of a Devils

**See Map H18**

see MAP H19

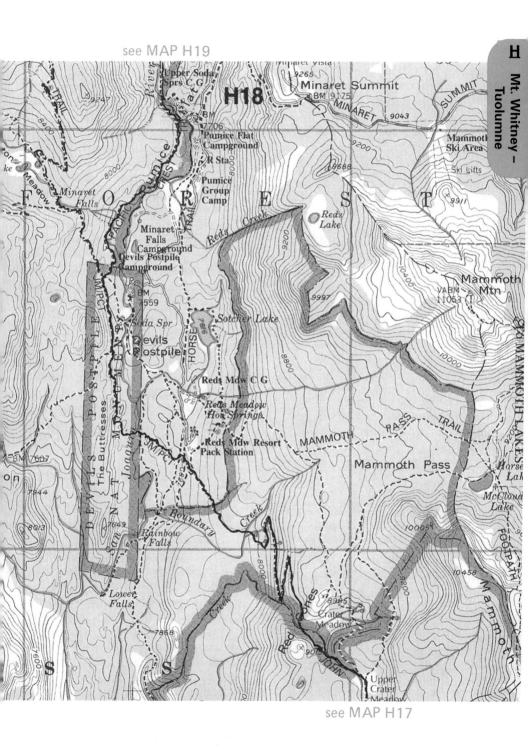

see MAP H17

Postpile lava flow, you can head ¼ mile east to the paved road, mentioned earlier, then hike a few yards north on it to the entrance to Reds Meadow Campground. In it you can get a free, luke-warm shower at the bathhouse by the campground's "hot" spring. From the lavaflow junction the alternate route climbs ¼ mile northwest to a ridge, from which you can take a short trail up to the glacially polished top of the Devils Postpile. The main trail skirts along the base of this columnar lava flow, reaching a junction in about ¼ mile, just beyond a junction with a trail from the top of the lava flow. If you were to continue straight ahead from this second junction, you'd reach the monument's small visitor center (with a phone) and its adjacent campground in about ⅓ mile. Instead, to regain the PCT, you turn left at the second junction, descend to a nearby bridge over the San Joaquin River, and in a minute reach a junction. From here, head 0.4 mile north to the PCT.

Back at the monument's east boundary, PCT purists immediately cross the San Joaquin River on a sturdy bridge, wind westward past two seasonal ponds, then make a struggling climb north through deep pumice to an intersection with the old, trans-Sierra Mammoth Trail (7710-1.0). This relatively unscenic one-mile slog was built to keep PCT equestrians away from the Postpile. Northbound, the old trail descends ¼ mile to meet the alternate route, while the PCT contours along pumice-laden slopes, soon reaching the end of the alternate route (7660–0.6). Here the John Muir and Pacific Crest trails, which have coincided through most of this hiking section, diverge for a few miles, becoming one tread again near Thousand Island Lake. On their divergence both quickly re-enter Ansel Adams Wilderness, though the PCT briefly leaves it in the Agnew Meadows area.

**Alternate route:** Briefly, the 12.9-mile JMT segment—the more popular of the two—climbs up to a trail junction near Minaret Creek, quickly crosses the creek (with adjacent campsites) and winds over to another junction by Johnston Meadow (more campsites), 1.4 miles from the PCT junction. The JMT climbs up past knee-deep Trinity Lakes, then later makes a three-stage descent to Shadow Lake, dropping to shallow Gladys and ideal Rosalie lakes along the way (respectively 6.1 and 6.8 miles from the PCT junction). **You can camp at either lake but not at Shadow Lake, except near its southwest shore. However, good-to-excellent, popular campsites abound in the ⅔-mile JMT stretch west of the lake, up along Shadow Creek. No campfires are allowed along this stretch, but stoves are okay.** From the creek the JMT climbs 1.9 miles up to a high ridge, then drops ¾ mile to the east end of Garnet Lake, which is off-limits to camping. Ruby Lake, about 1⅓ miles farther, offers one campsite, as does Emerald Lake, just beyond it. Emerald, however, is probably the best lake along this 12.9-mile route for swimming. **Finally, no camping is allowed near the east end of Thousand Island Lake.**

Back where the JMT and the PCT split, the pumice-lined PCT winds down to the distributaries of Minaret Creek (7590–0.6), which must be waded except in the late season, just below dramatic Minaret Falls. Still in pumice, the trail bends northeast and almost touches Middle Fork San Joaquin River before climbing north away from it over a lava-flow bench that overlooks Pumice Flat. In a shady forest of lodgepole pines and red firs, you make a brief descent to a bridge across the Middle Fork. From the far side of the bridge (7680–1.4), a trail heads just around the corner to the west end of Upper Soda Springs Campground. Beyond the bridge

**See Maps H18, H19, H20**

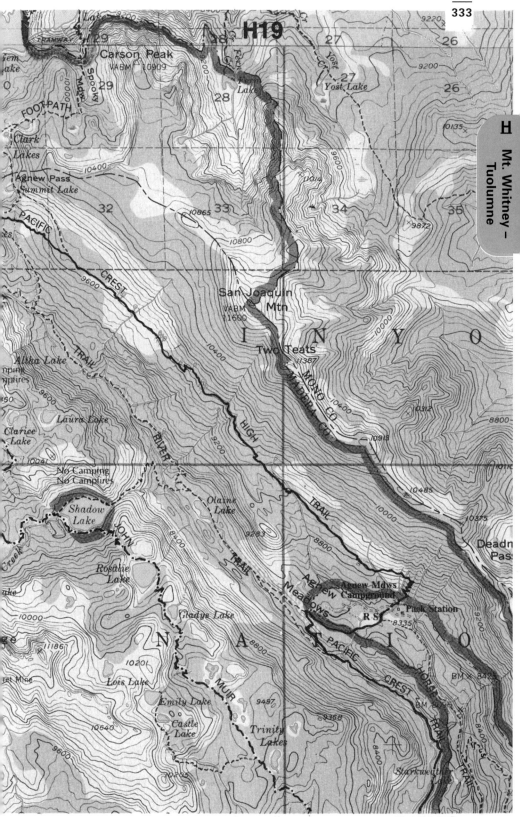

H19

Carson Peak
VABM 10909

Yost Lake

FOOTPATH

Clark
Lakes

Agnew Pass
Summit Lake

PACIFIC

CREST

San Joaquin Mtn
VABM 11600

I N Y O

Two Teats
11387

Alpha Lake

MONO CO.

Laura Lake

HIGH

Clarice
Lake

No Camping
No Campfires

Shadow
Lake

Olaine
Lake

TRAIL

Deadm
Pass

JOHN

Rosalie
Lake

Gladys Lake

Agnew Mdws
Campground

Agnew
Meadows

Pack Station

R S

Lois Lake

MUIR

PACIFIC

CREST

Emily Lake

TRAIL

9487

Castle
Lake

Trinity
Lakes

BM X 84

Starkweather

see MAP H18

you head upriver, having many opportunities to drop to nearby eating, drinking and chilly-swimming spots along the dashing Middle Fork. After crossing a permanent stream (7810–1.0), the trail bends from north to northwest and crosses a second stream (7910–1.1). Then, just past a small knoll, it reaches a junction (8000–0.2).

**Alternate route:** You can continue straight ahead, up river, having many camping opportunities before rejoining the PCT in 5.9 miles, at a point about ⅓ mile west of the Badger Lakes.

Leaving the river route, the PCT first parallels it northwest, then climbs via short switchbacks to a junction with the River Trail (8280–0.5). You start east up it and in 80 yards meet a fork. The left (east) fork goes 0.4 mile to Agnew Meadows Campground, from which you can walk 0.4 mile east on a winding dirt road, along which you'll find the PCT's resumption by a trailhead parking area. Taking the right (southeast) fork, you hike through a long, narrow trough before curving northeast around a meadow, almost touching the ranger's trailer (with a parking area) before reaching the **Agnew Meadows road (8360–0.9), which has water and an outhouse by a trailhead parking area.**

**Resupply access:** The main road to Reds Meadow lies ¼ mile east, and at that junction is the first of 10 stops made by shuttle buses from Mammoth Mountain Inn (see Supplies at start of this chapter).

From the Agnew Meadows road the PCT route follows the signed High Trail, which switchbacks upward for about 400 vertical feet before climbing northwest.

**Water access:** Creeks, creeklets and springs abound along the High Trail, for the volcanic-rock formations above us

store plenty of water, which they slowly release throughout the summer.

Views are relatively few until just before the boundary of Ansel Adams Wilderness (9680–2.8), and then the Ritter Range explodes on the scene, with Shadow Lake and the Minarets, both across the canyon, vying for your attention. Views and water abound over the next 2 miles of alternating brushy and forested slopes.

Your traversing route comes to a junction (9710–2.4) with a trail that climbs easily over Agnew Pass to good camps near the largest of the Clark Lakes, about 1.1 miles distant. Summit Lake, just before the pass, is good for swimming but a bit short on level camping spots. The High Trail, your route, now descends, crossing Summit Lake's seasonal outlet creek before climbing briefly to an intersection of a steep Middle Fork-Clark Lakes Trail (9500–0.8). Westward, your climb abates and you soon reach a de facto trail (9590–0.3), which you'll find just past a lakelet on your left.

**Side route:** This trail goes 0.2 mile southeast to good camps beside the largest of the Badger Lakes, which is the only one that is more than waist-deep. It is one of the best lakes in the entire Ansel Adams Wilderness.

Leaving the Badger Lakes area and the **last legal campsites on the PCT this side of Rush Creek,** you continue westward, passing a third trail to the Clark Lakes in ¼ mile. Soon you make a brief descent to a junction with the River Trail (9560–0.5), then climb moderately northwest before rambling southwest to a reunion with the John Muir Trail near the east end of spreading Thousand Island Lake (9840–1.0). **Camping is prohibited within ¼ mile of this lake's outlet, but is legal elsewhere.**

**See Map H20**

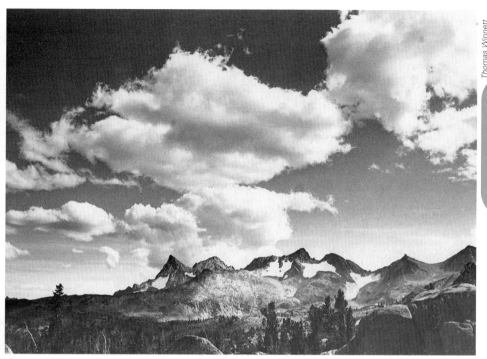

*Banner Peak (the leftmost), Mt. Ritter, and three unnamed peaks*

Particularly look along the lake's southeast shore.

The PCT climbs moderately through a thinning forest to two lakelets, reached just before Island Pass (10,200–1.8). The trail then traverses ⅓ mile to a ridge before descending to a sometimes obscure junction (9690–1.0).

From here a trail climbs 0.8 mile south to the tip of lower Davis Lake. Campsites by it are small and quite exposed, but the beauty of this lake and its surroundings makes them a worthy goal.

About 250 yards past the Davis Lakes Trail junction you reach the first of several Rush Creek forks. Along the ½-mile trail segment that ensues, the early-season hiker may have three wet fords to make. You may therefore want to keep your boots off until the last ford, just before a junction with the Rush Creek trail (9600–0.4).

**Resupply access:** This trail descends a lengthy 9.5 miles to popular Silver Lake, on well-traveled State Route 158 (June Lake Loop Road). As such, you will want to take it only for emergency reasons. While you can get supplies in the town of June Lake, the effort is not worth it.

In the past the Forks area had many small camps, which now would all be illegal because they are within 100 feet of a creek or a trail. A seasonal ranger, sometimes camped 200 yards southeast of the junction, can give you advice on where to camp in this vicinity.

Leaving the Forks, you quickly engage some short, steep switchbacks that you follow northwest up to a ridge, then cross it and ease up to a junction with the Marie Lakes Trail (10,030–0.8). The lakes' outlet creek, just beyond the junction, is best crossed at an obvious jump-across spot

**See Maps H20, H21**

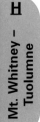

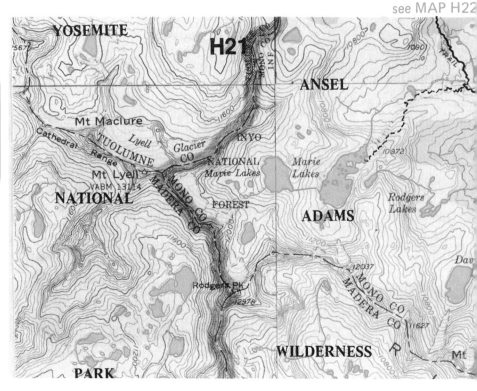

slightly downstream. After the ford the trail winds excessively in an oft-futile attempt to avoid the boulders and bogs of the increasingly alpine environment. Whitebark pines diminish in number and stature as you climb toward a conspicuous saddle—easily mistaken in early season for Donohue Pass. After a wet slog across the tundra-and-stone floor of your alpine basin, you veer southwest toward a prominent peak and ascend a sometimes obscure trail past blocks and over slabs to the real, signed, tarn-blessed Donohue Pass (11,056-2.6), where you leave Ansel Adams Wilderness.

The Yosemite high country unfolds before you as you descend northwest, partly in a long, straight fracture (southbound hikers take note). You then curve west to a sharp bend southwest, a few yards from which you can get a commanding panorama of Mt. Lyell, at 13,114 feet Yosemite's highest peak, and deep Lyell Canyon. Leaving the bend, you now descend southwest ½ mile to the north end of a boulder-dotted tarn that occasionally reflects Lyell and its broad glacier—the largest one you'll see in the Sierra. Contour along the tarn's west shore, then briefly climb southwest to a gap in a low ridge. Next, wind north and soon begin a steep northeast descent that ends at the north end of a small meadow, where you cross the Lyell Fork, usually via boulders (10,220–1.8). Immediately above this crossing the creek has widened almost to a narrow lake, and trekkers ascending in the opposite direction may assume (incorrectly) that they have reached the aforementioned tarn.

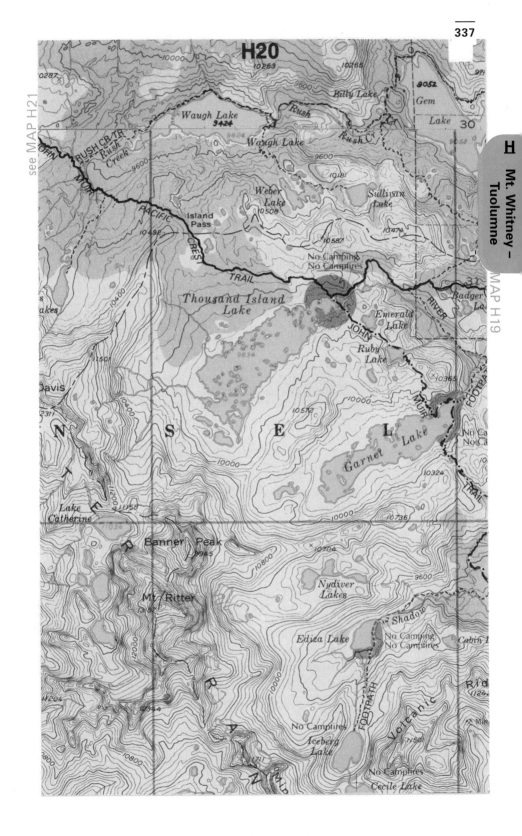

*Thomas Winnett*

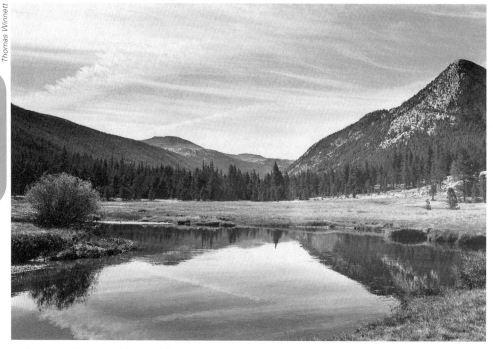

*Potter Point (right), and the Lyell Fork, Lyell Canyon*

A spacious, well-used camping area exists here among sparse tree cover, the first adequate site since the Rush Creek Forks area. In Yosemite National Park campfires are banned here and everywhere else above 9600 feet. Large campsites appear on a forested bench by another Lyell Fork crossing (9700–0.8), via a bridge.

Now you'll stay on the west bank of the river all the way to Tuolumne Meadows. Beyond the bench you make your last major descent—a steep one—partly across rock-avalanche slopes—down to the Lyell Fork base camp (9000– 1.4), at the southern, upper end of Lyell Canyon. This camp, a 3-hour trek from Highway 120, is a popular site with weekend mountaineers. Your hike to the highway is now an easy, level, usually open stroll along meandering Lyell Fork. **A major camping area is found at the**

junction (8880–2.8) **with a trail to Vogelsang High Sierra Camp.** Past the junction, occasional backward glances at receding Potter Point mark your progress north along trout-inhabited Lyell Fork. With the oft-looming threat of afternoon lightning storms, one wishes the trail would have been routed along the forest's edge, rather than through open meadow.

Typical of meadowy trails, yours is multitreaded. Numerous treads arise mainly because as the main tread is used, it gets deepened until it penetrates the near-surface water table and becomes soggy. Odds are great that you'll have to leave the tread at least once, thus helping to start a new one.

Shortly after Potter Point finally disappears from view—and beyond half a dozen campsites—you curve northwest, descend between two bedrock outcrops,

**See Maps H22, H23**

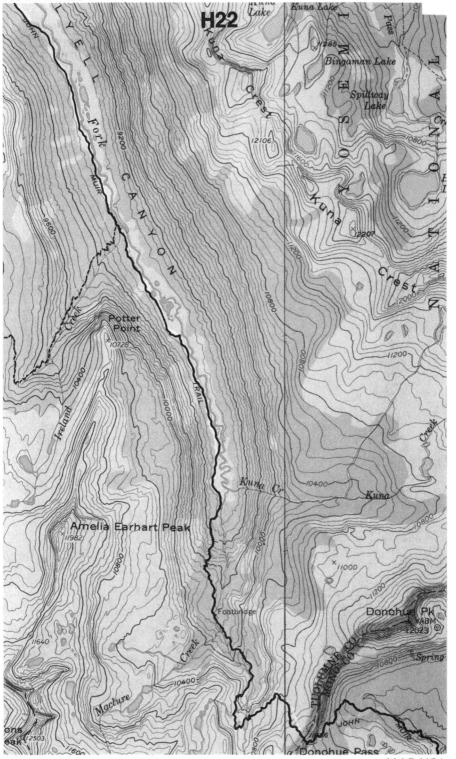

**H22**

and then contour west through alternating soggy meadows and lodgepole forests. Both abound in mosquitoes through late July, as does most of the Tuolumne Meadows area. Two-branched Rafferty Creek soon appears, its main branch can be crossed on a bridge. Just beyond it you meet the Rafferty Creek Trail (8710–4.4), part of the very scenic and very popular High Sierra Loop Trail. You continue west and soon meet another junction (8650– 0.7).

**Side route:** From here, a trail goes ¾ mile west to a junction immediately east of Tuolumne Meadows Campground. This has 25 sites for backpackers (and other nonmotorized park travelers). From that junction the left branch skirts around the campground's south perimeter while the

right branch quickly ends at the campground's main road. This road leads ½ mile west to Highway 120, and just southwest on it you'll find services.

Rather than head for the campground, you turn north and soon come to bridges across the Lyell Fork. A photo pause here is well worth it, particularly when clouds are building over Mts. Dana and Gibbs in the northeast. A short, winding climb north followed by an equal descent brings you to a sturdy bridge across the Dana Fork (8690– 0.7) of the Tuolumne River, this bridging being only 130 yards past a junction with an east-climbing trail to the Gaylor Lakes. Immediately beyond the bridge you meet a short spur trail to the Tuolumne Meadows Lodge.

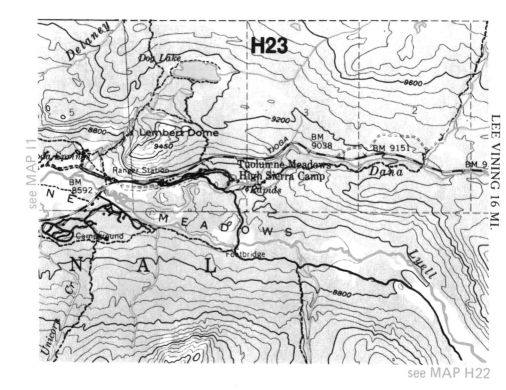

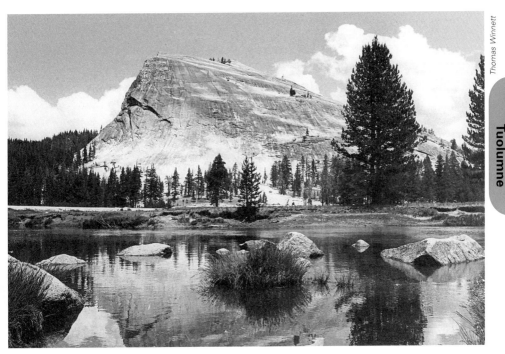

*Lembert Dome above Tuolumne River*

**Resupply access:** The lodge offers both showers and meals, but you probably will have to make a dinner reservation early in the day.

You parallel the Dana Fork downstream and soon hear the stream as it makes a small drop into a clear pool, almost cut in two by a protruding granite finger. At the base of this finger, about 8–10 feet down, is a hole in it, essentially an underwater arch, which is an extremely rare feature in any kind of rock. Just beyond the pool you approach the Lodge's road (8650–0.3), where a short path climbs a few yards up to it and takes one to the entrance of a large parking lot for backpackers. Now you parallel the paved road westward, passing the Tuolumne Meadows Ranger Station, and quickly reaching a junction. The main road curves north to the sometimes-noisy highway, but you follow the spur road west, to where it curves into a second large parking lot for backpackers. In its east end you'll find an office from which a summer ranger dispenses wilderness permits. The road past the lot diminishes to a wide trail before the time you arrive at this section's end, Highway 120 (8595–0.8), across from the start of the Soda Springs road. A campground, store and post office lie on Highway 120 just southwest of the Tuolumne River bridge.

**See Map H23**

# Recommended Reading and Source Books

(Some source materials are out of print)

## Pacific Crest Trail

Berger, Karen. 2001. *Hiking the Triple Crown*. Seattle: The Mountaineers Books.

Clarke, Clinton C. 1945. *The Pacific Crest Trailway*. Pasadena: The Pacific Crest Trail System Conference.

Croot, Leslie C. 2002. *Pacific Crest Trail Town Guide*. Sacramento: Pacific Crest Trail Association.

Go, Benedict. 2002. *Pacific Crest Trail Data Book*. Sacramento: Pacific Crest Trail Association.

Green, David. 1979. *A Pacific Crest Odyssey*. Berkeley: Wilderness Press.

Ross, Cindy. 1987. *Journey on the Crest: Walking 2600 Miles from Mexico to Canada*. Seattle: The Mountaineers Books.

Ryback, Eric. 1971. *The High Adventure of Eric Ryback*. San Francisco: Chronicle Books.

Schaffer, Jeffrey P., and Andy Selters. 2000. *The Pacific Crest Trail, Volume 2: Oregon and Washington*. Berkeley: Wilderness Press.

Semb, George, and Patricia Semb. 2000. *Day Hikes on the Pacific Crest Trail: California*. Berkeley: Wilderness Press.

Semb, George, and Patricia Semb. 2000. *Day Hikes on the Pacific Crest Trail: Oregon & Washington*. Berkeley: Wilderness Press.

## Backpacking, Packing, and Mountaineering

Back, Joe. 1994. *Horses, Hitches and Rocky Trails: The Packer's Bible*. Boulder, CO: Johnson Books.

Backcountry Horsemen of America. 1997. *Back Country Horsemen Guidebook*. Graham: Backcountry Horsemen of America (Box 1367, Graham, WA 98338-1367).

Darville, Fred, Jr. 1998. *Mountaineering Medicine*. Berkeley: Wilderness Press.

Drummond, Roger. 1998. *Ticks and What You Can Do About Them*. Berkeley: Wilderness Press.

Elser, Smoke, and Bill Brown. 1980. *Packin' In On Mules and Horses*. Missoula, MT: Mountain Press.

Ganci, Dave. 1993. *Desert Hiking*. Berkeley: Wilderness Press.

Graydon. Don, ed. 1997. *Mountaineering: The Freedom of the Hills*. Seattle: The Mountaineers Books.

La Chapelle, Edward R. 1985. *The ABC of Avalanche Safety*. Seattle: The Mountaineers Books.

Latimer, Carole. 1991. *Wilderness Cuisine*. Berkeley: Wilderness Press.

Letham, Lawrence. 2001. *GPS Made Easy: Using Global Positioning Systems in the Outdoors*. Seattle: The Mountaineers Books.

Steele, Peter, ed. 1999. *Backcountry Medical Guide*. Seattle: The Mountaineers Books.

Wilkerson, James, ed. 1986. *Hypothermia, Frostbite, and Other Cold Injuries*. Seattle: The Mountaineers Books.

Wilkerson, James, ed. 1993. *Medicine for Mountaineering & Other Wilderness Activities*. Seattle: The Mountaineers Books.

Winnett, Thomas, and Melanie Findling. 1994. *Backing Basics*. Berkeley: Wilderness Press.

# History

Brewer, William H. 1930 (1974). *Up and Down California in 1860-1864*. Berkeley: University of California Press.

Browning, Peter. 1991. *Place Names of the Sierra Nevada*. Berkeley: Wilderness Press.

Johnston, Verna R., and Carla J. Simmons. 1996. *California Forests and Woodlands: A Natural History*. Berkeley: University of California Press.

King, Clarence. 1872 (1997). *Mountaineering in the Sierra Nevada*. Yosemite: Yosemite Association.

Reid, Robert L. 1983. *A Treasury of the Sierra Nevada*. Berkeley: Wilderness Press.

# Geology

American Geological Institute. 1984. *Dictionary of Geological Terms*. New York: Doubleday.

Ernst, W. Gary, and Clemens A. Nelson. 1998. *Integrated Earth and Environmental Evolution of the Southwestern United States*. Boulder: Geological Society of America.

Harden, Deborah R. 1998. *California Geology*. Upper Saddle River, NJ: Prentice Hall.

McPhee, John. 1993. *Assembling California*. New York: Farrar, Straus and Giroux.

Schaffer, Jeffrey P. 1997. *The Geomorphic Evolution of the Yosemite Valley and Sierra Nevada Landscapes*. Berkeley: Wilderness Press.

Sharp, Robert P., and Allen F. Glazner. 1993. *Geology Underfoot in Southern California*. Missoula, MT: Mountain Press.

Shelton, John S. 1966. *Geology Illustrated*. San Francisco: W. H. Freeman.

# Biology

Barbour, Michael, Bruce Pavlik, Frank Drysdale, and Susan Lindstrom. 1993. *California's Changing Landscapes: Diversity and Conservation of California Vegetation.* Sacramento: California Native Plant Society.

Gaines, David. 1992. *Birds of Yosemite and the East Slope.* Lee Vining: Artemisia Press.

Gray, Mary Taylor. 1999. *Watchable Birds of California.* Missoula, MT: Mountain Press.

Havert, Bill, and Gary Gray. 1996. *Nature Guide to the Mountains of Southern California by Car & on Foot.* Earth Trails Publications.

Hickman, James C. 1993. *The Jepson Manual: Higher Plants of California.* Berkeley: University of California Press.

Horn, Elizabeth L. 1998. *Sierra Nevada Wildflowers.* Missoula, MT: Mountain Press.

Jameson, E. W., Jr., and Hans J. Peeters. 1988. *California Mammals.* Berkeley: University of California Press.

Johnston, Verna R., and Carla J. Simmons. 1996. *California Forests and Woodlands: A Natural History.* Berkeley: University of California Press.

Keator, Glenn, and Jeanne C. Koelling. 1978. *Pacific Coast Berry Finder.* Berkeley: Nature Study Guild (distributed through Wilderness Press).

Keator, Glenn, and Ruth M. Heady. 1981. *Pacific Coast Fern Finder.* Berkeley: Nature Study Guild (distributed through Wilderness Press).

Lederer, Rojer J. 1977. *Pacific Coast Bird Finder.* Berkeley: Nature Study Guild (distributed through Wilderness Press).

Niehaus, Theodore F., and Charles L. Ripper. 1976. *A Field Guide to Pacific States Wildflowers.* Boston: Houghton Mifflin.

Pavlik, Bruce M., Pamela C. Muick, Sharon Johnson, and Marjorie Popper. 1991. *Oaks of California.* Los Olivos, CA: Cachuma Press.

Russo, Ron, and Pam Olhausen. 1987. *Pacific Coast Mammals.* Berkeley: Nature Study Guild (distributed through Wilderness Press).

Sawyer, John O., and Todd Keeler-Wolf. 1995. *A Manual of California Vegetation.* Sacramento: California Native Plant Society.

Schoenherr, Allan A. 1995. *A Natural History of California.* Berkeley: University of California Press.

Sibley, David Allen. 2000. *The Sibley Guide to Birds.* New York: Alfred A. Knopf.

Stuart, John David, and John O. Sawyer. 2001. *Trees and Shrubs of California.* Berkeley: University of California Press.

Watts, Tom. 1973. *Pacific Coast Tree Finder.* Berkeley: Nature Study Guild (distributed through Wilderness Press).

Weeden, Norman F. 1996. *A Sierra Nevada Flora.* Berkeley: Wilderness Press.

# INDEX

## A

Acorn Canyon Trail, 164, 170
acorn-woodpecker, 77
Acton, 164, 181, 185
Advisory Council for the PCT, 3
Agnew Meadows, Campground
 and Pass, 330, 332-34
Agua Caliente Creek, 95, 97,
 102-05
Agua Dulce, 161, 164, 191, 194
Aguanga Fault, 98
airplane crashes, 183, 262
airports, 194
alkali flats, 284
Alkali Wash, 111
Aliso Spring, 180
alpine environment, 335
alluvial fans, 36, 87, 152, 215
alternate routes, 59
altitude sickness, 32
American Hiking Society, 263
American Long Distance Hikers
 Assoc. West, 11
Andreas Canyon, 116
Angeles Crest Highway, 164,
 171, 174-76
Angeles Forest Highway, 180
Angeles National Forest, 15,
 129, 165 (fire restrictions),
 170, 197, 214
animals. *See* wildlife
Annan Ranch, 197

Ansel Adams Wilderness, 16,
 330-34
Antelope Valley, 30, 45, 178,
 180, 191, 194, 203, 205, 207,
 211, 213, 215, 220
Antelope Valley Freeway, 188
antelopes, 191
Antsell Rock, 116
Anza, 100, 109
Anza, Captain Juan Bautista de,
 83, 106
Anza-Borrego Desert State Park,
 48, 65, 67, 79, 84-85, 87, 91,
 98, 105, 107, 109
Apache Peak, Spring and Trail,
 116
Appalachian Trail, 2-3, 6
Apple Canyon 116
archeological sites, 266
Army Corps of Engineers, 151
Arrastre Creek, 140
Arrastre (Deer Springs) Trail
 Camp, 136, 140
Arrastre Flat, 144
Arrowhead Lake, 311
Ash Meadow, 285
Aspen Meadow, 320
Atchison Topeka and Santa Fe,
 225
Atmore Meadows Campground,
 210
avalanches, 302, 315

## B

Backcountry Horsemen, 13
backpacking, 7-8, 12, 18-19
bacteria, 22
Badger Lakes, 334
Bakersfield, 229
Bald Mountain, 270
Baldwin Lake, 140-43
Balky Horse Canyon, 140
Bandido Campground, 176
Banner, 85
Banner Peak, 335
Banning, 128
Banning Fault, 97, 119
Bare Mountain Canyon, 177
Barrel Spring, 85, 88, 93, 95
Barton Flats camp area, 137
Baxter Pass Trail, 311
bearbagging and bearproof
 canisters, 28-29
Bear Campground, 210
Bear Creek, 321
Bear Diversion Dam, 321
Bear Gulch, 171
Bear Spring, 197-98
bears, black, 22, 23, 27-28, 257,
 280, 289, 303
bears, grizzlies, 144, 161
beaver dams, 147, 152
Beck Meadows, 276-79
bees, wasps, and yellowjackets,
 25

Belleville, 144
Bench Camp, 148
Bench Lake and Trail, 314
berry plants, 48
Bertha Peak and Ridge, 144
Big Arroyo, 292
Big Bear City, 128, 144-45
Big Bear Lake, 125, 126, 128, 144-46
Big Buck Trail Camp, 180
Big Dry Meadow, 282
Big Meadows, 137
Big Oak Spring, 199
Big Pete Meadow, 315
Big Tree Trail, 197
Bighorn Mine, 171
Bighorn Plateau, 304
bighorn sheep, 161, 174
bike path, 244-45
Bike Springs, 167
biodegradable soaps, 22
biology, 42-43. *See also* life zones; wildlife
biotic influences, 46
birds, 49-56, 77, 132, 140, 150, 187, 235, 245, 264, 279
Bird Spring Pass, 246-47
Bishop and Pass Trail, 301
Black Mountain Group Camp and Road, 119
blazes (trail markers), 21, 60
Blue Ridge, 170-71
Bobcat Canyon, 187, 189
Bonnie Bell fault, 131
books about the PCT, 1, 2, 5, 7-9, 12, 14
books and field guides on natural history, 49, 342-44 (refs.)
boots, 18
borax teams, 157, 167
Border Patrol, 69
Borrego Sink, 107
Borrego Springs, 67, 94
Boulder Oaks Campground and Store, 75
Bouquet Canyon, 199-200
Boy Scouts, 171-72, 181, 207
Brokeoff Mountain, 35
Brown Creek, 119
Brown Mountain, 277
Bubbs Creek and Trail, 301, 305
Buckhorn Flat Campground, 175
Bucks Lake Wilderness, 17
Bucksnort Mountain, 97, 105-06, 110, 111
Buena Vista Creek, 94
Bull Canyon, 112

Bullfrog Lake, 305
Bureau of Land Management (BLM), 15-17 (offices), 135-36, 229, 241
Burkhart Trail, 175
Burnham Canyon, 220
Burnt Rancheria Campground, 77-78
buses, 91, 164, 257, 301, 327, 334
Butterfield Stage Line, 83, 88, 98, 100

**C**

Cabazon, 101, 113, 123, 128
Cache Peak, 235-36
cacti, 91, 125, 251, 274
Cajon Canyon, 126, 157-59, 161, 164
Cajon Pass, 129, 161
Caliente Creek, 236
California Aqueduct, 153, 194, 201, 203, 215
California Dept. of Water Resources, 293
California Desert Protection Act, 246, 258
California Riding and Hiking Trail, 84, 132, 199
Cameron Canyon, 225
Cameron Valley, 80
Camp Pajarito, 176
campfire restrictions, 15, 101, 197, 214, 241, 257, 305, 320, 336
camping. *See also* wilderness permits
  location of site, 21-22
  restrictions on, 15, 165, 238, 305, 311, 320, 326, 334
  where prohibited, 153, 214, 293
Campo (town and creek), 67, 70
Cañada Verde, 95, 102
Canadian Zone, 125
Canebreak Creek, 253
Cane Canyon, 248
Caramba Trail, 117
Cardinal Mountain, 314
Caribou Creek, 144, 147
Carson, Kit, 98
Carson-Iceberg Wilderness, 16
Carson River canyon, 42
Cascade Valley Trail, 326
Castle Crags, 17, 35
Castle Rock Ranch, 69-70
Catclaw Flat, 134
Cathedral Peak, 34

cattle and grazing, 24, 77, 135, 229, 284, 293
Cedar Glen, 128
Cedar Glen Post Office, 148
Cedar Grove, 301
Cedar Spring Camp and Trail, 113
Cedar Springs Dam, 153
Chamise Boat-in Picnic Area, 154
Channel Islands, 126
chaparral, 51, 97, 100-02, 121, 157, 189
Chariot Canyon, 77, 81, 84-85
Charlotte Lake, 305
checklist for planning and packing, 18-19
Chicken Spring Lake, 288-89
Chief Lake, 326
Chihuahua Valley, 105
Chilao Flat/Waterman Mountain Trail, 176
children, 20
Chimney Creek and Campground, 263-64, 266
Chimney Peak Recreation Area and Wilderness, 16, 258, 264, 267
China Lake Naval Air Weapons Station, 259, 262
Cibbets Flat Campground, 77
Cienaga Canyon, 210
Cienaga Redonda Trail, 148
Cienaga Seca Creek, 140
Civilian Conservation Corps (CCC), 263, 276
Cinder Cone, 35
cinder cones, 42
Cirque Peak, 288
Civil War, 144
Clark Lakes, 334
cleaning, 22
clearcutting, 10, 47
Clearwater Fault, 199
Cleghorn Mountain Fault, 153, 156
Cleghorn Picnic Area, 154
Cleghorn Ridge, 156
Cleveland National Forest, 15, 69, 103, 129
Cleveland NF Descanso Ranger District, 82
climate change, 40, 44, 47. *See also* weather
clothing and shoes, 8, 31
Cloudburst Canyon and Summit, 176
Clover Meadow Trail, 274, 276

Coachella Valley, 113
Colby Meadow, 320
Colorado Desert, 65, 77, 83
Colorado River Aqueduct, 131
Combs Peak, 105
*Communicator* (PCTA publication), 10
companions, finding, 10
compass, 57-58, 258
Congress, 3, 191
Continental Divide Trail, 3, 6
Coon Creek and Camp, 137, 140
Cooper Canyon, 175-76
Corpsman Creek, 285
Coso Mountains, 284
Cottonwood Canyon, 82, 131, 202, 216
Cottonwood Creek, 75, 207, 218, 239
Cottonwood Lakes, 285
Cottonwood Pass, 271
cougars, 26, 257
Cow Canyon and Creek, 263, 279-80
Cow Spring Canyon, 214
Coyote Canyon, 105
Crab Flats Trail, 148
Crabtree Meadow, 57, 292
Crabtree Ranger Station, 293
Crag Creek, 274, 276
craters, 35. See also cinder cones
creosote bush, 46, 50, 206, 215
Crestline, 155
Crowder Canyon, 155, 158-59, 165
Crystal Lake Recreation Area, 174
Cucamonga Wilderness, 167
Cuyamaca Rancho State Park, 82, 84
Cuyamaca Reservoir, 81
Cypress Park Resort, 187

**D**

dams, 151-53, 161
Dana Fork, 340
Dark Canyon Campground, 118
Davis Lake and Trail, 334-36
Darwin Canyon, 320
Dawson Peak, 170
day-hiking the PCT, 7, 18
Death Canyon, 282
Death Valley, 172
Death Valley borax teams, 157
declination settings, 57-58
Deep Creek, 126, 148, 150-52
Deep Creek Hot Spring, 150

Deer Creek, 326
Deer Meadow, 314
Deer Mountain, 277
Deer Springs Trail, 118
dehydration, 195
Delamar Mountain and Spring, 146
dermatitis, 23, 250
Desert Divide, 97, 101, 105, 112-13
desert ecology, 48, 141, 150, 203
Desert Hot Springs, 121
desert survival, 195-96
Desert View Nature Trail, 77-79
Desolation Wilderness, 17
Devils Backbone, 170
Devil's Hole fishing area, 150
Devils Postpile National Monument, 35, 330-32
Devils Punchbowl, 40, 162, 174
Devil's Slide Trail, 100, 117-18
dinosaur, 271
dirt-bikers, 218
Doble Fault and Road, 142
Doble Gold Mine and Trail Camp, 143
dogs on the trail, 21, 101
Dollar Lake, 311
Dome Land Wilderness, 16, 263, 273
Donohue Pass, 336
Dove Spring, 245
Dowd Canyon, 200
Dragon Lake Trail, 311
Dragon Peak, 308
Duck Creek, 326
Duck Lake Trail, 326
ducks (trail marker), 21, 60
Dusy Branch, 315
Dutch Meadow, 285

**E**

Eagles Roost Picnic Area, 175
Earthquake Valley, 87
earthquakes, 42, 111, 231, 263, 270, 292. See also geology; San Andreas fault
Ebbetts Pass, 16
Echo Lake Resort, 41
ECONOmy Inn, 129, 159
ecosystems, 47-49, 56, 125. See also habitat; plants; wildlife
edaphic influences, 45-46, 137
Edwards Air Force Base, 232
Eldorado National Forest, 16
Elephant Butte, 232
elevations on the PCT, 43-44, 123, 140, 215

Elizabeth Lake and Canyon, 200-01
El Paso Mountains, 245, 258
Elsinore Fault, 95
Emerald Lake, 332
Emigrant Wilderness, 16
endangered species, 151
environmental issues, 22, 47-48, 281-82
equestrians, 6, 9, 12-13, 20. *See also* horses
  California Riding and Hiking Trail, 84, 132, 199
  organizations, 13
  reserved campgrounds, 84, 101, 150
  special trail directions, 102, 177, 258, 282, 330
  trail registers, 197
erosion, 42
Erwin Lake, 141
Escondido Canyon, 187-88
Escondido extrusive rocks, 35
Evolution Lake, Meadow and Valley, 320

**F**

Fairmont Reservoir, 203
Fawnskin, 128, 145
Federal Aviation Administration site, 79-80
federal agencies, 15
feet, taking care of, 20
fire, 22, 47-48, 69, 154, 157, 214, 251. *See also* campfire
  restrictions caused by humans, 148, 170, 171, 267-270, 274
  Clover Meadow Blaze (1980), 274
  in Southern California, 102, 113, 197
  Fire Safe Area, 241
  fuelbreaks, 116
  Manter Fire, 267
  Paloma Canyon, 181
  permits, 229, 257. *See also* wilderness permits
  Pines Fire, 81
  Willow Fire, 148
  Woodpecker Fire of 1947, 271
fish and fishing,
  Devil's Hole Fishing Area, 150
  endangered species, 187
  Kennedy Meadows, 274
  South Fork Kern River, 270, 273
  trout, 282

Whitewater Trout Farm, 132
Wild Trout Area, 148
Fish Creek Canyon PCT Trail
Camp, 206, 326
flash floods, 216, 220
Flathead Flats, 80
Florence Lake and Trail, 301-02,
320-321
Flume Canyon, 170
Fobes Saddle, 116
food. (*For food sources, see*
*supplies at beginning of each*
*section.*)
disposal, 22
natural sources used by Native
Americans, 125, 233, 250, 258
storage, 15
protecting from bears, 28-29,
289, 303
fording streams, 21, 30, 257,
302-03, 323
Forester Pass, 303, 305
Fork springs, 129, 136
Forest Service, 5, 93, 95, 181,
191, 229. *See also* land-use
battles
Forest Service offices, 15
Fountainhead Spring, 177
Fred Canyon, 75
Fremont Valley, 236, 245
Fresno, 301
Fryer Canyon, 185
Fuller Ridge, 97, 118-19
Fuller Ridge Trailhead Remote
Campsite, 119
fungi, 47

**G**

gabbro, 34
garbage, 22
Gamble Spring Canyon, 220
Garces Overlook, 154
Garlock Fault, 227, 231
Garnet Lake, 332
Garnet Peak, 79, 81, 83
Garnet Ridge and Valley, 113,
116
gas stoves, 165, 197
gates, 20
Gaylor Lakes, 340
geologic time, 37-39, 162
geology, 33-42, 79, 84, 97-98,
111, 126, 132, 142, 152, 156,
158, 162, 185, 187, 188, 199,
205, 231, 270, 311, 314, 330.
*See also* earthquakes; glaciation; rock types
getting lost, 20

Giant Forest, 304
*Giardia*, 18, 24, 196
glaciation, 33, 41-42, 46, 47,
293-94, 336
Glacier Creek, 314
Gladys Lake, 332
Glen Pass, 303, 305, 308
gneiss, 36, 75, 132, 142
Gobber's Knob, 170
Goddard Divide and Canyon,
315, 320
Gold Canyon, 131-32
gold mines, 85, 87, 141, 144,
180, 232, 267. *See also* mines
gold rush, 167
Golden Oaks Spring, 230, 235
Golden Spike Ceremony, 4
Golden Trout Creek, 288
Golden Trout Wilderness, 16,
30, 257, 274, 281-82, 289
Gomez Meadow, 281-82, 284
Goodale Pass Trail, 326
Granada Canyon of the
Tuolumne River, 41
Granite Chief Wilderness, 17
Granite Mountain, 87
granitic rock (granite), 34, 36,
87, 97, 136, 185, 231, 232
Grapevine Canyon and Spring,
93
Grapevine Mountain, 91
Grass Mountain, 200
Grass Valley Creek, 155
Great Western Divide, 270, 288-
89, 304
Green Valley and Ranger Station,
194, 200
Grinnell Mountains, 140
grizzly bears, 28
groundwater, 30, 67. *See also*
water
Grouse Meadow, 314-15
Guffy Campground, 159, 164,
170
Guitar Lake, 294
gun clubs. *See* hunting; rifle
ranges
Guyot Flat, 292

**H**

habitats, 47-49. *See also* life
zones; wildlife
Haiwee Trail, 276
Hamp Williams Pass, 236
Harris Grade, 241
Hatchery Canyon, 132
Hauser Wilderness, 15, 68-69,
73-75

health risks, 18, 20-23, 31-32
Heart Bar Creek, 136-37
Heart Lake, 321
Helen Lake, 315
Helendale Fault, 142
Hell for Sure Pass Trail, 320
heritage trails, 2-3
Hesperia and Hesperia Lake
Park, 128, 151, 152
high-altitude sickness.
*See* altitude sickness
High Sierra Loop Trail, 338
High Trail, 334
Highway 58, 191, 228-30
Highway 120, 338, 341
Highway 173, 152
Hiker's Oasis (The Bears), 109
Hilgard Creek, 321
history of book, xi
history of PCT, 1-6
Hitchcock Lakes, 294
hitchhiking, 194, 225, 257, 285,
301
Holcomb Creek, Valley, and
Trail Camp, 144, 146-48
Hook Creek, 128
Hoover Canyon, 93
horned toad, 158
Horse Canyon, 111, 248-49
Horseshoe Lake, 327
Horseshoe Meadow, 258
horses, 6, 9, 12, 20.
*See also* equestrians
California Riding and Hiking
Trail, 84
campgrounds reserved for, 84,
280
corrals, 75, 101, 128, 147, 181,
194, 215, 280, 282, 284
hitching posts, 189
pack stations, 330where
banned, 13, 332
where to buy feed, 128, 189,
194, 215
wild, 221
Horsethief Canyon, 157
horsethieving, 157
host homes, 189, 194
hot springs, 98, 100, 121, 150,
332. *See also* Mono Hot
Springs
Hot Springs Fault and
Mountain, 105
Hughes Lake, 202
Humboldt-Toiyabe National
Forest, 16
hunting, 27, 122, 141
hypothermia, 31-32

**I**

Ice Age, 39
ice axe for icy conditions, 116, 119, 257, 302
icons used in this book, 59
Idyllwild, 100, 113, 117
igneous rock, 33-35
illness and injuries, 20, 23
Independence, 301
Indian Flats, 97
Indian Wells Canyon, 259
Indian Wells Valley, 245
Indians. *See* Native Americans
insects, 24-25, 203, 205
Interstate 15, 161
intrusive rock, 33-34, 97
Inyokern, 259
Inyo Mountains, 284
Inyo National Forest, 16, 279
iodine tablets, 24, 196. *See also* water
Isabella Lake, 229, 242
Islip Saddle, 174

**J**

Jacks Creek Canyon, 253
Jackson Flat Group Campground, 171
Jawbone Canyon, 236
Jenkins, James Charles, i, 12, 259-60
Joe Devel Peak, 289
John Muir Trail, 57, 292-93, 295, 298, 304, 314, 321, 326, 334
John Muir Wilderness, 16, 330
Johnston Meadow, 332
Joshua Tree National Park, 116
Joshua Tree Spring, 263
Joshua trees, 51, 126, 192, 203-06, 215
Julian, 67, 85, 88
Junction Peak, 304
Jupiter Mountain, 200

**K**

Kamp Anza Kampground, 100, 108-09
Kaweah Peaks Ridge, 281, 292
kayak rentals, 229
Kearsarge Pass Trail, 301, 305
Kearsarge Lakes and Pinnacles, 305
Kelso Creek, 248
Kelso Valley, 236

Kennedy Meadows and Campground, 257, 273-74, 279, 303
Kern County, 215, 262
Kern Peak, 282-84
Kern Plateau, 255, 266, 271-73, 282, 288
Kern River, 229, 233, 255, 270-79, 288, 304
Kernville, 229, 273
Kiavah Dome Land, 16
Kiavah Wilderness, 246, 253
Kings Canyon National Park, 16, 28, 302, 305, 320
Kings-Kern Divide, 304
Kings River, 305, 313-14
Kitchen Creek, 75
Kitching Peak, 134
Klamath National Forest, 17

**L**

Laguna/El Prado Campground, 81
Laguna Mountains, 65, 69, 74-80
Laguna Rim Trail, 81
Lake Arrowhead, 126, 148, 150
Lake Edison, 301, 321
Lake Hemet, 116
Lake Henshaw, 95
Lake Hughes, 194, 202
Lake Hughes Truck Trail, 201
Lake Italy Trail, 321
Lake Marjorie, 314
Lake McDermand, 320
Lake Morena County Park, 70
Lake South America Trail, 305
Lake Tahoe Basin Management Unit, 17
Lake Virginia, 326
Lamel Spring, 171
Lamont Peak, 264
Lancaster, 194
Landers Creek, 239-41
land-use issues, 3-4, 75, 87, 93, 191, 211. *See also* private property; Tejon Ranch
La Posta Creek, 77
Lassen Volcanic National Park, 17
Le Conte Canyon, 314
"leave-no-trace" hiking, 22
legend for the map, 61
Lembert Dome, 341
length of the PCT, 4, 43
length of trip, 7, 15
Leona Divide Truck Trail, 200

Liebre Mountain, 191, 210-11, 215
Liebre Mountain Truck Trail, 210
life zones, 43-46, 80, 97, 125, 150, 335
lightning, 21, 30, 47-48, 250, 338
Lightning Ridge Nature Trails, 171
lightweight backpacking, 7
Lyell Canyon and Fork, 336-40
Lily Spring, 174
limestone, 36, 37, 126
Lion Peak and Spring, 113
Little Horsethief Canyon, 157
Little Jimmy Campground and Spring, 174
Little Oak Canyon Creek, 216
Little Pete Meadow, 315
Little San Bernardino Mountains, 116, 121
Live Oak Spring, 112-13
Lou Beverly Lake, 321
Lyell Canyon and Fork, 336
Lyme disease, 229
Lytle Creek, 167
lizards, 130, 205, 267
llamas, 9
locator map showing the PCT in California, *xii*
lodgepole pine, 47, 55
logging, 10, 47-48, 281
Lone Pine (town), 257, 285
Lone Pine Canyon, 167
Los Angeles, City of, 192
Los Angeles Aqueduct, 191-92, 202, 206, 216-18, 233
Los Angeles Dept. of Water and Power, 216-18, 284
Los Caballos Campground, 84
Los Padres gold mines, 180
Lost Valley Spring, 105
Lower Morris Meadow, 77
low-impact hiking, 21
Lyme disease, 130, 229
Lyell Canyon and Fork, 338-40
Lytle Creek Ridge, 158

**M**

Mace Meadows, 239
Magic Mountain Amusement Park, 211
Magic Mountain Fault, 185
mailing tips, 14
maintenance of trail, 10
Mammoth Lakes, 301-02, 326-27
Mammoth Mountain, 330

Mammoth Pass, 327
map legend, 61
mapping the PCT, 3
maps, *xii*, 5, 57-61
Marble Mountain, 37, 46
Marble Mountain Wilderness, 17
Marie Lake, 299, 321
Marie Lakes Trail, 335
Marion Mountain Trail and Camp, 118
marmots, 23, 24
Martindale Canyon, 198-99
Mason Valley Track Trail, 84
Mather Pass, 314
Mattox Canyon Ford, 181, 184-85
Maxwell Truck Trail and Camp, 207-08
Mayan Peak, 236, 244
McCloud Lake, 327
McClure Meadow, 320
McGee Pass Trail, 326
McIvers Spring, 249-251
meadow ecology, 47, 320
meningoencephalitis, 150
Mesa Wind Farm, 123, 126, 131
Messenger Flats Campground, 181, 184
metamorphic rocks, 36-37, 97, 126, 187, 262
Mexican border, 65, 69
mileages, 4-5, 62-63
military installations, 180, 232, 259. *See also* NASA
Mill Canyon, 181, 183-85
Mill Creek Summit and Ranger Station, 180, 184
Minaret Creek, 332
Minarets, 301, 327, 334
Mineral King, 292
mines and mining towns, 47, 85, 87, 142-44, 171, 180, 207, 232, 242, 245, 267
Mint Canyon, 189, 197
Mission Creek and Camp, 125, 132-37
Mojave (town), 195, 229
Mojave Desert, 30, 126, 129, 150, 157, 161, 164, 191-96, 207, 213, 215, 232
Mojave River, 126, 150
Mokelumne Wilderness, 16
Monache Meadows, 255, 276-77
Mono Creek and Hot Springs, 301, 321, 323
Mono Lake, 192
Mono Pass Trail, 321

Montezuma Valley, 93
Monument Peak, 79-80
Morena Butte, 73
Morena Village, 67
Mormon history, 157, 167, 141, 203
Mormon Rocks, 162, 165, 167
Morris Peak, 259
Morris Ranch, 113
mosquitoes, 24-26
motocross, 147-48, 220
motorcycles, 207, 279, 281
Mott Lake, 323
Mount Baden-Powell, 140, 161, 164, 170-73
Mount Baden-Powell Trail, 171
Mount Baldy, 121, 140
Mount Barnard, 304
Mount Clarence-King, 311
Mount Gleason, 180, 187, 197, 213
Mount Gleason Young Adult Conservation Corps Center, 180
Mount Guyot, 292
Mount Hawkins, 174
Mount Hitchcock, 292, 294
Mount Jenkins, I, 235, 241, 259, 262
Mount Laguna, 67
Mount Laguna Post Office, 79
Mount Langley, 277, 281, 285
Mount Lyell, 336
Mount Muir, 295
Mount Palomar Observatory, 95
Mount Ritter, 335
Mount San Antonio, 121, 157-58, 167, 170-71
Mount Shasta, 35
Mount Wilson, 121, 213
Mount Whitney, 38, 235, 253, 257, 277, 281, 295, 301
Mount Whitney Trail junction, 298
Mount Williamson, 197
Mount Williamson Trail, 174
Mt. Young, 292, 304
mountain bikes, 10, 100
Mountain High Ski Area, 170
Mountain Leagues, 2
mountain lions 26, 257
movie settings, 189
Muir, John, 21, 161, 315-16
Muir Pass, 315
Muir Trail Ranch, 320
Mulkey Meadows and Pass, 285
Munz Canyon, 200
Murray Canyon, 116

Myrick Canyon, 203

**N**

NASA space shuttle center, 220
National Forest Adventure Pass, 129, 164, 196
National Park offices, 15
National Scenic Trail, 191
National Trails System Act, 2-4
National Wilderness Preservation System, 246, 270
Native Americans, 77, 84, 98, 100, 151, 157, 233, 246, 264-65, 281
  archeological site, 265-66
  diet and food sources, 125, 233, 250, 258
  Tule River Indian Reservation, 281
nature centers and/or trails, 165, 171, 189
Nelson Ridge, 142
Noble Canyon Trail 5E04, 81
*Nolina parryi*, 261, 262
North Fork Fish Canyon, 209
North Fork Saddle, 185
North Fork Saddle Ranger Station, 164
North Lake, 301, 320

**O**

Oak Canyon, 113
Oak Creek Canyon, 220-21
Oasis Spring, 81
ocotillo shrubs, 91
off-highway or off-road-vehicles (OHVs, ORVs or RVs), 123, 230, 242-44
OHV center, 239
Olancha Pass, 280-82, 284
Olancha Peak, 235, 253, 277-79, 281, 284
Onion Valley, 301
Onyx (town), 229, 257
Onyx Peak, 140
Oregon Skyline Trail, 1
organizations relevant to the PCT, 9-13
Oriflamme Canyon and Mountain 81-84
Owens Lake, 284
Owens Peak, 199-200, 235, 241, 253, 262-63, 267
Owens Peak Wilderness, 46, 258, 263
Owens Valley, 192, 258

**P**

pack, weight of, 7
pack animals, 9, 20
Pacific Crest Trail. *See also* land-use issues; trail angels
  completion, 187, 213
  history, 1-6
  high and low elevations, 123, 125, 140, 220, 215, 263, 305
  host homes, 189
  internet mail list, 91
  land-use battles, 75. *See* private property
  maintenance, 20
  quotas, 18, 295, 302
  registers, 11, 131, 194, 215, 246, 262, 273, 295
  sign problems, 303-04
  Southern Terminus, 69
Pacific Crest Trail Association (PCTA), *ix*, 10-11
  as source of info on trail conditions, 31
  lobbying efforts of, 11, 189
  publications, 9-10
  registers, 11, 131, 194
Pacific Crest Trail System Conference, 2, 9-10
Pacific Ocean, 161, 211
packing, 7, 18-19. *See also* checklist, clothing
Painted Lady, 308
Palisade Basin, Creek, and Peaks 314
Palm Canyon, 113
Palm Springs, 101, 113, 140
Palmdale, 188
parking restrictions, 129, 165, 196. *See also* National Forest Adventure Pass
partners, finding, 10
Peninsular Ranges, 97-98
Penny Pines reforestation program, 81
Penrod Canyon, 111, 113
permits, 11, 15-17, 18-19, 68, 101, 129, 164-65, 196-97, 229, 257, 302
pesticides, 47
pets, 21
physiographic influences, 44-45
pikas, 23
Pinchot Pass, 313
Pine Canyon, 214
Pine Creek, 267, 273
Pines-to-Palms Highway, 107, 109, 111, 113

Pink Motel, 131
Pinto Mountain Fault, 135
Pinyon Mountain, 245
pinyon pines, 125, 141, 227, 234, 249-50, 258
Pioneer Mail Trailhead Picnic Area, 77, 81
pioneers, 165, 167, 203. *See also* Mormon history
Pitney Canyon, 220
Piute Mountains, 227, 238, 241
Piute Pass Trail, 301, 320
plague, 25
planning a trip, 7-17. *See also* parking; water sources
  packing checklist, 19
  season and weather conditions, 29-30, 301
plants and plant communities, 46-56, 77, 80, 102, 135, 137, 141, 188, 227, 264, 266-67, 274-76. *See also* chaparral; Joshua trees; trees; yucca
  chia, 258
  creosote bush, 46, 50, 206, 215
  diseases, 47
  edaphic effects, 137
  ecosystem diversity, 125
  in drought conditions, 121
  *Nolina parryi*, 261, 262
  Poodle Dog Bush, 250
  xerophytic, 274
Plumas National Forest, 17
plutons and plutonism, 34, 37-38, 126
Pocket Meadow, 323
poison oak, 23
Poligue Canyon, 145
pollution, 22, 161-62. *See also* water
Portal Ridge, 202-03
Potter Point, 338
post offices, 14
Potomac Heritage Trail, 3
power plants, 153
precipitation. *See* rain
prickly-pear cactus, 274
prickly poppy, 253
private property, 3-4, 132, 140, 153, 191-92, 230, 235, 238, 273 *See also* land-use issues; Tejon Ranch
Purple Lake, 326
Putney Canyon

**Q**

Quail Lake, 191
quotas, 18, 295, 302

**R**

rabies, 25
radiocarbon dating, 37, 207
Rae Lakes, 308
Rafferty Creek and Trail, 338
raft trips, 229
railroad, 162, 165, 225, 231. *See also* Southern Pacific Railroad
rain. *See also* rain shadow
  impact on life zones, 80
  precipitation patterns, 33, 93, 301
  preparation for, 21, 29-32
Rainbow Falls, 326, 330
raingear, 31
rain shadow, 79, 93
Ralston Peak, 167
Ranchita, 94
Ranchos del Campo and del Reyo, 69, 70
rangers, 303
rattlesnakes, 26-27, 69, 135, 150
Red Buttes Wilderness, 17
Red Cones, 330
Red Rock Canyon State Park, 245
Red Rock Water Tank, 210
Red Spur, 292
Reds Meadow, 301-02, 326-27, 330-32
Reds Meadow Pack Station, 330
reforestation programs, 81
registers, 11, 131, 194, 215, 246, 262, 273, 295
resupply centers, 57, 59
reverse-bearing compasses, 58
Ridgecrest, 259, 273
rifle ranges, 141
risks, v, 8, 18, 58
Ritter Range, 334
River Trail, 334
rivers and stream crossings, 21, 30, 257, 302-03, 323
Robin Bird Spring, 236
rockfall, 42
rock climbers, 270
Rock Creek and Ranger Station, 288-89, 292
rock types, 33-42, 45, 79, 97, 126, 162, 187, 231, 262, 311
Rockhouse Basin, 41, 271
rodents, 23, 25
Rodriguez Canyon and Truck Trail, 87-88
Rodriguez Spur Truck Trail, 81, 85
Rogue River National Forest

Rosalie Lake, 332
Rose Lake, 321
Rosemarie Meadow, 321
Round Valley Trail Camp, 118
Ruby Lake, 332
Rush Creek, 334-35, 338
Russian wilderness, 17
RV parks, 185-87

**S**

Sacatara Creek, 216
Saddle Junction, 100, 117
safety, v, 18-22, 27, 195
Sageland, 242
Sally Keyes Lakes, 321
Salton Sea, 109, 140
San Andreas fault, 38, 40, 119,
    121, 125-26, 158, 162, 167,
    170, 200, 203, 227
San Bernardino (city), 129, 159
San Bernardino Mountains, 97,
    118, 125-29, 146
San Bernardino National Forest,
    15, 111, 122, 129, 136
San Bernardino Valley, 121, 167
San Felipe Creek, 88
San Felipe Valley, 65, 67, 87, 93
San Francisquito Canyon and
    Camp, 194, 200
San Francisquito Fault, 199
San Gabriel Mountains, 121,
    126, 152, 158, 161-62, 164,
    172, 185, 202, 205, 213
San Gabriel River, 171
San Gabriel Valley, 121
San Gorgonio Mountain, 87, 98,
    105, 118, 121, 134, 136, 140,
    158
San Gorgonio Pass, 98, 100, 113,
    117, 119, 121, 123, 125-159
San Gorgonio River, 118, 123,
    170, 171
San Gorgonio Wilderness, 15,
    43, 125, 132, 136, 140, 144,
    165
San Jacinto Mountains, 15,
    97-100, 111-12, 118, 123
San Jacinto Peak, 87, 98, 105,
    111, 117-18, 121, 134, 137
San Jacinto Peak Trail (aka Deer
    Springs Trail), 118
San Jacinto River, 118, 122
San Jacinto Wilderness, 100,
    116-17
San Joaquin River, 320, 330, 332
San Ysidro Creek, 95
Sand Canyon, 233
sandstone, 126, 188

Sandy Meadow, 304
Santa Ana River, 136, 140
Santa Clara Divide, 181
Santa Clara River, 186-187
Santa Fe Trail pioneers, 165
Santa Monica Mountains, 211
Santa Rosa Mountains, 15, 85,
    98, 105, 112, 123, 140
Santa Rosa Summit, 111
Sapphire Lake basin, 320
Saragossa Spring, 144
Saugus, 194
Sawmill Campground, 208
Sawmill Canyon, 206-07
Sawmill Mountain and Truck
    Trail, 207-09, 213
Sawmill Pass Trail, 313
Sawtooth Mountains Wilderness,
    15, 79
Sawtooth Peak, 292
Scissors Crossing, 91
Scodie Mountain, 246-49, 258
scorpions, 25
sedimentary rocks, 35-36, 162,
    188
Selden Pass, 299, 321
Sentenac Cienaga, 88, 94
Senger Creek, 321
serpentine (serpentinite rock),
    45
Serrano Campground, 145
Seven Pines Trail, 118
setting a schedule, 8
*Sequoia gigantea*, 43, 46
Sequoia National Forest, 246,
    279
Sequoia National Park, 16, 28,
    229, 257, 289, 302-03, 305
Seven Pines Trail, 118
Shadow Lake, 332
Shake Canyon, 208
Sharknose Ridge, 285
Shasta-Trinity National Forest,
    17
Sheep Mountain Wilderness, 15,
    170, 165, 173
Shepherd Pass Trail, 304
sheepherders, 282
shoes, 8, 303
shortcuts, 20
showers, 301, 340
shuttle services, 195, 301,327,
    334
Siberian Pass Creek, 289
Sierra Club,
    founders, 305
    trail angels, 88, 91
    volunteers, 123, 131, 262

Sierra Mammoth Trail, 332
Sierra National Forest, 16
Sierra Nevada, 227
Sierra Pelona, 187, 197, 211
Silver Divide, 326
Silver Lake, 335
Silver Moccasin Trail, 172
Silver Pass Creek, 323
Silver Pass Lake, 326
Silverwood Lake State Recreation
    Area, 153-56
Sixty Lake Basin Trail, 308
ski areas, 170-71, 301, 330
Sky River, 235
skin rashes, 23
Skunk Cabbage meadows, 116
Smithsonian Institute, 295
smog, 47, 161, 170, 202
snakes, 65. *See also* rattlesnakes
snow,
    obscuring the trail, 21, 60, 302
    precipitation patterns, 33, 44
    preparation for, 116, 119, 21,
        257, 302
    seasons, 30-31, 125, 257
Snow Canyon, 121-22
Snow Creek and Snow Creek
    Road, 98, 118-19, 122-23
snowpack, 30-31, 44, 293
snow pillow, 293
soil types, 46
Soledad Canyon, 181, 184-86
Soledad Mountain, 232
solo hiking, 20, 27
Sonora Pass, 41
Sonoran Zone, 125
Sotcher Lake, 330
South Fork Kern River Valley,
    233
South Lake, 301
South Portal Canyon, 200
South Sierra Wilderness, 274,
    279, 281
Southern Pacific Railroad, 123,
    187, 225
Southern Terminus of PCT, 69
space shuttles, 233
Spanish explorers, 83, 102, 167,
    258
Spanish Needle and Creek, 263-
    64
spotted fever, 130, 229
Spunky Canyon and
    Campground, 199-200
Squaw Lake, 326
squirrels, 23
stage stations, 83, 88, 98, 100
Stanislaus National Forest, 16

Stephenson Peak, 79
Storm Canyon, 81
storms. *See* thunderstorms;
  weather
Strawberry Cienaga, 118
Strawberry Junction Trail Camp,
  118
Strawberry Valley, 118
Stubbe Canyon Creek, 123, 130
Sugarloaf Mountain, 136
Sullivan's Curve, 162, 165
Summit Lake, 334
Summit Valley, 129, 152-53
sun exposure, 21, 22, 196
Sunrise Highway, 81-82,
Sunset Sage Trail, 109
supplies, 57
Swarthout Valley, 170
Sweet Ridge, 235
swimming, 150, 195, 273, 332

**T**

Table Mountain and Truck Trail,
  109-10
Taboose Pass Trail, 314
Tahoe National Forest, 17
Tahquitz Valley and Trail, 116-17
Tamarack Road, 123
Tawny Point, 304
Tayles Hidden Acres, 137
Tehachapi (town), 194-95, 221,
  225, 229, 231
Tehachapi Mountains, 191-92,
  200, 211, 218, 220, 227
Tehachapi Pass, 202, 227, 230
Tehachapi Post Office, 225
Tejon Ranch, 4, 191, 213-14
Telescope Peak, 172
temperature, 44
Ten Thousand Foot Ridge, 136
Terwilliger, 97, 100, 109-10
Terwilliger Road, 107, 109
Teutang Canyon, 132
The Roughs, 288
The Thumb, 326
Thomas Mountain, 105, 111, 113
Thomas Mountain Fault, 116
Thousand Island Lake, 332, 334
Three Points, 172, 214
Throop Peak, 173
thru-hikers, 5, 7-9, 257
thunderstorms, 21
Tibbets Creek canyon, 41
tick paralysis, 130
ticks, 25, 104, 129-30, 183,
  229-30
Timberline Lake, 293
Tip Top Mountain, 141-42

toilet practices, 22
trailhead quotas, 18
trail angels, 88, 91,109, 164, 194
trail junctions, 60, 81
trail maintenance.
  *See* maintenance
trail markers, 2, 21, 60
Trail Pass and Trail, 279, 285
Trail Peak, 285
Transition Zone, 125, 161
Transverse Ranges, 40, 126, 162
trash disposal, 22
trees, 43, 46-48, 80, 161, 266,
  289, 292, 321. *See also* fire;
  Joshua trees
  bristlecone pines, 207
  foxtail pine, 280-81
  junipers, 266, 267
  limber pines, 171
  oak, 236
  pinyon pines, 125-26, 233,
  249-50, 258, 267-70
  plantations, 185, 207
Trinity Alps, 17
Trinity Lake, 332
Tule Canyon, 106-07
Tule Spring, 107-08
Tully Hole, 326
Tunnel Spring Trail, 112-13
Tuolumne Meadows and facili-
  ties, 298, 301-02, 338-341
Twin Lakes, 313
Twin Lakes Campground, 327
Tyndall Creek and Frog Ponds,
  304-05
Tylerhorse Canyon, 218, 220

**U**

ultralight backpacking, 7-8
ultraviolet radiation, 21, 32
United States Border Patrol, 69
United States Bureau of Land
  Management. *See* Bureau of
  Land Management
United States Department of
  Agriculture, Forest Service. *See*
  Forest Service
United States National Park
  system. *See* National Parks
uplift, 38
Upper Crater Meadow, 301
Upper Shake Campground,
  207-08, 215
Upper Soda Springs
  Campground, 332
Upper Vidette Meadow, 305
uranium contamination, 131,
  258

**V**

Valle de San Jose, 105
Vallecito Valley, 79, 83
vandalism, 82, 167
Van Dusen Canyon, 144, 147
Vasquez Rocks/Vasquez Rocks
  County Park, 185, 187-89,
  197
Vermilion Resort, 301, 303
Victorville, 142, 164
Vidette Meadow, 305
visitor centers, 171, 332. *See also*
  nature centers
Vogelsang High Sierra Camp,
  338
Volcan Mountain, 84, 93
volcanism, 33-35, 37, 40, 42,
  330, 334
volunteers, 10

**W**

Walker Pass and Campground,
  227-29, 253, 259, 298
walking sticks, 26, 257
Wallace Creek, 304
Wanda Lake, 315, 320
Warm Spring, 150
Warner Springs, 65, 67, 79, 97
Warner Springs Post Office, 95,
  103
Warner Springs Ranch, 100
waste disposal, 22
waterborne microscopic
  organisms, 24
Waterhole Trail Camp, 239
water crossings, 21
water dangers, 21, 23
water sources, 59. *See also* dehydration; giardia. [*Note:* water
  information appears throughout each description of the
  sections of the PCT, with a
  summary in the introduction
  to each section.]
  contamination of, 21, 22, 130,
  167, 181, 229, 258
  finding sources of, 10, 164,
  196, 257
  groundwater sources,
  in drought years, 129, 196,
  257
  irrigation sprinklers, 203
  needed for survival, 195-96
  purification of, 24, 196, 229
  Sierra Club trail angels, 88, 91
  tanks, 207-10
Waterfall Canyon, 230, 233

Waterhole Trail Camp, 239
weather, 29-31. *See also* flash
   floods; lightning; rain; snow
   mild climate zone, 298, 301
   preparation for adverse conditions, 8, 21, 116, 119, 257-58
   rain shadow, 79
   storms and thunderstorms, 21,
   29, 257
weathering, 42
Web addresses that might be
   useful, 15-16
weight of pack, 8, 18. *See also*
   backpacking; ultralight backpacking
Weldon Peak, 238
West Palm Springs Village, 100,
   123, 128, 129
White Water, 113
White's Motel, 195
Whitewater (town), 213
Whitewater Canyon, 132-34
Whitewater River, 123, 125, 129,
   132
Whitewater Trout Farm, 132
Whitney Creek, 292
Whitney Meadow, 289
Whitney Portal, 292, 295,
   301-02
wilderness areas, 15, 246
wilderness classification, 284
wilderness permits, 11, 15-17,
   18-19, 68, 101, 129, 164-65,
   196-97, 229, 257, 302, 340
wildflowers. *See* plants and plant
   communities
Wildlands Conservancy, 135
wildlife, 22, 23-29, 48-56, 77,
   135, 150, 158, 161, 196, 203,
   235-36, 257, 264. *See also*
   bears; birds; insects;
   rattlesnakes; ticks, etc.
   animal ranges, 49
   beaver dams, 147
   bighorn sheep, 235-36
   cougars/mountain lions, 26,
   257
   deer, 48
   endangered, 151
   grizzly bears, 28
   in desert area, 126
   kit fox, 196
   lizards, 130, 205, 267
   llamas, 9
   marmots, 23, 24
   pikas, 23
   pronghorn antelope, 191
   tule elk, 236

Williamson Rock, 175
Willow Spring, 244-45
wind, 31, 229, 305
wind farms/wind-turbines, 20,
   123, 126, 131, 221, 225, 231-
   32, 235
Windy Gap and Spring, 174
Winston Peak, 176
women hikers, 22
Woodpecker Meadow and Fire,
   271
Woods Creek, 311, 313
Wright Creek, 304
Wright Mountain, 170
Wrightwood, 129, 164, 170
Wyleys Knob, 245-46

**Y**

Yellow Jacket Spring, 245, 249
Yosemite National Park, 16, 28,
   41, 302, 338
yucca-feeding ground sloth, 203
yuccas, 53, 203, 241

**Z**

zip codes of post offices, 14

3/15 a

8/18 (19) 6/18